Immunology of the Gut

The Ciba Foundation for the promotion of international cooperation in medical and chemical research is a scientific and educational charity established by CIBA Limited – now CIBA-GEIGY Limited – of Basle. The Foundation operates independently in London under English trust law.

Ciba Foundation Symposia are published in collaboration with Elsevier Scientific Publishing Company, Excerpta Medica, North-Holland Publishing Company, in Amsterdam.

Elsevier/Excerpta Medica/North-Holland, P.O. Box 211, Amsterdam

Immunology of the Gut

Ciba Foundation Symposium 46 (new series)

In memory of the late Joseph Heremans

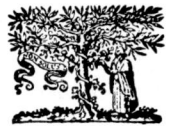

1977

Elsevier · Excerpta Medica · North-Holland
Amsterdam · Oxford · New York

© *Copyright 1977 Ciba Foundation*

All rights reserved. No part of this publication may be reproduced or transmitted in any form or by any means, electronic or mechanical, including photocopying and recording, or by any information storage and retrieval system, without permission in writing from the publishers.

ISBN Excerpta Medica 90 219 4052 3
ISBN Elsevier North-Holland, Inc. 0-444-15246-6

Published in March 1977 by Elsevier/Excerpta Medica/North-Holland, P.O. Box 211, Amsterdam and Elsevier North-Holland, Inc., 52 Vanderbilt Avenue, New York, N.Y. 10017.

Suggested series entry for library catalogues: Ciba Foundation Symposia.
Suggested publisher's entry for library catalogues: Elsevier/Excerpta Medica/North-Holland

Ciba Foundation Symposium 46 (new series)
384 pages, 69 figures, 46 tables

Library of Congress Cataloging in Publication Data

Symposium on Immunology of the Gut, London, 1976.
    Immunology of the gut.

    (Ciba Foundation symposium; new ser., 46)
    Symposium held Apr. 26-28.
    Bibliography: p.
    Includes indexes.
    1. Immunologic diseases--Congresses. 2. Immunoglobulin A--Congresses. 3. Intestines --Congresses. 4. Immune response--Congresses. I. Title. II. Series: Ciba Foundation. Symposium; new ser., 46.
RC582.S95   1976   616.3'4'079   76-30326
ISBN 0-444-15246-6

Printed in The Netherlands by Van Gorcum, Assen

Contents

P. J. LACHMANN Introduction 1

J. J. CEBRA, R. KAMAT, P. GEARHART, S. M. ROBERTSON and J. TSENG The secretory IgA system of the gut 5
Discussion 22

A. J. HUSBAND, H. J. MONIÉ and J. L. GOWANS The natural history of the cells producing IgA in the gut 29
Discussion 42

P. PORTER, S. H. PARRY and W. D. ALLEN Significance of immune mechanisms in relation to enteric infections of the gastrointestinal tract in animals 55
Discussion 67

P. BRANDTZAEG and K. BAKLIEN Intestinal secretion of IgA and IgM: a hypothetical model 77
Discussion 108

S. AHLSTEDT, B. CARLSSON, S. P. FÄLLSTRÖM, L. Å HANSON, J. HOLMGREN, G. LIDIN-JANSON, B. S. LINDBLAD, U. JODAL, B. KAIJSER, A. SOHL-ÅKERLUND and C. WADSWORTH Antibodies in human serum and milk induced by enterobacteria and food proteins 115
Discussion 129

T. LEHNER Immunological responses to bacterial plaque in the mouth 135
Discussion 150

G. MAYRHOFER Sites of synthesis and localization of IgE in rats infected with *Nippostrongylus brasiliensis* 155
Discussion 175

B. M. OGILVIE and D. M. V. PARROTT The immunological consequences of nematode infection 183
Discussion 195

P. B. BEESON   Role of the eosinophil   203
  Discussion   213

J. F. SOOTHILL   Genetic and nutritional variations in antigen handling and disease   225
  Discussion   236

A. J. KATZ and F. S. ROSEN   Gastrointestinal complications of immunodeficiency syndromes   243
  Discussion   254

M. SELIGMANN   Immunobiology and pathogenesis of alpha chain disease   263
  Discussion   275

M. B. PEPYS, M. DRUGUET, H. J. KLASS, A. C. DASH, D. D. MIRJAH and A. PETRIE   Immunological studies in inflammatory bowel disease   283
  Discussion   297

A. FERGUSON and T. T. MACDONALD   Effects of local delayed hypersensitivity on the small intestine   305
  Discussion   319

C. C. BOOTH, T. J. PETERS and W. F. DOE   Immunopathology of coeliac disease   329
  Discussion   341

General discussion
  Homing of T blasts   347
  The induction of tolerance to orally administered antigens   350
  Immunization with *Escherichia coli* hybrids   355
  Antigen entry in gut   356
  The intestinal bacterial load   360
  Gut not a primary lymphoid organ   361
  Future work   362

Index of contributors   367

Subject index   369

Participants

Symposium on Immunology of the Gut, held at the Ciba Foundation, London, 26th–28th April 1976

Chairman: P. J. LACHMANN MRC Group on Mechanisms in Tumour Immunity, Laboratory of Molecular Biology, The Medical School, Hills Road, Cambridge CB2 2QH

S. AHLSTEDT Research and Development Laboratory (Pharmacology), Astra Läkemedel AB, S-151 85 Södertälje, Sweden

C. ANDRÉ INSERM Unité de Recherches de Physiopathologie Digestive, Hôpital Edouard-Herriot, Pavillon H, 69374 Lyon Cedex 2, France

P. B. BEESON Veterans Administration Hospital, 4435 Beacon Avenue South, Seattle, Washington 98108, USA

J. BIENENSTOCK Department of Medicine, McMaster University, Hamilton, Ontario L8S 4J9, Canada

C. C. BOOTH Department of Medicine, The Royal Postgraduate Medical School, Du Cane Road, London W12 OHS

P. BRANDTZAEG Institute of Pathology, Immunohistochemical Laboratory, Rikshospitalet, Oslo 1, Norway

J. J. CEBRA Mergenthaler Laboratory for Biology, Johns Hopkins University, Baltimore, Maryland 21218, USA

A. J. S. DAVIES Chester Beatty Research Institute, Fulham Road, London SW3 6JB

D. J. EVANS Department of Histopathology, The Royal Postgraduate Medical School, Du Cane Road, London W12 OHS

ANNE FERGUSON Gastro-Intestinal Unit, Western General Hospital, Crewe Road, Edinburgh EH4 2XU

J. L. GOWANS   MRC Cellular Immunology Unit, Sir William Dunn School of Pathology, Oxford OX1 3RE

Mme J. HEREMANS 99 Tiensestraat, B-3000 Leuven, Belgium

J. V. JONES   Department of Rheumatology, Rush-Presbyterian-St Luke's Medical Center, 1753 West Congress Parkway, Chicago, Illinois 60612, USA

T. LEHNER   Department of Oral Immunology and Microbiology, Guy's Hospital, London SE1 9RT

G. MAYRHOFER   MRC Cellular Immunology Unit, Sir William Dunn School of Pathology, Oxford OX1 3RE

BRIDGET M. OGILVIE   National Institute for Medical Research, Mill Hill, London NW7 1AA

DELPHINE M. V. PARROTT   Department of Bacteriology and Immunology, Western Infirmary, Glasgow G11 6NT

M. B. PEPYS   Department of Immunology, Royal Free Hospital, Pond Street, London NW3 2QG

N. F. PIERCE   Department of Medicine, The Baltimore City Hospitals, 4940 Eastern Avenue, Baltimore, Maryland 21224, USA

P. PORTER   Unilever Research Laboratories, Colworth House, Sharnbrook, Bedfordshire MK44 1LQ

F. S. ROSEN   Immunology Division, The Children's Hospital Medical Center, 300 Longwood Avenue, Boston, Massachusetts 02115, USA

G. SCHMIDT   Max-Planck-Institut für Immunbiologie, 78 Freiburg-Zahringen, Stübeweg 51, Germany

M. SELIGMANN   Department of Immunology, Research Institute on Blood Diseases, Hôpital Saint-Louis, 75475 Paris Cedex 10, France

J. F. SOOTHILL   Department of Immunology, Institute of Child Health, 30 Guilford Street, London WC1N 1EH

J. P. VAERMAN   Faculté de Médecine, Unité de Médecine expérimentale, UCL 7430, Avenue Hippocrate 75, B-1200 Bruxelles, Belgium

R. G. WHITE   Department of Bacteriology and Immunology, Western Infirmary, Glasgow G11 6NT

Editors: RUTH PORTER (*Organizer*) and JULIE KNIGHT

Introduction

P. J. LACHMANN

MRC Group on Mechanisms in Tumour Immunity, Laboratory of Molecular Biology, The Medical School, Cambridge

The area that this symposium is going to work over is an extensive one. I was taught at medical school that the absorptive area of the intestine alone was the size of a tennis court, though I cannot vouch for this being true. It is the overlapping fields of gastroenterology in its widest sense—to include even dental caries, in which perhaps not all gastroenterologists regard themselves as practitioners—that have been brought together with immunology in this symposium. Immunological mechanisms can be thought of as protecting the *milieu intérieur* from the *milieu extérieur*, at any rate as far as macromolecules are concerned. The mechanisms for doing this have to apply not only to the normal, sterile tissues of the body, which are protected from most macromolecules except for the insect's sting and the doctor's needle, but also to regions like the gut and to some extent the respiratory tract where the *milieu extérieur* has succeeded in getting inside the *milieu intérieur* and where foreign molecules in the form of both food and microorganisms exist in quantities which, compared with the quantities that immunologists usually deal in, are astronomical.

It is interesting here to draw a distinction between the respiratory tract and the gut. The respiratory tract is protected from antigenic material by a number of mechanical barriers, but once antigenic material gets down to the lung it is almost as antigenic there as when it is introduced parenterally. In the gut, on the other hand, there is no mechanical protection; and in parts of the gut, at any rate, foreign macromolecules are present in large quantities; but in this site they are not antigenic to any substantial extent. Therefore it is not surprising that specialized immunological mechanisms have evolved around areas like the respiratory tract and particularly the gut to deal with these special situations, and these special mechanisms are concerned intimately with the secretory immunoglobulins and especially with IgA. This is the particular immunoglobulin with the characterization of which Joe Heremans was intimately involved, and his absence, through his premature death, makes not only this meeting but the whole immunological community very much the poorer. Others are going to discuss IgA—its production, its functions and the cells that make it. The other limb of the immune response, cell-mediated immunity, will not be left out, and I am relieved to see that even complement will have a mention!

The interactions of immunology and clinical medicine have always been very much two-way. It is not just that work on immunology has expanded the field of medicine but also very much that studies of individual patients, the subtle experiments of nature, have made considerable contributions to our understanding of immunology. By no means the worst example of this is the role that studies of multiple myeloma and myeloma proteins have had in increasing our knowledge of immunoglobulin structure, function and genetics, and IgA and IgG, both of which are to be discussed, give good examples of this. It is still a very active field and we shall hear in some detail about the current status of the work on alpha chain disease, that extraordinary situation where partial immunoglobulin molecules are produced and secreted.

The study of immunity deficiency is a second good example of the two-way interaction, and here too work is still very active. We shall hear not only about the effects of primary immune deficiencies, of the sort where the immunodeficient child develops infections; but also about the paradoxical situation, which is now being increasingly appreciated, where minor forms of immune deficiency may become manifest not in increased sensitivity to infection as much as in increased liability to produce allergic diseases due to inappropriate immunological reactivity.

In their turn, studies of immunology have led to great advances both in the understanding and the prevention of disease. Perhaps prophylactic immunization against infection is still the major man-made change in the pattern of morbidity throughout the world, and it is to be hoped that in this area there is still much progress to be made. One could imagine, for example, that a vaccine against dental caries might have almost as much effect on morbidity in the world as a vaccine against cholera, though perhaps not as much as a vaccine against hookworm or malaria (although the latter is not directly relevant to the gut). To develop effective prophylactic immunization one has to understand the processes by which immunological mechanisms bring about immunity. This is a curiously complex topic in which much interest has been taken again in the past few years after a period when there was relatively little work devoted to it. The mechanisms seem to be different for all the major classes of pathogenic organisms. One might say that they are understood badly for bacteria, and worse for worms! We are going to hear about both these topics—about immunity to the pathogenic variants of the normal gut flora, and about immune mechanisms directed towards nematodes, where there remains the long-standing question of whether the IgE system does have any useful function, and if it does, whether it is in relation to nematodes in the gut.

One major understanding which has come from the study of the immunology of infection is that the same mechanisms which give rise to immunity can also give rise to allergic tissue damage and can themselves contribute to the manifestations of the very infectious diseases against which they also provide protection. This is true both of overt infectious disease (it has, for an example in the gut, been claimed that the diarrhoea of shigella dysentery is largely allergic in nature) and also of diseases that are not obviously infectious at all. For example, brain damage in subacute sclerosing panencephalitis is now recognized as being due to allergic reactions to measles virus infection. The extent to which mechanisms of this kind may be involved in inflammatory bowel disease is a subject of great importance, and this is also to be discussed in the symposium.

Such allergic reactions are not restricted to antigens of infectious organisms, and a consideration of disease caused by allergic manifestations to dietary antigens will be a fitting conclusion to a meeting where I am sure there will be plenty for us all to mark, learn and inwardly digest!

The secretory IgA system of the gut

JOHN J. CEBRA, RAMESH KAMAT, PATRICIA GEARHART, STELLA M. ROBERTSON and JEENAN TSENG

Department of Biology, The Johns Hopkins University, Baltimore, Md.

Abstract Most commonly, humoral immunity manifested in the gastrointestinal tract of mammals is due to the presence of secretory IgA antibodies. Antibody specificities have been detected in the secretory IgA of gut secretions to a wide range of naturally occurring viral and bacterial components and to test antigens such as chemically modified proteins. Much of the IgA found in gut secretions is synthesized and secreted locally by the abundant plasma cells of the lamina propria. Development of methods for establishing local protective immunity in the gut requires knowledge of the origins of these plasma cells and of the whereabouts of their precursors when they are susceptible to antigen-driven proliferation and/or maturation.

The Peyer's patches have been shown to contain a population of B lymphocytes especially rich in precursors for IgA plasma cells and in cells which can repopulate gut lamina propria with such IgA plasma cells. The Peyer's patches also appear to 'sample' gut antigens, in that small amounts of antigens are passed intact through their dome epithelial cells.

Recent experiments bearing on the origins, differentiation and maturation, antigen sensitivity, migration and lodging of precursors for gut IgA plasma cells are discussed. We use the following three systems: (1) congenic transfer of cells from different murine lymphoid cell sources or mixtures of these (CB20 → BALB/c or BALB/c → CB20) and the use of allo-antisera to IgA allotypic determinants to assess their potential to impart an adoptive IgA antibody response to the recipient and to repopulate its histocompatible lamina propria with IgA plasma cells; (2) clonal precursor analysis (the method of Klinman) both to enumerate antigen-sensitive cells in different tissues of mice and to evaluate their potential to generate plasma cells making particular isotypes and idiotypes of antibodies; (3) use of pairs of Thiry-Vella loops in rabbits, each member either bearing or lacking a Peyer's patch, and quantitation of antibodies of each isotype and of total secretory IgA to assess the response of each loop with the time after local immunization. The results from all three systems provide strong evidence for the importance of Peyer's patches in supplying cells responsible for local humoral immunity and suggest both a differentiative pathway for IgA precursors and their whereabouts when antigen may cause the expansion of a population of specific cells.

Most commonly, humoral immunity manifest in the gastrointestinal tract of mammals is due to the presence of secretory immunoglobulin A (sIgA) antibodies. Thus, in order to devise effective immunization procedures leading to the establishment of local protective immunity in the gut, one must gain some knowledge of the following: (1) the origins and locations of the cells responsible for the synthesis and secretion of sIgA; (2) the stages at which they and/or their precursors are susceptible to antigen-driven proliferation and their whereabouts when such specific expansion may be possible after both primary and secondary challenge; (3) the interactions these cells must undergo with other cell types or with humoral factors—antigens, mitogens, hormones, etc.—before their maturation to IgA plasma cells; and (4) the migration routes and any tissues of temporary domicile favoured by the cellular progenitors of the gut IgA response and any selective lodging properties that they may develop *en route* to intestinal lamina propria. Observations to be presented by ourselves and by Dr Ahlstedt later in this symposium (Ahlstedt *et al.*, pp. 115–129) suggest that an understanding of these aspects of the development of humoral immunity in the gut may also be germane to the appearance of sIgA antibodies in other secretory (exocrine) tissue. Of course, another process relevant to the occurrence of sIgA antibodies in the gut that is not directly related to the generation of a local IgA response involves the passage of the IgA antibodies across an epithelial cell barrier into the intestinal or glandular lumen, and this will be considered later by Dr Brandtzaeg (Brandtzaeg & Baklien, this volume, pp. 77–108).

Our ability to formulate these particular areas of inquiry pertinent to the development of humoral immunity in the gut follows directly from a series of basic observations made during the past 17 years, many by Professor Joseph Heremans and his colleagues. The Heremans group isolated that isotype of immunoglobulin (Ig) from human serum which we now call IgA and defined some of its characteristic properties, such as its lower isoelectric point and higher sugar content relative to other Igs and its propensity to occur in a number of polymeric forms (Heremans *et al.* 1959). Using immunohistochemical methods we were then able to show the synthesis of the IgA isotype by a class of human or rabbit plasma cells different from those making IgG or IgM (Bernier & Cebra 1965; Cebra *et al.* 1966). This separate population of IgA cells assumed greater significance when considered with the finding by Hanson, Tomasi and colleagues from their two groups that the concentration of IgA in human milk and other exocrine secretions was considerably greater than that of any other isotype of Ig (Hanson, 1960, 1961; Tomasi & Zigelbaum 1963; Tomasi *et al.* 1965). The Tomasi group characterized the human sIgA as some sort of polymer of serum IgA containing 'extra' antigenic sites (Tomasi *et al.* 1965) which were later found to occur on a separate polypeptide now called secretory component (SC) (South *et al.* 1966). Yet another distinct polypeptide, called J chain, was later found in sIgA, IgM and polymeric serum IgAs (Halpern & Koshland 1970). Shortly after the isolation of human sIgA (Tomasi *et al.* 1965) we were able to purify its homologue from rabbit milk (Cebra & Robbins 1966) and deduce from it the molecular weight and polypeptide chain composition of sIgA: four pairs of heavy (α) and light (L) polypeptides + one SC (mol.wt. = 60–70 000) + one J chain (mol.wt. = 15 000) (Cebra & Small 1967; O'Daly & Cebra 1971). In a comprehensive study the Heremans group went on to show that IgA either predominated over all other Ig isotypes in secretions or at least was more concentrated in secretions than in serum from all of many mammalian species examined (Heremans & Vaerman 1971). The rabbit represents a rather extreme case of IgA distribution since the concentration of this isotype, which is the major one in secretions, is about 20-fold higher in milk and 5–10 fold higher in intestinal secretions than in serum (Cebra & Robbins 1966; Robertson & Cebra 1976). An appreciation of the protective role of sIgA in the gut lumen has evolved in parallel with the molecular characterization. Although sIgA antibodies appear neither to react with Fc receptors of any cell type—and therefore do not 'opsonize'—nor to activate complement starting with Cl (Eddie *et al.* 1971), they do appear to be effective simply by complexing with antigen in the gut or at other mucosal surfaces. Thus sIgA antibodies can specifically neutralize toxins, prevent viral attachment to host target cells, and diminish adherence of bacteria to mucosal surfaces and hence the probability of colonization by them (see Ogra *et al.* 1975; Smith *et al.* 1966; Gibbons 1974; Freter 1970).

The local synthesis of much of the sIgA in secretions was inferred from the finding by Tomasi's group of many IgA plasma cells in the interstitium of human salivary glands (Tomasi *et al.* 1965) and by Heremans and his colleagues that human gut mucosa contained up to 200 000 IgA plasma cells per mm^3 in the lamina propria (Crabbé *et al.* 1965), or an estimated 7.5×10^{10} of such cells in the entire gut (Heremans 1975). The lamina propria of the rabbit intestine contains a similarly large number of IgA plasma cells (Crandall *et al.* 1967). Reflecting the 10–20 fold difference in IgA concentration between secretions and serum, these IgA cells are markedly compartmentalized in lamina propria and exocrine tissue—where they comprise 85% of all plasma cells—away from most IgG and IgM plasma cells which are found in spleen and peripheral lymph nodes in the company of only 2–5% IgA cells (Crandall *et al.* 1967; Cebra *et al.* 1966). In an effort to deduce how this compartmentalization of IgA plasma cells was achieved in the rabbit, we sought a source for cells which could repopulate the gut lamina propria of lethally irradiated animals among a variety of lymphoid tissues. Among the tissues tested were Peyer's patches, which are situated in the mucosa of the small bowel and are quite distinct from the IgA plasma cell-rich surrounding lamina propria. The histology of mammalian Peyer's patches, especially those of the rabbit, has been thoroughly described (Faulk et al. 1971; Waksman et al. 1973). Large follicles of B lymphocytes, containing many dividing cells in the deeper and lateral regions of each, are characteristic of this lymphoid tissue. Smaller, thymus-dependent areas rich in T lymphocytes occur between the B cell follicles and closer to the dome epithelium.

Using the allotypic determinants present on the L chains of rabbit Igs as markers of cellular origin, we were able to show that Peyer's patches and appendix were enriched sources of cells which could repopulate the gut lamina propria of lethally irradiated rabbits with IgA plasma cells (Craig & Cebra 1971). Relative to peripheral lymph nodes, blood or spleen, Peyer's patches contained many more immediate precursors of IgA plasma cells as judged by the pokeweed mitogen-stimulated appearance of IgA plasma cells *in vitro* upon microculture of cells from the different sources and by the number of IgA plasma cells generated in spleens of recipients of the various cell populations (Craig & Cebra 1971; Jones et al. 1974; Craig & Cebra 1975). A sub-population of Peyer's patch lymphocytes was identified which bore no detectable *endogenous* membrane IgM but did carry as surface markers L chain and Fab (α) determinants associated with IgA (Craig & Cebra 1975; Jones & Cebra 1974). We were able to isolate this sub-population of cells, which usually comprised $<10\%$ of Peyer's patch lymphocytes, by fluorescence-activated cell sorting (Jones et al. 1974). Almost all of the immediate precursors for IgA plasma cells were found in this sub-population (Jones et al. 1974). A similar small minority of B lymphocytes with surface IgA has been detected in mouse Peyer's patches (McWilliams et al. 1974; Guy-Grand et al. 1974) although the potential of this sub-population has not been evaluated.

An 'antigen sampling' role has also been ascribed to the Peyer's patches, since macromolecules and even bacteria may pass through or by their dome epithelial cells and arrive intact in the midst of B lymphocyte areas (Bockman & Cooper 1973; Carter & Collins 1974). Heremans and his colleagues have made the very important observation that oral administration of either sheep erythrocytes or ferritin to germ-free mice results in the sequential appearance of IgA antibody-forming cells to the former in mesenteric nodes and then spleen and the appearance of ferritin-binding IgA cells after 30 days in gut lamina propria (Crabbé et al. 1969; Bazin et al. 1970). Gowans and his group and others (Guy-Grand et al. 1974; Gowans & Knight 1964; Griscelli et al. 1969; McWilliams et al. 1975) have shown that a small population of rapidly dividing lymphocytes in rat thoracic duct lymph or in mouse and rat mesenteric lymph nodes can accumulate in the gut lamina propria. Some of these thoracic duct cells bear surface IgA and some may contain specific cytoplasmic IgA antibodies (Williams & Gowans 1975; Pierce & Gowans 1975). It is tempting to suggest that IgA precursors have their first encounter with antigen in the Peyer's patches. Thus we arrive at a consideration of the areas for inquiry suggested at the start by directing our attention to the antigen-sensitivity and immunological potential of Peyer's patch cells themselves.

DO PEYER'S PATCHES CONTAIN ANTIGEN-SENSITIVE B LYMPHOCYTES?

Attempts to stimulate the appearance of antibody-forming plasma cells in Peyer's patches by a wide variety of antigens and immunization schedules have consistently failed (see Henry *et al.* 1970; Coppola *et al.* 1972). Similarly, efforts to adoptively transfer an antibody response with patch cells alone have been unrewarded (Katz & Perey 1973; Knudson *et al.* 1975). However, transfers of mixtures of appendix cells with autologous thymocytes into X-irradiated rabbits or of patch cells with spleen cells into syngeneic, cyclophosphamide-suppressed mice led to an increased number of IgM antibody-producing cells over that observed when appendix or patch cells were omitted from the inoculum (Ozer & Waksman 1972; Coppola *et al.* 1972). A more recent example of such 'synergism' with patch cells involved their adoptive transfer to syngeneic, X-irradiated mice along with bone marrow cells and a resulting anti-sheep erythrocyte response including some IgA antibody-producing cells (Knudson *et al.* 1975). Because of the experimental design the tissue source of the antibody-producing cells could not be ascertained. Finally, attempts to elicit an *in vitro* IgM response to sheep erythrocytes with Peyer's patch cells alone have been successful with cells of rabbit origin (Henry *et al.* 1970) and likewise for mouse cells, except that there is some controversy about the need for accessory, adherent peritoneal cells (Kagnoff & Campbell 1973) or not (Jones *et al.* 1976).

We proposed that much of the difficulty in demonstrating the expression of a primary antibody response by patch cells—especially an IgA antibody response—encountered using either an adoptive transfer or an *in vitro* assay was due to the failure to maintain either viable recipients or cultures sufficiently long enough. Thus we have adoptively transferred lymphoid cells into sublethally irradiated (600 R) syngeneic mice to assess both their potential to respond to antigen and their time-course of response, and into similarly irradiated congenic recipients differing in Ig allotype from the cell donors to establish the origin of any antibody-producing cells. In our first experiments

TABLE 1

Time-course of PFC response in recipients of Peyer's patch cells

Day of assay	No. of animals	Mean plaques/spleen			
		IgM	IgG1	IgG2	IgA
7	2	740	0	0	0
10	3	633	443	N.D.	516
12	4	690	2120	4240	1200
15	2	310	3040	N.D.	740
19	3	520	612	814	570

DBA/2J → DBA/2J.
10^7 Peyer's patch cells + 10^7 thymus cells.

10^7 Peyer's patch cells, 10^7 spleen cells or 3×10^7 peripheral lymph node cells (excluding cells from mesenteric nodes) from normal DBA/2 mice were transferred along with 10^7 syngeneic thymus cells into X-irradiated DBA/2 recipients. After 24 hours the mice were challenged with 5×10^8 sheep erythrocytes given intraperitoneally. The recipients were sacrificed from 7–19 days after challenge and their spleens were assayed for IgM, IgG1, IgG2, and IgA antibody-producing cells (PFC) by the Jerne plaque assay technique. Table 1 shows that by day 7 the Peyer's patch cell recipients expressed only IgM PFC. From day 10 onwards IgA and IgG PFC were also detected. Cells expressing either of these isotypes reached a maximum number around day 12–15 and declined thereafter. Table 2 shows that the IgA PFC detected 12 days after antigenic challenge are only observed in recipients of patch cells plus thymocytes and not in mice receiving mixtures of cells from other sources or thymocytes alone. In order rigorously to ascertain the source of the IgA PFC and to rule out the possibility that the response obtained in sub-lethally irradiated syngeneic recipients is due to host B cell regeneration followed by some undefined interaction with donor cells, we did congenic transfers using CB20 mice (Lieberman et al. 1974) as the presumptive B cell donors and BALB/c as the thymocyte

TABLE 2

Comparison of PFC responses in recipients of lymphocytes from different sources

Type of transfer	Day of assay	No. of animals	Mean plaques/spleen			
			IgM	IgG1	IgG2	IgA
10^7 spleen + 10^7 thymus	12	3	884	3730	2940	6
3×10^7 lymph node + 10^7 thymus	12	3	504	3190	2610	5
10^7 Peyer's patch + 10^7 thymus	12	4	690	2120	4240	1200
10^7 thymus	12	2	57	0	0	0

DBA/2J → DBA/2J.

TABLE 3

PFC response by recipients of Peyer's patch or peripheral lymphoid cells in a congenic transfer

Type of transfer	Day of assay	No. of animals	Mean plaques/spleen				$\frac{Ig2^b}{IgA} \times 100$ spleen plasma cells
			IgM	IgG1	IgG2	IgA	
10^7 CB20 PP^a + 10^7 BALB/cJ thymus	7	2	2490	0	0	0	N.D.
10^7 CB20 PP + 10^7 BALB/cJ thymus	10	3	630	950	0	610	100
2×10^7 CB20 LN + 10^7 BALB/cJ thymus	10	3	700	106	0	0	N.D.

^{a}PP, Peyer's patch cells; LN, lymph node cells.

donors and recipients. These two strains are histocompatible (H-2^d) but their Ig molecules can be distinguished by allotypic markers. For instance, alloantisera can be raised which specifically distinguish the IgA molecules of the two congenic strains which express allelic C_α genes (Ig-2^a and Ig-2^b for BALB/c and CB20 respectively) (Herzenberg 1964). Table 3 shows that cell transfers between such mice resulted in IgA PFC by day 10 only when Peyer's patches were the source of donor B cells. At this time, essentially all of the IgA plasma cells in recipients' spleens also carried the donor IgA allotype marker, as judged by staining with fluorochrome coupled anti-alpha chain and anti-Ig-2^b. Thus Peyer's patches of the donor were the source of the antibody-forming IgA plasma cells and do contain antigen-sensitive cells capable of generating IgA plasma cells while spleen and peripheral nodes appear to contain many fewer of such cells. The results also suggest that Peyer's patches share with other lymphoid tissue the potential to generate IgM, IgG1 and, at least in the DBA/2 strain, IgG2 plasma cells.

ENUMERATION OF FREQUENCY OF ANTIGEN-SENSITIVE PRECURSORS IN PEYER'S PATCHES AND ASSESSMENT OF THEIR POTENTIAL TO EXPRESS VARIOUS Ig ISOTYPES

To enumerate the precursor frequency in different lymphoid populations we have employed the technique of clonal analysis developed by Klinman and his colleagues (Klinman 1969) and evaluated the clonal precursor cells (CPC) sensitive to the phosphorylcholine (PC) determinant, since considerable information is available concerning splenic CPC reactive with this hapten (Gearhart et al. 1975). Briefly, mice to be used for scoring CPC were carrier-

TABLE 4

Frequency of anti-phosphorylcholine (PC) precursors

Donor	Total no. cells analysed	Total clones/ 10^5 B cells	No. clones/10^5 B cells with T15 idiotype	% anti-PC response represented by T15 idiotype
Spleen	630×10^6	2.28 ± 1.78	1.77 ± 1.63	74 ± 28
Peyer's patch	94×10^6	3.13 ± 1.14	1.23 ± 0.84	39 ± 15

primed with *Limulus* haemocyanin 6–8 weeks before cell transfer. They were then lethally irradiated (1300 R) and one day later were injected with limiting doses of the lymphoid cells to be tested. After 16 hours the mice were sacrificed and their spleens were sliced into 1.0 mm cubes. The spleen fragments were individually cultured in Dulbecco's modified Eagle's medium with 10% agammaglobulinaemic horse serum in the wells of microtitre plates along with an optimum concentration of PC conjugated to haemocyanin through a tri-peptide spacer (5×10^{-7} M in PC). At intervals culture fluid was removed from the wells and fresh medium was added. The fluids from the wells were individually assayed for anti-PC antibody, isotype of anti-PC antibody and for the presence of a common idiotype of anti-PC antibody from BALB/c mice (prototype myeloma protein TEPC 15) (Potter & Lieberman 1970) using radioimmunoassays. If the appropriate, limiting dilutions of lymphocytes are delivered to the scoring animal, then the total amount of antibody and its isotype(s) and idiotype in a positive spleen fragment can be considered to be the product of a single clone and to reflect that potential of a single precursor expressible in the CPC assay by its progeny (Klinman 1969; Gearhart *et al.* 1975). Table 4 compares the frequency of anti-PC CPC with and without the potential to express TEPC 15 idiotype in spleen and Peyer's patches. The frequency of CPC in both these tissues, based on B cell content, is similar to that previously observed for spleen (Gearhart *et al.* 1975). The lower frequency of CPC in patch cells that express the TEPC 15 idiotype than in spleen is conspicuous and provides a hint that the two cell sources may be subject to different mixtures of naturally occurring PC-determinants which may selectively expand out different sub-populations of anti-PC precursor cells. Table 5 compares the CPC from the two tissues with respect to isotypes of anti-PC antibodies expressed by their clonal progeny. The CPC of splenic origin predominantly generate clones which make only IgG1, IgM and IgG1 or IgM, IgG1 and IgA anti-PC. The population of CPC from Peyer's patches is conspicuously different in that their resultant clones produce IgM and IgA or only IgA anti-PC with a very high incidence. Fig. 1 graphically illustrates

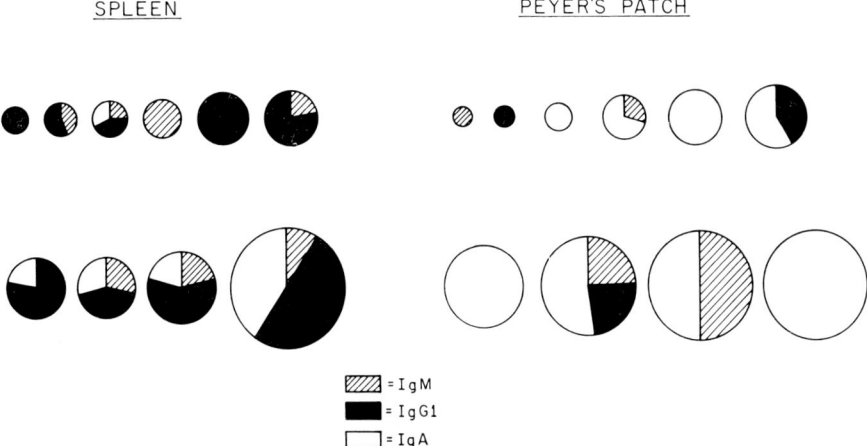

FIG. 1. Anti-phosphorylcholine (PC) response of B lymphocyte-derived clones expressing the TEPC 15 idiotype marker. The area of each circle represents the size of the clone estimated from total output of product antibody. The sectors shown in some circles represent the proportion of total antibody present as a particular isotype (IgA, IgM, IgG1). The clones depicted were chosen to be representative of much larger samples derived from both spleen and Peyer's patch.

this difference in populations of CPC as well as the relative sizes of the clones generated by the two cell sources as judged by their total output of anti-PC antibody (proportional to area of circles). There seems to be no correlation between clone size and isotype(s) expressed. Thus the Peyer's patches are as rich a source of antigen-sensitive CPC as the spleen but their potential to generate clones making IgA antibodies is far greater. The Peyer's patches are known to differ from other lymphoid tissue in some or all of the following characteristics: (1) T lymphocyte areas segregated away from B cell follicles;

TABLE 5

Isotype distribution

Heavy chain class	% B cell clones with TEPC 15 idiotype	
	Spleen	Peyer's patch
μ	10	6
$\gamma 1$	16	6
α	2	46
$\mu, \gamma 1$	26	3
$\gamma 1, \alpha$	6	8
μ, α	4	26
$\mu, \gamma 1, \alpha$	36	8

(2) no organized antigen-trapping reticulum; (3) excessive numbers of suppressor T lymphocytes; (4) deficiency in accessory cells; (5) extensive B lymphocyte proliferation without *in situ* maturation to plasma cells (see: Faulk et al. 1971; Waksman et al. 1973; Bockman & Cooper 1973; Kagnoff & Campbell 1974; Kamin et al. 1974). Thus one unique feature of the Peyer's patch may be that it provides an environment that permits B cell division—at least in part antigen-driven—without providing those interactions necessary for maturation to plasma cells. One might suppose therefore that the patch B cell population contains cells that, on the average, are more divisions removed from the pre-B or 'virgin' B cell than those of any other lymphoid tissue. Such cells may be more likely to generate clones which express IgA. Whether, in addition to permitting such B cell divisions, the milieu of the Peyer's patch can also influence the course of differentiation (perhaps gene rearrangement) or development (gene expression) is still conjectural.

However, having demonstrated that Peyer's patches contain antigen-senstitive precursors for IgA plasma cells and that they are enriched sources of precursors for clones which express IgA, we must consider their role in populating the lamina propria of gut mucosa. We have already discussed observations by others that dividing cells from mesenteric nodes and thoracic duct lymph appear to selectively lodge in gut (p. 10). However, such short-term selective accumulation in gut has not been shown for cells of Peyer's patches. Our own studies related above have clearly shown that allogeneic patch cells contained a sub-population of B cells that could fully repopulate intestinal lamina propria with IgA plasma cells. We have now examined such repopulation in mice histocompatible with the donated cells in a system which permitted unequivocal assignment of the B cell source of IgA plasma cells.

REPOPULATION OF HISTOCOMPATIBLE INTESTINAL MUCOSA WITH IgA PLASMA CELLS FROM CONGENIC DONORS

As before, our lymphoid cell donors were CB20 mice and the recipients were sub-lethally (600 R) X-irradiated BALB/c congenic mice. Each animal received either 10^7 patch cells or 2×10^7 peripheral lymph node cells from CB20 mice either with or without 10^7 BALB/c thymocytes. The addition of exogenous thymus cells appeared to have no effect on the repopulation observed. The recipients were sacrificed at various times after cell transfer. Spleens were rendered into single-cell suspensions for replicate cell monolayer preparation by cyto-centrifugation (Dore & Balfour 1965) and random cryostat sections of the small intestine were made. Each film and section was consecutively stained with fluorescein (F)-labelled anti-α and rhodamine (R)-labelled anti-Ig-

TABLE 6

Relative repopulation of spleen and gut lamina propria by donor-derived IgA plasma cells

Cell source[a]	Day	Exp. no.	% Ig-2^b/α in spleen[b]	Relative α+ area of gut analysed[c]	Average % Ig-2^b/α in gut[d]
PP	6	1	0	–	0
PP	6	1	0	–	0
PP	7	2	0	–	N.D.
PP	7	2	0	–	N.D.
PP	8	3	93	517	42
PP	10	2	100	498	47
PP	10	2	N.D.[a]	693	49
PP	10	2	N.D.	967	48
PP	12	1	100	2391	58
PP	14	3	90	375	96
PLN	10	2	15	662	21
PLN	10	2	N.D.	486	15
PLN	10	2	N.D.	498	9
PLN	14	3	45	423	36

[a] PP, Peyer's patch cells; PLN, peripheral node cells; N.D., not done.
[b] % of Ig-2^b plasma cells of total IgA plasma cells. About 200–400 and 20–100 IgA plasma cells were present per 2×10^5 nucleated cells in spleens of recipients of PP and PLN cells respectively.
[c] About 20 plasma cells comprise 100 units of area.
[d] Determined from area measurements.

2^b (anti-CB20 IgA allotype). Differential cell counts were made on the monolayers. Fields of the gut sections were randomly chosen on the basis of content of F anti-α-staining cells alone and these were photographed first and then rephotographed under filter conditions permitting visualization of any R anti-Ig-2^b positive cells. Each set of transparencies from a single field was magnified, projected in turn onto the same tracing paper, and the areas of α and Ig-2^b positive cells were recorded. The latter cells were always a sub-set of the former. The IgA and allotype positive areas were measured using a planimeter and the extent of repopulation was expressed as the percentage of the total α-positive area which was Ig-2^b allotype positive. Table 6 indicates that very few, if any, donor-derived IgA cells appear in spleen or gut through days 6–7. However, by day 8–10 there is a sudden appearance of donor IgA plasma cells in lamina propria of patch cell recipients, when they comprise about 40–50% of the total IgA cell population. By day 14 almost all gut IgA cells of patch cell recipients are of donor origin. The peripheral nodes seem considerably less effective at recolonizing recipients with IgA plasma cells and contribute only 10–20% of such cells by day 10 and 36% by day 14. Of course, as donor-derived cells are repopulating the gut, the host's own cells are diminishing in number. Our finding that almost complete replacement of intestinal IgA cells occurs by 14 days in Peyer's patch cell recipients is consistent with a previous estimate, based on a different measurement, of 4.7 days as the half-life of mouse IgA cells in lamina propria (Mattioli & Tomasi 1973). By 14 days the host cells should have endured three half-lives and should have diminished to about 12% of their original number. Thus comparison of different cell sources for their potential to repopulate by other methods should be more meaningful at early times (days 8–10) when the host compartment is still substantial and hence provides a more accurate internal standard.

Peyer's patch cells can certainly repopulate gut lamina propria with IgA plasma cells. However, it is still not known whether they must temporarily reside in other tissues before gaining their propensity to lodge in lamina propria or whether they pass directly to the gut, there to mature into plasma cells. Another property of these IgA precursors which has not yet been evaluated is whether they can divide after lodging in the lamina propria and before maturation into plasma cells. A truly 'local' secondary response would seem to require such a reserve potential for antigen-stimulated division.

On the basis of some of the principles deduced by ourselves and others we have attempted to devise a model system for evaluating the role of Peyer's patches after the introduction of antigen into the gut lumen (Robertson & Cebra 1976).

A MODEL SYSTEM FOR THE STUDY OF INDUCTION OF HUMORAL IMMUNITY IN THE GUT

Many investigators have been able to stimulate the appearance of specific IgA antibodies in mammalian secretions (Blackman et al. 1974; Montgomery et al. 1974; Yardley et al. 1976). Particularly, Hanson and his colleagues have been able to correlate the appearance of IgA antibody-secreting cells in human milk with colonization of mothers' guts with a distinctive serotype of E. coli (Goldblum et al. 1975). Most of these studies suffer from the drawbacks that it is technically difficult to identify the precise tissues where B lymphocytes respond to antigen and to directly implicate Peyer's patches in this response. Thus, sites of earliest response of B cells to antigen could include: (1) Peyer's patches; (2) lamina propria; (3) mesenteric lymph nodes; (4) spleen and other lymphoid tissues reached by antigen via the bloodstream after absorption by the gut.

Using rabbits we have constructed a series of animals having two 20-cm isolated ileal loops (Thiry-Vella), each bearing or lacking a Peyer's patch, by

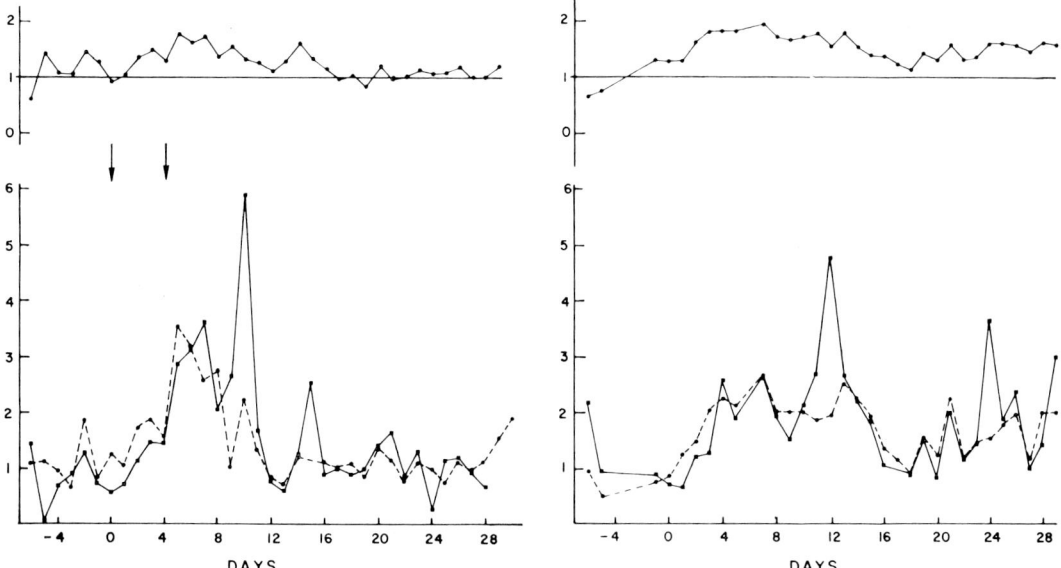

FIG. 2. Analysis of daily loop secretions of rabbit 1 (containing Peyer's patches) which received two doses of antigens, DNP-KLH and *Salmonella typhimurium*, into the loops on day 0 and day 4 (↓). Data for the stimulated loop (SL) are shown on the left and the control loop (CL) on the right. Symbols: – • – – • –, specific IgA anti-DNP activity as determined by ^{125}I anti-α in the radioimmunoassay (RIA) at a 1/600 sample dilution; ——•——, total anti-DNP activity as determined by ^{125}I anti-Fab in the RIA at a 1/600 sample dilution. The relative sIgA concentration (•——•) was determined at a 1/3000 sample dilution by ^{125}I anti-Fab and anti-α BAC in the RIA. The value of '1' for the SL is 1.6 mg sIgA/ml secretions; for the CL, 2.3 mg/ml. The specific anti-DNP activity has been normalized by a factor which reflects the daily fluctuation of total sIgA.

the method used by Yardley and his group (Keren *et al.* 1975). These loops, though isolated, still maintain their mesenteric attachment and thus their neurovascular supply. Seven days after surgery, antigens—2,4-dinitrophenylated keyhole limpet haemocyanin (DNP-KLH) (400 µg) and heat-killed *Salmonella typhimurium* LT-2 Zinder (4×10^7)—were introduced into one of the loops (distal) and saline was introduced into the other control loop (proximal). After 12 hours the remaining antigens were flushed out of the loops with air and the introduction of antigen was repeated at the desired times. The secretions of the loops were collected at intervals and the total sIgA, total antibody and total IgA antibody concentrations were measured by radioimmunoassay using appropriate insoluble antigens (Elson & Taylor 1974; Klinman & Taylor 1969). The specific serum response was also monitored. Fig. 2 shows that a specific IgA anti-DNP response could be elicited by two applications of the mixture of antigens into the distal loop on days 0 and 4 (Robertson & Cebra 1976). The

TABLE 7

Absolute concentrations of anti-DNP antibodies and of sIgA in the intestinal loop fluids

Animal	Loop	Peyer's patch[c]	Pre-immune levels		Maximum response levels	
			Total IgA (mg/ml)	Anti-DNP (μg/ml)	Total IgA (mg/ml)	Anti-DNP (μg/ml)
1	SL[a]	+	3.1	33	4.5	138-216
	CL[b]	+	3.4	51	6.8	147
2	SL	+	1.7	16	2.2	87
	CL	+	1.1	27	2.7	49-86
3	SL	+	3.1	22	4.8	60
	CL	+	>5	27	>5	80
4	SL	+	2.9	6	4.1	25-36
	CL	+	5	15	>5	72
5	SL	—	3.7	5	>5	10
	CL	—	3.2	4	5.5	14
6	SL	—	2.7	23	>5	44
	CL	—	2.8	17	4.7	36
7	SL	—	5.4	5	>5	24
	CL	+	>5	13-34	3.4-6.5	34-42
8	SL	+	1.5	4	5.6	45
	CL	—	0.072	7.7	0.43-0.96	44

[a] SL, stimulated loop.
[b] CL, control loop.
[c] +, Peyer's patch present in loop; —, Peyer's patch absent from loop.

time-course of appearance of anti-DNP antibodies was somewhat variable but often showed an early rise (days 4–8) followed by a slight decline and then another modest rise to a rather constant level, which occurred later (days 12–20). Most often, the change in antibody concentration with time followed the same course in secretions of the distal (immunized) and proximal (control) loop. Almost all the anti-DNP present in the secretions was IgA and this was in the form of dimers and higher polymers. Immunohistochemical staining showed plasma cells making anti-DNP in the lamina propria of the loops. Throughout the 20–40 days during which loop secretions could be monitored, no rise in serum anti-DNP titres of any isotype could be detected. The maximum concentration of IgA anti-DNP often rose 5–10 fold over pre-stimulation values to 100–200 μg/ml (Table 7). However, if the loops lacked Peyer's patches, the increase in anti-DNP in secretions was either slight or did not occur at all (Table 7). We believe that this model system implicates the Peyer's patch in the response to antigens impinging on the gut mucosa. The observations are consistent with antigen-stimulated B cell division in the patch follicles followed by departure of these cells via the mesenteric nodes, through the circulation and back to the lamina propria of all sections of the gut. The possibility of temporary residence of these cells in mesenteric nodes and further antigen-driven proliferation and maturation before further emigration is also consistent with our findings.

We have tried to provide some recent findings pertinent to the stimulation of humoral immunity in the gut and to sharpen the areas of inquiry we posed at the outset as relevant to this process. I am sure that subsequent contributors to this symposium will further elucidate the mechanisms for both the eliciting and the functioning of gut immunity.

ACKNOWLEDGEMENTS

We would like to thank Drs Michael Potter and Elizabeth Mushinski for generously providing breeding stock for the initiation of our CB20 mouse colony, Drs J. H. Yardley and D. F. Keren and Ms Gertrude Brown for aiding in the construction of ileal loops in rabbits and Dr Norman Klinman for aiding in the splenic focus assay.

The work described in this paper was supported by grants from the National Institute of Allergy and Infectious Diseases of the United States (AI-09652) and the National Science Foundation (GB38798). Patricia Gearhart is supported by a Helen Hay Whitney Foundation postdoctoral research fellowship. Stella M. Robertson is supported by Training Grant no. T01 HD00139-08.

References

AHLSTEDT, S., CARLSSON, B., FÄLLSTRÖM, S. P., HANSON, L. Å., HOLMGREN, J., LIDIN-JANSON, G., LINDBLAD, B. S., JODAL, U., KAIJSER, B., SOHL-ÅKERLUND, A. & WADSWORTH, C. (1977) Antibodies in human serum and milk induced by enterobacteria and food proteins, this volume, pp. 115-129

BAZIN, H. G., LEVI, G. & DORIA, F. (1970) Predominant contribution of IgA antibody-forming cells to an immune response detected in extra-intestinal lymphoid tissues of germ-free mice exposed to antigen by the oral route. *J. Immunol. 105*, 1049-1051

BERNIER, G. & CEBRA, J. J. (1965) Frequency distribution of α-, γ-, κ-, and λ-polypeptide chains in human lymphoid tissues. *J. Immunol. 95*, 246-253

BLACKMAN, U., GRABOFF, S. R., HAAG, G. E., GOTTFELD, E. & PICKETT, M. J. (1974) Experimental cholera in chinchillas: the immune response in serum and intestinal secretions to *Vibrio cholerae* and cholera toxin. *Infect. Immun. 10*, 1098-1104

BOCKMAN, D. E. & COOPER, M. D. (1973) Pinocytosis by epithelium associated with lymphoid follicles in the bursa of Fabricius, appendix, and Peyer's patches. An electron microscopic study. *Am. J. Anat. 136*, 455-477

BRANDTZAEG, P. & BAKLIEN, K. (1977) Intestinal secretion of IgA and IgM: a hypothetical model, this volume, pp. 77-108

CARTER, P. B. & COLLINS, F. M. (1974) The route of enteric infection in normal mice. *J. Exp. Med. 139*, 1189-1203

CEBRA, J. J., COLBERG, J. E. & DRAY, S. (1966) Rabbit lymphoid cells differentiated with respect to α-, γ-, and μ-heavy polypeptide chains and to allotypic markers AA1 and AA2. *J. Exp. Med. 123*, 547-558

CEBRA, J. J. & ROBBINS, J. B. (1966) γA-Immunoglobulin from rabbit colostrum. *J. Immunol. 97*, 12-24

CEBRA, J. J. & SMALL, P. A. (1967) Polypeptide chain structure of rabbit immunoglobulins. III. Secretory γA-immunoglobulin from colostrum. *Biochemistry 6*, 503-512

COPPOLA, E. D., ENEIN, A. A., KOPYCINSKI, C. F. & DE LUCA, F. (1972) Synergism between Peyer's patch cells and spleen cells in humoral antibody production. *J. Immunol. 108*, 831-833

CRABBÉ, P. A., CARBONARA, A. O. & HEREMANS, J. F. (1965) The normal human intestinal mucosa as a major source of plasma cells containing gamma A-immunoglobulin. *Lab. Invest. 14*, 235

CRABBÉ, P. A., NASH, D. R., BAZIN, H., EYSSEN, H. & HEREMANS, J. F. (1969) Antibodies of the IgA type in intestinal plasma cells of germ-free mice after oral stimulation or parenteral immunization with ferritin. *J. Exp. Med. 130*, 723-744

CRAIG, S. W. & CEBRA, J. J. (1971) Peyer's patches: an enriched source of precursors for IgA-producing immunocytes in the rabbit. *J. Exp. Med. 134*, 188-200

CRAIG, S. W. & CEBRA, J. J. (1975) Rabbit Peyer's patches, appendix, and popliteal lymph node B lymphocytes: a comparative analysis of their membrane immunoglobulin components and plasma cell precursor potential. *J. Immunol. 114*, 492-502

CRANDALL, R. B., CEBRA, J. J. & CRANDALL, C. A. (1967) The relative proportions of IgG-, IgA-, and IgM- containing cells in rabbit tissues during experimental trichinosis. *Immunology 12*, 147-158

DORE, C. F. & BALFOUR, B. M. (1965) A device for preparing cell spreads. *Immunology 9*, 403-405

EDDIE, D. S., SHULKIND, M. L. & ROBBINS, J. B. (1971) The isolation and biological activities of purified secretory IgA and IgG anti-*Salmonella typhimurium* 'O' antibodies from rabbit intestinal fluid and colostrum. *J. Immunol. 106*, 181-190

ELSON, C. J. & TAYLOR, R. B. (1974) The suppressive effect of carrier priming on the response to a hapten carrier conjugate. *Eur. J. Immunol. 4*, 682-687

FAULK, W. P., MCCORMICK, J. N., GOODMAN, J. R., YOFFEY, J. M. & FUDENBERG, H. H. (1971) Peyer's patches: morphologic studies. *Cell Immunol. 1*, 500-520

FRETER, R. (1970) Mechanism of action of intestinal antibody in experimental cholera. II. Antibody-mediated antibacterial reaction at the mucosal surface. *Infect. Immun. 2*, 556

GEARHART, P. J., SIGAL, N. Y. & KLINMAN, N. R. (1975) Heterogeneity of the BALB/c anti-phosphorylcholine antibody response at the precursor cell level. *J. Exp. Med. 141*, 56-71

GIBBONS, R. J. (1974) Bacterial adherence to mucosal surfaces and its inhibition by secretory antibodies, in *The Immunoglobulin A System* (Mestecky, J. & Lawton, A. R., eds.), pp. 315-325 (*Adv. Exp. Med. Biol. 45*), Plenum Press, New York

GOLDBLUM, R. M., AHLSTEDT, S., CARLSSON, B., HANSON, L. Å., JODAL, U., LIDIN-JANSON, G. & SOHL-ÅKERLUND, A. (1975) Antibody-forming cells in human colostrum after oral immunization. *Nature (Lond.) 257*, 797-799

GOWANS, J. L. & KNIGHT, E. J. (1964) The route of re-circulation of lymphocytes in the rat. *Proc. R. Soc. Ser. B Biol. Sci. 159*, 257-282

GRISCELLI, C., VASSALLI, P. & MCCLUSKEY, R. T. (1969) The distribution of large dividing lymph node cells in syngeneic recipient rats after intravenous injection. *J. Exp. Med. 130*, 1427-1451

GUY-GRAND, D., GRISCELLI, C. & VASSALLI, P. (1974) The gut-associated lymphoid system: nature and properties of the large dividing cells. *Eur. J. Immunol. 4*, 435-443

HALPERN, M. S. & KOSHLAND, M. E. (1970) Novel subunit in secretory IgA. *Nature (Lond.) 228*, 1276-1278

HANSON, L. Å. (1960) The serological relationship between human milk and blood plasma. *Int. Arch. Allergy 17*, 45-69

HANSON, L. Å. (1961) Comparative immunological studies of the immune globulins of human milk and of blood serum. *Int. Arch. Allergy 18*, 241-267

HENRY, C., FAULK, W. P., KUHN, L., YOFFEY, J. M. & FUDENBERG, H. H. (1970) Peyer's patches: immunologic studies. *J. Exp. Med. 131*, 1200-1210

HEREMANS, J. F. (1975) The secretory immune system. A critical appraisal, in *The Immune System and Infectious Diseases* (Neter, E. & Milgrom, F., eds.), pp. 376-385, Karger, Basel

HEREMANS, J. F. & VAERMAN, J. P. (1971) Biological significance of IgA antibodies in serum and secretions, in *Progress in Immunology I* (Amos, B., ed.) (*First International Congress of Immunology*), pp. 875-890, Academic Press, New York

HEREMANS, J. F., HEREMANS, M. T. & SCHULTZE, M. E. (1959) Isolation and description of a few properties of β_{2A}-globulin of human serum. *Clin. Chim. Acta 4*, 96

HERZENBERG, L. A. (1964) A chromosome region for gamma 2a and beta 2A globulin H chain isoantigens in the mouse. *Cold Spring Harbor Symp. Quant. Biol. 29*, 455-462

JONES, P. P. & CEBRA, J. J. (1974) Restriction of gene expression in B lymphocytes and their progeny. III. Endogenous IgA and IgM on the membranes of different plasma cell precursors. *J. Exp. Med. 140*, 966-976

JONES, P. P., CRAIG, S. W., CEBRA, J. J. & HERZENBERG, L. A. (1974) Restriction of gene expression in B lymphocytes and their progeny. II. Commitment to immunoglobulin heavy chain isotype. *J. Exp. Med. 140*, 452-469

JONES, T. L., WILKS, C. F. & COPPOLA, E. D. (1976) Antibody response to antigen stimulation by mouse Peyer's patch cells *in vitro*. *Fed. Proc. 35*, 863 (abstr. 3625)

KAGNOFF, M. F. & CAMPBELL, S. (1973) Functional characteristics of Peyer's patch lymphoid cells. *J. Exp. Med. 139*, 398-406

KAMIN, R. M., HENRY, C. & FUDENBERG, H. H. (1974) Suppressor cells in the rabbit appendix. *J. Immunol. 113*, 1151-1161

KATZ, D. H. & PEREY, D. Y. E. (1973) Lymphocytes in Peyer's patches of the mouse: analysis of the constituent cells in terms of their capacities to mediate functions of mature T and B lymphocytes. *J. Immunol. 111*, 1507-1513

KEREN, D. F., ELLIOTT, H. L., BROWN, G. D. & YARDLEY, J. H. (1975) Atrophy of villi with hypertrophy and hyperplasia of Paneth cells in isolated (Thiry-Vella) ileal loops in rabbits. *Gastroenterology 68*, 83-93

KLINMAN, N. R. (1969) Antibody with homogeneous antigen binding produced by splenic foci in organ culture. *Immunochemistry 6*, 757-759

KLINMAN, N. R. & TAYLOR, R. B. (1969) General methods for the study of cells and serum during the immune response: the response to dinitrophenyl in mice. *Clin. Exp. Immunol. 4*, 473-487

KNUDSON, K. C., FRANCE, C. M., COPPOLA, E. D., MILLER, H. C. & JONES, T. L. (1975) Interaction between cells of Peyer's patches and cells of bone marrow origin in the immune response. *J. Immunol. 114*, 1428-1430

LIEBERMAN, R., POTTER, M., MUSHINSKI, E. B., HUMPHREY, W. & RUDIKOFF, S. (1974) Genetics of a new IgV_H (T15 idiotype) marker in the mouse regulating natural antibody to phosphorylcholine. *J. Exp. Med. 139*, 983-1001

MATTIOLI, C. S. & TOMASI, T. B. (1973) The life span of IgA plasma cells from the mouse intestine. *J. Exp. Med. 138*, 452-460

MCWILLIAMS, M., LAMM, M. E. & PHILLIPS-QUAGLIATA, J. M. (1974) Surface and intracellular markers of mouse mesenteric and peripheral lymph node and Peyer's patch cells. *J. Immunol. 113*, 1326-1333

MCWILLIAMS, M., PHILLIPS-QUAGLIATA, J. M. & LAMM, M. E. (1975) Characteristics of mesenteric lymph node cells homing to gut-associated lymphoid tissue in syngeneic mice. *J. Immunol. 115*, 54-58

MONTGOMERY, P. C., COHN, J. & LALLY, E. T. (1974) The induction and characterization of secretory IgA antibodies, in *The Immunoglobulin A System* (Mestecky, J. & Lawton, A. R., eds.) (*Adv. Exp. Med. Biol. 45*), pp. 453-462, Plenum Press, New York

O'DALY, J. A. & CEBRA, J. J. (1971) Chemical and physiochemical studies of the component polypeptide chains of rabbit secretory immunoglobulin A. *Biochemistry 10*, 3843-3850

OGRA, P. L., MORAG, A. & BEUTNER, K. R. (1975) Amplification of local immune responses with active immunization, in *The Immune System and Infectious Diseases* (*4th Int. Convoc. Immunol.*) (Neter, E. & Milgrom, F., eds.), pp. 322-333, Karger, Basel

OZER, H. & WAKSMAN, B. H. (1972) Appendix and γM antibody formation. V. Appendix and thymus cell synergism in the direct and indirect plaque-forming cell responses to sheep erythrocytes in the rabbit. *J. Immunol. 109*, 410-412

PIERCE, N. F. & GOWANS, J. J. (1975) Cellular kinetics of the intestinal immune response to cholera toxoid in rats. *J. Exp. Med. 142*, 1550-1563

POTTER, M. & LIEBERMAN, R. (1970) Common individual antigenic determinants in five of eight Balb/c IgA myeloma proteins that bind phosphorylcholine. *J. Exp. Med. 132*, 737-751

ROBERTSON, S. M. & CEBRA, J. J. (1976) A model for local immunity. *La Ricerca in Clinica e in Laboratorio 6*, suppl. 3, 105-119

SMITH, C. B., PURCELL, R. H., BELLANTI, J. A. & CHANOCK, R. M. (1966) Protective effect of antibody to parainfluenza type 1 virus. *N. Engl. J. Med. 275*, 1145-1152

SOUTH, M. A., COOPER, M. D., WALLHEIM, F. A., HONG, R. & GOOD, R. A. (1966) The IgA system. I. Studies of the transport and immunochemistry of IgA in the saliva. *J. Exp. Med. 123*, 615-627

TOMASI, T. B., JR. & ZIGELBAUM, S. D. (1963) The selective occurrence of γA globulins in certain body fluids. *J. Clin. Invest. 42*, 1552-1560

TOMASI, T. B., JR., TANS, E. M., SOLOMON, A. & PRENDERGAST, R. A. (1965) Characteristics of an immune system common to certain external secretions. *J. Exp. Med. 121*, 101-124

WAKSMAN, B. H., OZER, H. & BLYTHMAN, H. E. (1973) Appendix and γM-antibody formation. VI. The functional anatomy of the rabbit appendix. *Lab. Invest. 28*, 614-626

WILLIAMS, A. F. & GOWANS, J. L. (1975) The presence of IgA on the surface of rat thoracic duct lymphocytes which contain internal IgA. *J. Exp. Med. 141*, 335-345

YARDLEY, J. H., KEREN, D. F. & HAMILTON, S. R. (1976) The local and systemic immune response to cholera toxin in rabbits with chronically isolated (Thiry-Vella) ileal loops. *Gastroenterology 70*, 953

Discussion

Soothill: How secure is your evidence that the Peyer's patch is relevant to the IgA response in the experiments with ileal loops?

Cebra: The general finding in about 20 rabbits is that if there is an IgA response, it is manifest in the secretions of both loops, and the time-courses are almost identical. If the loop receiving antigen lacks a patch, there is no response in either loop, or a minimal response in both; but if the loop receiving antigen bears a patch, the response tends to be higher in both loops, though not as high in the control loop as when both loops have a patch. The overall net increase in IgA antibodies when both loops have a patch is 10-fold, sometimes 20- or 25-fold, from about 20 μg/ml of background antibody to 200 μg/ml. If neither loop contains a patch, there is 10–20 μg/ml of antibody before stimulation which may rise to 30 or 35 μg/ml with antigen.

Porter: So the segmental immunization reported by Ogra & Karzon (1969) is really determined by where you do the immunization within a loop preparation? I assume they must have been applying antigen high up in the intestine, away from the Peyer's patch region?

Booth: No; Ogra used colonic segments.

Cebra: It is possible that one can, in the absence of a patch, stimulate a local immune response. One unanswered question is whether the cells that arrive in the lamina propria have a residual potential for antigen-driven proliferation. Such a potential would be necessary for a true secondary response. It has been shown that a small fraction of antigen can pass intact through gut epithelium in areas lacking a patch (Walker *et al.* 1972), so I would not rule out stimulation in the absence of a patch. However, I think our results show that a patch is essential for effective stimulation.

Soothill: Have you shown that this is not simply a result of the particular region of the bowel you are dealing with?

Cebra: No. In our choice of sites for stimulation we have favoured loops from the distal ileum, which is richer in patches and is known to play a role in stimulation by certain gut organisms that accumulate proximal to the ileal-caecal valve (Carter & Collins 1974).

Soothill: The result could be an effect of organisms present acting as adjuvants?

Cebra: Yes. In fact, there could be an enhanced response due to the salmonellae given with the antigen. We are now giving the antigen without salmonella organisms.

Lehner: A possible adjuvant effect is important, but it depends on the sequence of adding adjuvant to the antigen; this certainly applies to lipopolysaccharides (Johnson *et al.* 1956; Lagrange & Mackaness 1975). Have you tried to give lipopolysaccharide first and then antigen? This would not increase the humoral antibody response but might cause suppression.

Cebra: We have not done this but we are doing various extensions of this experiment, involving the use of LPS and varying the order of addition, and also we are assessing the effect of carrier-priming in a hapten–protein system. You are probably partly right in thinking that LPS is affecting the response. At least three-quarters of the animals show an increase in total IgA in the loop as well as the increase in specific antibody. We think this increase in IgA concentration may have something to do with the bacteria we put in the loop.

Gowans: Your evidence that you get a similar antibody response in both loops when you give antigen into only one loop contradicts other evidence in sheep which shows clearly that the highest concentration of specific antibody is found in the challenged loop (Husband & Lascelles 1974). I will be reporting similar results in rats (p. 39). How do you reconcile these differences?

Cebra: Pierce & Gowans (1975) have shown that antigen can influence IgA cell lodging. Probably at least two factors are involved in determining the magnitude of the response in different segments of the gut. One is a random lodging of B lymphocyte precursors of IgA plasma cells in the lamina propria after stimulation and emigration of cells from the patch through the mesenteric lymph nodes. The other factor might be a selective accumulation and/or proliferation of cells at sites adjacent to antigens or antigen-bearing material in the gut. Most of our rabbits are immunized two to four times, and immunization is still going on when we see the first responses. Perhaps by using small amounts

($<$400 µg) we are not detecting as big a role for local antigen in determining sites of IgA secretion as others have found.

Gowans: Did you study the time-course of the response? Is there any time at which the response is highest in the loop with a patch?

Cebra: The overall response may be less in the non-immunized loop but it follows very much the same time-course.

Porter: I want to take up the question of the class of antibodies. In your studies with *Trichinella* infections in rabbits (Crandall *et al.* 1967) you showed that the first cells in the response were IgM cells. Our work in the pig (Allen & Porter 1973) shows that in the early local immune response of the intestine to bacterial antigens, or in normal bacterial colonization in the developing pig, IgM cells far outnumber IgA cells over the first 4–5 weeks of life. The early antibody response is largely IgM. McNeish has similar findings in relation to *Escherichia coli* infections in infants in which IgM was the chief immunoglobulin (McNeish *et al.* 1975). Of course, IgM is a major secretory immunoglobulin. Your precursor cells in the loop experiments are probably µ-negative in their surface characteristics. If you had looked at your antibody response in the loops in terms of IgM, might you have found different characteristics of the response?

Cebra: Perhaps. There is always the possibility of inactivation and degradation of IgM antibodies before assay; if IgM antibodies are more susceptible we might have missed them in assaying the loop secretions. Had we looked at antibody-forming cells in the lamina propria, which we are doing now (which is harder because one cannot disperse lamina propria cells and do plaque-forming cell analysis), we might have seen significant numbers of IgM antibody-forming cells in the gut.

Let me try to reconcile two kinds of data in my paper. I spoke of immediate precursors for IgA plasma cells. These are important in the earliest phase of the IgA response. This early IgA response could even be regarded as a secondary response by patch cells that may be many divisions away from 'virgin' antigen-sensitive cells and may have been primed by naturally occurring antigens. I think that these immediate precursors are surface IgA-positive cells that can generate large clones of IgA plasma cells. The antibody responses seen later (days 10, 12, 15 after stimulation) are probably derived from µ-bearing cells that give rise to the µ plus α clones. Such µ+ cells may also be abundant clonal precursors in the Peyer's patches. In other words, I think antigen-sensitive cells may be at different stages of maturity in the patches. One doesn't know the importance of T cell interactions in influencing the expression of IgA by clonal progeny of µ+ antigen-sensitive cells originating in the patch or in selectively stimulating maturation of the daughters derived from α+ cells. The time-sequence and relative numbers of IgM and IgA antibody-forming cells may vary, depending on the amount of T cell cooperation.

Porter: In your adoptive transfer studies did your μ-negative cells give rise predominantly to IgA producers?

Cebra: Yes. Plasma cells derived from μ-negative Peyer's patch cells found in either spleen or gut lamina propria of allogeneic rabbit recipients predominantly were IgA producers. Probably the precursors of these cells are equivalent to those cells in mouse Peyer's patches that generate clones which produce only IgA. However, other precursors found in mouse Peyer's patches can give rise to clones expressing IgM and occasionally IgGl as well as IgA. It is probable—although not formally shown—that these latter precursors bear IgM on their surface.

Pierce: You mentioned a biphasic antibody response in your loops. Was the second phase of that response similar in magnitude to the first, and equal in both loops? Have you an explanation for this observation?

Cebra: We often but not always see the biphasic response. If one phase is missing it is usually the earlier one. An explanation may be derived from our clonal precursor analysis: at any given time one has in the patch an assortment of cells having equal proliferative potential; any can give rise to, say, a thousand antibody-secreting cells. Some of these cells in the patch are differentiated to the point where they can provide clones expressing only IgA, and I think these are responsible for the earliest phase of the secretory IgA response. These precursors could be regarded as secondary cells, even though they have not been deliberately primed. Other antigen-sensitive cells which probably bear IgM occur in the Peyer's patches and these may be even more abundant than the precursors which generate clones expressing only IgA. These go through further divisions after antigen stimulation before producing daughters that make IgA. I would postulate that these cells account for the later phase of the secretory IgA response. It also seems possible that the development of maximal expression of a secretory IgA response is dependent on the time-course of the generation of cooperating T cells.

Gowans: You have never shown that μ-bearing cells are the precursors of cells which eventually make IgA, have you?

Cebra: No, not formally, but we have shown that a high proportion of antigen-sensitive cells from the patch reactive with the phosphorylcholine determinant can generate clones which produce IgM and IgA. Assaying with the DNP rather than the phosphorylcholine determinant, the picture is a little different (P. J. Gearhart & J. J. Cebra, unpublished work 1976). Almost half of the clones derived from the spleen or patch contain some cells which express IgM. However, there are hardly any clonal precursors for DNP in the unimmunized mouse which generate clones making only IgA. Almost all of the derivative clones expressing IgA also make IgM or IgM plus IgG1. While we have not shown in these assays that μ-bearing cells go on to make IgA, there is a strong suggestion that some of their daughter plasma cells do.

Pierce: Have you any evidence of a third or fourth wave or is this response in the loops only biphasic, not multiphasic? Secondly, you gave antigen repeatedly. Do you time these responses in relation to the first dose of antigen or the last? Is it possible that the biphasic response is related to the schedule of multiple doses?

Cebra: The phases of the response do not seem to be related to the timing of antigen doses, since the last antigen administration is usually at the beginning of the response and most of our observations have been made after stimulation on days 0 and 4. It is not clear if there are subsequent waves of secretory IgA responses because the system gets rather 'noisy' later.

Pepys: Have you any data on a delta-like heavy chain on the Peyer's patch cells, in view of the work showing that delta is a major heavy chain isotype on such cells in mice (Vitetta *et al.* 1975)?

Cebra: No.

Parrott: In your adoptive transfer experiments, you always added thymocytes, evidently because there are not enough T cells in Peyer's patches. If you took Peyer's patches from germ-free mice or from mice of other ages, would you need to add the thymocytes?

Cebra: For the adoptive transfer of a sheep red blood cell response you can leave out the thymocytes; there are sufficient T cells in the patch. However, if you remove the T cells from the Peyer's patch cell population, there is no appreciable adoptive antibody response transferred with the residual cells. If T cells from a primed animal are added to a Peyer's patch cell inoculum, more IgA PFC cells arise in the spleens of the recipients and these appear sooner than in recipients of patch cells alone. We feel that there is a T cell-dependence of the expression of the IgA plaque-forming cells (PFC) and part of the delay in the appearance of IgA PFC until 10–12 days after cell transfer might be due to the necessity for generating sufficient T cells. We are now investigating the role of suppressor and cooperating T cells in this adoptive transfer system.

White: You mentioned the dome epithelium and the implication seemed to be that antigens were entering through this epithelium. Where is the antigen? You said that there is no antigen-retaining reticulum in Peyer's patches. Is the antigen associated with antibody?

Cebra: The work I quoted was that of Bockman & Cooper (1973) and of Walker *et al.* (1972). When ferritin or peroxidase has been introduced into the gut lumen the active protein has been found in vesicles in dome epithelial cells, and presumably must be transported through these cells since the proteins are also found among the patch lymphoid follicles. Very quickly thereafter the active proteins may be found trapped in the reticulum of draining mesenteric lymph nodes. I don't know what the mechanism is by which protein is transported across the dome epithelial cell. Perhaps the mechanism is similar to that found in studies by Rodewald (1975) on transport of maternal immunoglobulin across the absorptive gut epithelium of newborn mice and rats. There appears to be a membrane-bound receptor for immunoglobulin which becomes bound to membrane within vesicles upon endocytosis. After trans-cellular passage the immunoglobulin is ejected on the basal side of the cell by a reversal of endocytosis.

Cells that can take up antigen have been observed scattered through the patch (Faulk *et al.* 1971), so I would not exclude any trapping of antigen there, but there is no organized antigen-trapping reticulum in the patches. I know of no studies concerning the role of antibody in transport of antigen into the patch or in trapping it there.

Evans: You mentioned the difficulties of dispersing lamina propria cells for plaquing studies. Methods have been described for doing plaquing on sections (Berenbaum & Stringer 1970). Have you found these to be impractical on intestine?

Cebra: We have not been able to make the plaquing method work for gut sections because of non-specific lysis. We want to follow the cells after adoptive transfers to the lamina propria and we have resorted to an immunohistochemical method.

Parrott: Your main thesis is that the Peyer's patches populate the whole of the lamina propria. Dr Crabbé did beautiful studies (Crabbé *et al.* 1970) showing that there are more IgA cells in the villi close to the Peyer's patches than in more distant villi, and we (Parrott & Ferguson 1974) have pointed out that there are just a few lymphatic connections directly from Peyer's patches to those near villi where you can show with labelled cells that a few cells go straight through.

Cebra: I am familiar with these histological studies (Crabbé *et al.* 1970) and agree that lateral migration of IgA precursors directly from patches into the adjacent lamina propria may be an alternative means of populating the lamina propria. However, I believe that most observations support the lymph/blood circulation route as the major one leading to population of lamina propria.

References

ALLEN, W. D. & PORTER, P. (1973) The relative distribution of IgM and IgA cells in intestinal mucosa and lymphoid tissue of the young unweaned pig and their significance in ontogenesis of secretory immunity. *Immunology* 24, 493-504

BERENBAUM, M. C. & STRINGER, I. M. (1970) The localization of haemolytic antibody in sections of lymphoid organs: an improved method. *Immunology* 18, 85-90

BOCKMAN, D. E. & COOPER, M. D. (1973) Pinocytosis by epithelium associated with lymphoid follicles in the bursa of Fabricius, appendix, and Peyer's patches. An electron microscope study. *Am. J. Anat.* 136, 455-477

CARTER, P. B. & COLLINS, F. M. (1974) The route of enteric infection in normal mice. *J. Exp. Med.* 139, 1189-1203

CRANDALL, R. B., CEBRA, J. J. & CRANDALL, C. A. (1967) The relative proportions of IgG-, IgA- and IgM-containing cells in rabbit cells during experimental trichinosis. *Immunology* 12, 147-158

CRABBÉ, P. A., NASH, D. R., BAZIN, H., EYSSEN, H. & HEREMANS, J. F. (1970) Immunohistochemical observations on lymphoid tissues from conventional and germ-free mice. *Lab. Invest.* 22, 448-457

FAULK, W. P., MCCORMICK, J. N., GOODMAN, J. R., YOFFEY, J. M. & FUDENBERG, H. H. (1971) Peyer's patches: morphologic studies. *Cell. Immunol.* 1, 500-520

HUSBAND, A. J. & LASCELLES, A. K. (1974) The origin of antibody in intestinal secretion of sheep. *Aust. J. Exp. Biol. Med. Sci.* 52, 791

JOHNSON, A. G., GAINES, S. & LANDY, M. (1956) Studies on the O antigen of *Salmonella typhosa*. V. Enhancement of antibody response to protein antigens by the purified lipopolysaccharide. *J. Exp. Med.* 103, 225-246

LAGRANGE, P. H. & MACKANESS, G. B. (1975) Effects of bacterial lipopolysaccharide on the induction and expression of cell-mediated immunity. II. Stimulation of the efferent arc. *J. Immunol.* 114, 447-451

MCNEISH, A. S., EVANS, M., GAZE, H. & ROGERS, K. B. (1975) The agglutinating antibody response in the duodenum in infants with enteropathic *E. coli* gastroenteritis. *Gut* 16, 727-731

OGRA, P. L. & KARZON, D. T. (1969) Distribution of poliovirus antibody in serum, nasopharynx and alimentary tract following segmental immunization of lower alimentary tract with polio vaccine. *J. Immunol.* 102, 1423-1432

PARROTT, D. M. V. & FERGUSON, A. (1974) Selective migration of lymphocytes within the mouse small intestine. *Immunology* 26, 571

PIERCE, N. F. & GOWANS, J. L. (1975) Cellular kinetics of the intestinal immune response to cholera toxoid in rats. *J. Exp. Med.* 142, 1550-1563

RODEWALD, R. (1975) Intestinal transport of peroxidase-conjugated IgG fragments in the neonatal rat, in *Materno-fetal Transmission of Immunoglobulins* (Hemmings, W. A., ed.), pp. 137-153, Cambridge University Press, London

VITETTA, E. S., MCWILLIAMS, M., PHILLIPS-QUAGLIATA, J. M., LAMM, M. E. & UHR, J. W. (1975) Cell surface immunoglobulin. XIV. Synthesis, surface expression and secretion of immunoglobulin by Peyer's patch cells in the mouse. *J. Immunol.* 115, 603-605

WALKER, W. A., CORNELL, R., DAVENPORT, L. M. & ISSELBACHER, K. J. (1972) Macromolecular absorption: mechanism of horseradish peroxidase uptake and transport in adult and neonatal rat intestine. *J. Cell Biol.* 54, 195-205

The natural history of the cells producing IgA in the gut

A. J. HUSBAND, H. J. MONIÉ and J. L. GOWANS

MRC Cellular Immunology Unit, Sir William Dunn School of Pathology, University of Oxford

Abstract The IgA-secreting cells in the lamina propria of the small intestine are derived from large lymphocytes which enter the blood by way of the thoracic duct and then migrate into the gut where they complete their differentiation into plasma cells. Three aspects of this cellular traffic have been examined in rats.
1. The cells in thoracic duct lymph which give rise to IgA-secreting cells in the lamina propria are among those which carry surface IgA. Blast cells lacking surface immunoglobulin migrate mainly into the Peyer's patches and do not contribute to the IgA response.
2. Studies on a secondary antibody response to cholera toxoid, in which the challenge was given into a Thiry-Vella loop, showed that the antibody-containing blast cells in thoracic duct lymph were derived from Peyer's patches. The mesenteric nodes contributed little, if anything, to the cellular response in the lymph.
3. The idea that secretory component is a signal for the emigration of large lymphocytes from the blood into the lamina propria lacks experimental support. Secretory component does not bind to the IgA on the surface of thoracic duct cells. On the other hand, antigen in the gut may play an important part in immobilizing large lymphocytes in the lamina propria once they have migrated.

Immunity against potentially harmful microorganisms and macromolecules which may enter by way of the gut is provided by antibodies which are secreted into the intestinal lumen. The plasma cells which synthesize these antibodies are unusual in two ways: they are situated locally in the lamina propria of the intestine and not in lymphoid tissue; and in man and most animal species the predominant class of immunoglobulin which they synthesize is IgA. There is now evidence that the population of IgA-secreting cells in the gut is maintained by a traffic of large lymphocytes which enter the blood by way of the thoracic duct and then migrate from the blood into the intestinal lamina propria where they complete their differentiation into plasma cells (Gowans & Knight 1964; Guy-Grand *et al.* 1974: Pierce & Gowans 1975). This paper is concerned with three aspects of the generation and delivery of this remarkable local immunity: (1) the nature of the cells in thoracic duct lymph which migrate into the gut, (2) the origin of these cells, and (3) the factors which may influence their accumulation in the lamina propria.

Although IgA antibodies play an important protective role against enteric pathogens and their products it must be emphasized that both the small and large intestine of normal animals contain large numbers of IgA-secreting plasma cells. The antigens against which these antibodies are directed have not been identified but the density of plasma cells does not appear to be related in a simple way to the bacterial load in different parts of the intestine: the bacterial content of the large gut is considerably higher than that of the small, but this is not reflected in the density of plasma cells in the respective laminae propriae. Possibly, the absorption of sensitizing doses of dietary proteins constitutes a potential hazard against which the secretion of specific IgA antibodies is the normal response. The complex abnormalities sometimes associated with selective IgA deficiencies also suggest that the full range of function undertaken by IgA has probably not yet been uncovered. This paper is only indirectly concerned with the functions of IgA antibodies but it is necessary to point out that the cells in the gut which synthesize them are being continually generated in normal, healthy animals. The present experiments have been carried out on inbred strains of rats, raised under specific pathogen free conditions but later held in a conventional animal room for various periods before study. Unless otherwise stated the rats were not intentionally immunized.

ORIGIN OF INTESTINAL IgA-SECRETING CELLS FROM THORACIC DUCT LYMPHOCYTES

The thoracic duct collects lymph by way of the intestinal lymphatics from the whole intestinal bed, that is, from the large and small gut and from its associated lymphoid tissue, the mesenteric lymph nodes and the Peyer's patches (Fig. 1). In the absence of intentional immunization, both the small and large lymphocytes in thoracic duct lymph are derived almost exclusively from the intestinal bed. This has been established in rats by comparing the cell output from the thoracic duct with that from the intestinal lymphatics (Mann & Higgins 1950; G. Mayrhofer & J. L. Gowans, unpublished). The large lymphocytes, which make up less than 10% of all the cells in thoracic duct lymph, are formed by cell division in the intestinal lymphoid tissue because very few of them normally recirculate from the blood back into the lymph (Gowans & Knight 1964), and because they virtually all become labelled *in vivo* following a continuous 12-hour infusion of tritiated thymidine (Gowans 1959).

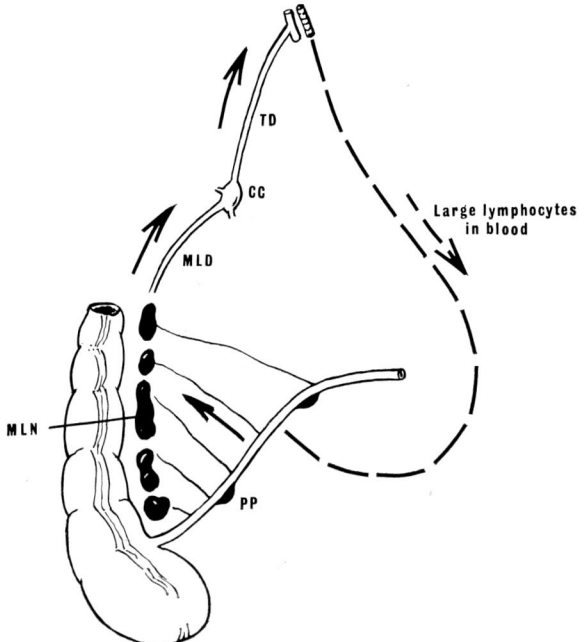

Fig. 1. The migration of large lymphocytes from the blood into the lamina propria of the small intestine and their origin from the lymphatic bed drained by the thoracic duct (TD). CC: Cisterna chyli; MLD: mesenteric (intestinal) lymph duct; MLN: mesenteric lymph nodes; PP: Peyer's patch.

Large lymphocytes in thoracic duct lymph, unlike the small, can be labelled by a brief incubation *in vitro* with radioactive precursors of DNA. The identification of such labelled cells by autoradiography after transfusion into syngeneic rats established that at least some of the plasma cells in the lamina propria of the intestine are derived from DNA-synthesizing lymphocytes which normally enter the blood by way of the thoracic duct. It was therefore proposed that the large lymphocytes were attracted into the lamina propria by the antigens which had originally provoked their formation in the intestinal lymphoid tissue (Gowans & Knight 1964), a view which will be reconsidered later. The subsequent discovery that the predominant class of immunoglobulin synthesized by intestinal plasma cells is IgA (Crabbé *et al.* 1965) led to the obvious conclusion that the large lymphocytes in thoracic duct lymph are the precursors of the IgA-synthesizing cells in the gut and this point has now been established (Guy-Grand *et al.* 1974; Pierce & Gowans 1975). Table 1 shows the results of a transfusion experiment in which large lymphocytes from the thoracic duct

TABLE 1

Proportion of labelled donor thoracic duct lymphocytes which contained internal IgA in gut of recipient rats

	% labelled cells with internal IgA in lamina propria	
	1	2
Jejunum	72 (72)	70 (91)
Ileum : upper	84 (49)	64 (142)
: lower	77 (74)	67 (143)
Colon : ascending	50 (48)	66 (29)

Donor thoracic duct lymphocytes labelled *in vitro* with tritiated thymidine (1 h, 37°C, 0.5μCi/ml, specific activity 5 Ci/mmole). Total of $2-8 \times 10^8$ cells given i.v. to each of two syngeneic rats which were killed 24 h later. Autoradiographs exposed for 14 days. Total number of labelled cells counted in gut sections in parenthesis; table shows % of these which also contained IgA by immunofluorescence. Technique for observing double label in Williams & Gowans (1975).

were identified in the intestine of syngeneic recipients both by their radioactive label and by their content of cytoplasmic IgA. It can be seen that about 70% of all the labelled cells in the lamina propria of the small intestine, and possibly a somewhat smaller proportion in the large intestine, also contained IgA. Labelled cells not containing IgA may have produced it at a later time or some may have been T blasts.

The fate of large lymphocytes has also been studied by estimating the distribution of radioactivity among the organs of rats after an intravenous transfusion of syngeneic thoracic duct cells previously labelled *in vitro* with a radioactive precursor of DNA (Hall *et al.* 1972). Fig. 2 illustrates a series of experiments of this kind which confirm that the tissue in which the greatest proportion of injected radioactivity accumulates is the small intestine (about 20–40% of the injected activity) and that a much smaller fraction localizes in the large intestine. Fig. 2 makes the additional point that a large fraction of the radioactive label appears in the urine, indicating that many of the transfused cells had died. This may merely reflect the damage sustained by the cells during handling *in vitro* or, possibly, that a proportion of the large lymphocytes are at the end of their lifespan and normally die in the lymph or in the blood.

Studies on the fate of DNA-synthesizing cells teased from lymph nodes are more difficult to interpret since the extent to which they reflect the population which normally migrates into the lymph is not known. However, large lymphocytes from mesenteric lymph nodes are second only to those from the thoracic duct in the proportion which localizes in the lamina propria (Griscelli

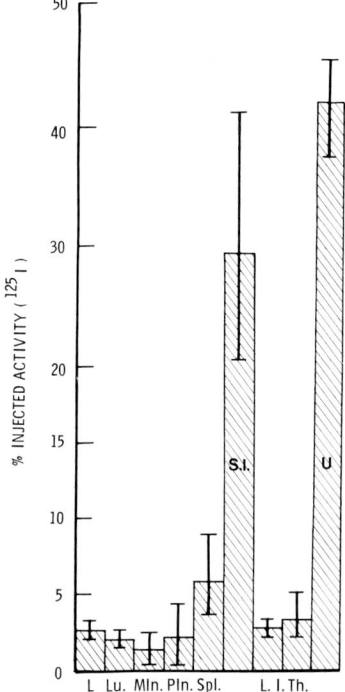

FIG. 2. Proportion of injected radioactivity recovered in whole organs of AO strain rats 24 h after an i.v. injection of syngeneic thoracic duct cells ($0.3-1.6 \times 10^8$) labelled *in vitro* with [^{125}I]iododeoxyuridine (^{125}IUdR) (1 h, 37°C, 0.1 μCi/ml). Mean and range for 5 recipients. Liver (L), lungs (Lu), mesenteric lymph nodes (Mln), inguinal, axillary, brachial and cervical nodes (Pln), spleen (Spl), small intestine (S.I.), large intestine (L.I.), thyroid (Th) and urine (U).

et al. 1969); large lymphocytes from peripheral nodes elsewhere show no predilection for the lamina propria (Griscelli *et al.* 1969). Paradoxically, DNA-synthesizing cells from Peyer's patches are reported not to home to the gut (Guy-Grand *et al.* 1974; McWilliams *et al.* 1975) although, as will be discussed later, Peyer's patches are the major source of the gut-seeking lymphocytes. The nature of the lymphocytes from bronchus-associated lymphoid tissue which populate the lamina propria is not known (Rudzik *et al.* 1975*b*).

The transfusion experiments make it clear that some IgA-secreting cells in the lamina propria are derived from precursors in thoracic duct lymph but they do not precisely identify them. The problem is complicated by the possibility that cells in the lymph not in DNA synthesis may also be precursors and by the heterogeneity of the blast cells themselves. These complications have been partially resolved by studying the distribution of surface and internal IgA

TABLE 2

Homing to the intestine of DNA-synthesizing large lymphocytes from the thoracic duct. Fate of all labelled blasts compared with that of subpopulation of blasts which lacked surface Ig

	% injected radioactivity recovered in intestine after transfusion of:			
Experiment	Undepleted TDL[a]		Depleted TDL[b]	
	S.I.	L.I.	S.I.	L.I.
1	32.1	3.6	42.8	4.6
2	40.6	4.7	32.0	3.3
3	43.8	5.5	37.5	4.0

[a] Normal thoracic duct lymphocytes (TDL) from inbred AO or PVG/c strain rats.
[b] TDL depleted of all cells carrying surface Ig by rosetting with sheep erythrocytes coated with rabbit $F(ab')_2$ anti-rat Fab and spinning through Isopaque/Ficoll (Parish & Hayward 1975; Mason 1976). About 10^8 normal or depleted TDL which had been labelled *in vitro* with tritiated thymidine (1h, 37°C, 0.5 µCi/ml, specific activity 5Ci/mmole) given i.v. to syngeneic recipients. Recipients killed at 24 h and whole small (S.I.) or large (L.I.) intestine incinerated on sample oxidizer and radioactivity (c.p.m.) measured by scintillation counting.

among rat thoracic duct lymphocytes. About half the large lymphocytes in thoracic duct lymph and also about half of those which label *in vitro* with tritiated thymidine contain considerable amounts of cytoplasmic IgA. Cells with internal IgA may account for up to 5% of all the lymphocytes in lymph from conventional rats but cells containing immunoglobulin of other classes are very rare. All the lymphocytes which contain cytoplasmic IgA also carry surface IgA which is not acquired by absorption from the lymph; a further 1–5% of all the cells carry surface IgA but lack internal IgA and these are mainly small lymphocytes (Williams & Gowans 1975). Similar values have been obtained for mouse thoracic duct cells by Guy-Grand *et al.* (1974). The cells in lymph carrying surface immunoglobulin of all classes can be efficiently removed by rosetting them with appropriately prepared sheep erythrocytes and then separating the rosettes from the non-rosetting cells by spinning through Isopaque/Ficoll (Parish & Hayward 1974; Mason 1976). Table 2 indicates that about the same proportion of blast cells in both the depleted and undepleted populations migrate into the intestine. However, autoradiography showed that the labelled cells which had originally lacked surface immunoglobulin accumulated predominantly in the T areas of Peyer's patches and to some extent in the villi at their margins; the few which were found in the lamina propria did not contain IgA. T blasts from the auricular nodes of mice (Parrott & Ferguson 1974) and from the thoracic duct of rats (Ford 1975), activated by oxazolone and a graft-versus-host reaction respectively, also migrate into the T areas of Peyer's patches but not into the lamina propria. It is not clear whether T blasts which have been normally activated by gut antigens show a greater tendency to migrate into Peyer's patches than those generated by other means; nor is their function known.

It can be concluded from these experiments that the blast cells in thoracic duct lymph which home into the lamina propria are those which carry IgA on their surface but it has yet to be established whether the small lymphocytes with surface IgA but not in DNA synthesis are also part of the precursor population.

THE ORIGIN OF IgA-CONTAINING CELLS IN LYMPH

The presence of IgA-containing cells in thoracic duct lymph can be interpreted in the light of the studies of Morris and his colleagues (Hall & Morris 1963; Hay *et al.* 1972) on the cellular response in efferent lymph which follows regional stimulation with antigen: the cells with internal IgA arise in intestinal lymphoid tissue in response to antigenic stimulation from the gut and are then released into the thoracic duct lymph. The study of a specific response to a defined antigen has made this interpretation more certain and has enabled the origin of the lymph-borne precursors of the intestinal IgA response to be determined. The candidates for the tissue of origin are clearly either the Peyer's patches and/or the mesenteric lymph nodes (Fig. 1).

Pierce & Gowans (1975) showed that when rats which had been primed intraperitoneally with cholera toxoid were given an intraintestinal boost with fluid toxoid, a wave of antitoxin-containing large lymphocytes (ACC) appeared in the thoracic duct lymph. They were first detected about two days after challenge and their numbers increased rapidly during the next 1–2 days to reach a maximum of about 200 000 ACC/h; at the height of the response 1% of all thoracic duct lymphocytes were ACC, of which about 80% contained IgA. In rats which had been primed orally, the intraintestinal boost produced ACC which contained IgA exclusively (Table 3).

A proportionally smaller ACC response in thoracic duct lymph was observed when the boosting dose of toxoid was given into the lumen of a Thiry-Vella loop (Markowitz *et al.* 1964) which had been constructed from about one-quarter of the total length of the small intestine (Fig. 3). On the other hand, no response was obtained after challenging loops from which the Peyer's patches had been removed surgically some time previously (Fig. 3). In other animals the long chain of mesenteric lymph nodes was removed and time allowed for the torn lymphatics to regenerate so that the normal flow of lymph from the intestine into the thoracic duct was re-established. A normal ACC response to challenge with cholera toxoid could be generated from Thiry-Vella loops prepared in such lymphatectomized animals (Fig. 3).

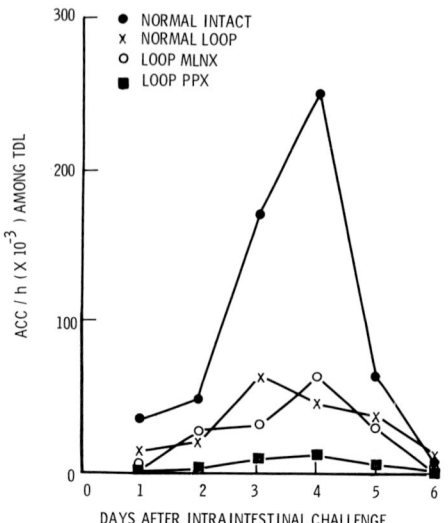

FIG. 3. Output of antitoxin-containing cells (ACC) in thoracic duct lymph after intraintestinal challenge with 1.0 mg of fluid cholera toxoid in rats primed 14 days previously with 0.1 mg of toxoid in CFA intraperitoneally. Challenge into duodenum of 5 normal intact rats (●); and challenge into Thiry-Vella loops of either 8 normal rats (×), of 4 rats from which the mesenteric lymph nodes (MLN) had been removed surgically (○), or of 3 rats in which the loops lacked Peyer's patches (PP) (■).

TABLE 3

Ig class of cholera antitoxin in thoracic duct lymphocytes (TDL) after intraintestinal challenge of primed rats

Immunization		No. rats	Ig class in ACC % ACC with internal:		
Primary	Secondary		IgA	IgM	IgG2
Intraperitoneal	Oral or intraduodenal	5	82 (76-88)	0	9 (6-14)
Oral		2	100 (99, 100)	0	0.5 (1, 0)

Rats primed with either 0.1 mg cholera toxoid in CFA i.p. or 25-40 mg toxoid in drinking water over 8-16 days. Challenge with either 5 mg toxoid orally or 1 mg intraduodenally 14 days after priming. Thoracic duct cannulated 3 days after challenge and lymph collected for 24 h. Ig class in TDL by autoradiography after incubation with ^{125}I-rabbit F(ab')$_2$ anti-rat Ig; internal cholera antitoxin by immunofluorescence. Values are mean and range. (From Pierce & Gowans 1975.)

TABLE 4

Effect of a thoracic duct fistula on the appearance of antitoxin-containing cells (ACC) in gut after intraduodenal challenge with cholera toxoid in primed rats

Rat	Immunization	Density of ACC in lamina propria (mean/mm^3 × 10^{-3} ± S.E.)		
		Jejunum	Ileum	Colon
Normal (6)	Primary only	0.7 ± 0.1	2.0 ± 0.5	3.1 ± 1.1
Normal (5-7)	Secondary	10.3 ± 2.0	14.9 ± 2.1	5.7 ± 1.3
With TD fistula (6-7)	Secondary	2.0 ± 0.6	2.8 ± 0.6	7.2 ± 1.0

Rats primed i.p. with 0.1 mg cholera toxoid in complete Freund's adjuvant and challenged intraduodenally with 1 mg of fluid toxoid 14 days later. In one group of rats a thoracic duct fistula was established just before challenge. Observations 19 days after priming. Number of rats in parenthesis. (From Pierce & Gowans 1975.)

These experiments show that the IgA antibody-containing large lymphocytes in thoracic duct lymph were derived from Peyer's patches. We had considered the possibility that although the precursors may have been discharged from Peyer's patches, their induction by antigen might have occurred upstream in the mesenteric nodes where antigen-trapping would probably be more efficient. In the event, the mesenteric nodes apparently contributed little to the response and engagement with antigen must have occurred in the Peyer's patches.

The wave of ACC which appeared in the lymph of primed rats after intraduodenal challenge with cholera toxoid was followed about two days later by the accumulation of IgA-containing ACC in the lamina propria of the small intestine (Pierce & Gowans 1975). This intestinal accumulation of ACC did not occur if a thoracic duct fistula had been established just before challenge: the density of ACC in the jejunum and ileum of rats with thoracic duct fistulae was not significantly different from the density observed in rats which had received primary immunization only (Table 4). Thus, the ACC which accumulated in the lamina propria were derived *exclusively* from lymph-borne cells. This conclusion does not refute the claim that cells from bronchus-associated lymphoid tissue may contribute to IgA production in the lamina propria (Rudzik et al. 1975b). It does, however, show that an immune response triggered in the intestine itself is delivered entirely by cells derived from the intestinal lymphoid mass.

The first evidence for the origin from Peyer's patches of IgA-secreting cells was provided by Craig & Cebra (1971). They showed that suspensions of cells teased from Peyer's patches gave rise to IgA-containing cells in the intestine and spleen of irradiated allogeneic rabbits. The splenic localization was probably an artefact of allogeneic transfer (Rudzik *et al.* 1975*a*) but the experiments clearly revealed the potentiality of cells from Peyer's patches in comparison with lymphoid tissue elsewhere. The precursors in Peyer's patches were among the cells with IgA on their surface (Jones & Cebra 1974). In view of all the evidence for the origin of IgA-secreting cells from Peyer's patches it is surprising that blast cells from Peyer's patches do not home into the gut (Guy-Grand *et al.* 1974). If this is not a consequence of cell damage during handling *in vitro* then it must be assumed that the lymph-borne precursors of the response only enter into DNA synthesis after their release from the Peyer's patches into the lymph, although this seems unlikely.

The mechanism of the remarkable class commitment shown by cells in Peyer's patches remains unexplained. It is not known whether Peyer's patches accumulate IgA precursors from the general recirculating pool of B lymphocytes or whether the environment of the Peyer's patches dictates their differentiation, perhaps from B cells initially carrying surface IgM. In any event, Peyer's patches have the capacity to accumulate IgA memory cells from elsewhere, because intraintestinal challenge produced a brisk secondary response of ACC in the lymph in rats which had been primed intraperitoneally, a route which does not engage lymphoid tissue in the intestinal bed (Pierce & Gowans 1975).

FACTORS AFFECTING THE MIGRATION OF LARGE LYMPHOCYTES INTO THE LAMINA PROPRIA

In discussing the factors which affect the localization of large lymphocytes in the intestine it is necessary first to consider the extent to which this migration shows selectivity. On a weight basis the spleen sequesters almost as great a proportion of an injected dose of labelled large lymphocytes as the small intestine. On the other hand, if one asks—into what organ or tissue do most of the large lymphocytes pass in order to execute their function?—then it is clear that the small intestine is overwhelmingly the dominant organ (Fig. 2). The large intestine attracts only a small fraction of all gut-localizing cells (Fig. 2); its behaviour is also anomalous in that a thoracic duct fistula did not prevent the accumulation of ACC in the colon in rats primed and challenged with cholera toxoid (Table 4). Plasma cells in the large gut may turn over relatively slowly or the large and small intestine may differ in the mechanisms by which plasma cells are generated or localized.

In the original work on the homing of large lymphocytes (Gowans & Knight 1964) it was suggested that antigen might play an important part in determining their localization in the gut. It would seem sensible to accumulate plasma cells in those areas of the intestine where the target for the secreted antibody is

TABLE 5

Antigenic challenge into Thiry-Vella loops prepared in rats primed intraperitoneally with cholera toxoid. Selective accumulation of antitoxin-containing cells (ACC) in challenged loop

	Loop challenged:		
	Proximal (4)	Distal (6)	
	ACC/cm	ACC/cm	IgA-containing cells/cm
Duodenum	13 (10-16)	15 (7-22)	2094 (1638-2569)
Proximal loop	69 (62-89)	15 (10-21)	822 (693- 921)
Distal loop	16 (12-20)	73 (52-121)	730 (662- 870)
Ileum	16 (8-26)	18 (12-25)	1122 (988-1265)

Proximal and distal Thiry-Vella loops (Markowitz *et al.* 1964) prepared from equal lengths of mid-third of small gut. Continuity re-established by joining jejunum to lower ileum. Loops made 10 days after priming with 0.1 mg cholera toxoid in complete Freund's adjuvant, i.p. Challenge into one loop with 1 mg fluid toxoid 4 days after surgery. Antitoxin-containing cells (ACC) and IgA-containing cells in gut 6 days after challenge scored by immunofluorescence in measured lengths of gut sections cut at 4 μm thickness. Number of rats in parenthesis.

present. Pierce & Gowans (1975) showed that ACC taken from the thoracic duct after challenging primed animals with cholera toxoid could be identified in large numbers in the intestine of normal recipients, whether or not they had been given antigen at the time of transfusion. On the other hand, it was found that in the primed animal itself, the greatest concentration of ACC in the lamina propria always occurred in that region of the intestine which had been challenged with antigen.

Similar evidence for the influence of antigen on the localization of specific antibody-producing cells in the lamina propria has come from studies on Thiry-Vella loops. Rats were primed intraperitoneally with cholera toxoid and two separate loops were prepared from the small intestine 10 days later. A challenge of toxoid was then given into one loop only and the number of ACC was counted in both loops six days later. Table 5 shows that the greatest number of ACC occurred in the loop which received antigen despite the fact that the loops themselves contained fewer total IgA cells than normal small intestine. Similar findings have been reported for responses in Thiry-Vella loops in sheep (Husband & Lascelles 1974).

The idea that antigen plays any part in the localization of large lymphocytes in the intestine is thought to be discredited by the observation that they will home selectively into neonatal or embryonic intestine which is presumptively antigen-free (Halstead & Hall 1972; Parrott & Ferguson 1974). How then is it possible to reconcile these observations with experiments which show that antigen dictates the area in the gut in which most specific antibody-forming cells accumulate? The dilemma could be resolved if two independent processes are at work. First, some property intrinsic to the small intestine favours the emigration of large lymphocytes into the lamina propria; and second, there is an antigen-dependent immobilization of the cells once they have emigrated. This implies that if the specific antigen is not present in the lamina propria the cells may leave it, re-enter lymphatics and pass by way of the thoracic duct back into the blood. In conventional animals such a recirculation of large lymphocytes would not be observed (Gowans & Knight 1964) because the antigens which gave rise to their formation are naturally present in the gut. The experiments in which ACC homed into the intestine whether or not cholera toxoid was present in the gut (Pierce & Gowans 1975) are incomplete since localization was only studied at one time-interval (5 hours) after transfusion. The same objection applies to studies on neonatal gut where the accumulation of cells in the lamina propria was only studied up to 8 hours after transfusion (Halstead & Hall 1972). The lymphatic obstruction which has been described in grafts of embryonic gut placed under the capsule of the kidney (Ferguson & Parrott 1972) may not allow cells which have emigrated into the lamina propria to leave it again.

The proposed immobilization of large lymphocytes in the lamina propria by antigen can be readily tested but even if it proves to be correct it would leave unexplained the mechanism of the initial migration from the blood which probably occurs through small venules. In anatomical terms it is reasonable to suppose that the signal for migration is provided by the vascular endothelium and that the first event is probably the adherence of the lymphocytes to it. A number of workers have considered the possibility that secretory component, synthesized by the intestinal epithelial cells, may provide the signal for migration because it might combine with the lymphocytes which carry IgA on their surface. This is not an attractive hypothesis because there is no evidence that secretory component is available either in the lamina propria or, more important, in the vascular endothelium. Further, our colleague H.-J. Gross has shown that secretory component does not, in fact, bind to the surface of rat thoracic duct lymphocytes: ^{125}I-labelled rabbit secretory component bound avidly to the internal IgA in fixed smears of rat thoracic duct large lymphocytes but it failed to bind to the surface of living large lymphocytes in suspension, possibly implying that the IgA on their surface is monomeric. The hypothesis is further weakened by the observation that migration of large lymphocytes into the gut is unperturbed by pre-treating animals with antibodies directed against either secretory component or IgA (McWilliams et al. 1975). For the moment, the molecular basis for the emigration of large lymphocytes into the lamina propria of the small intestine remains unsolved.

References

CRABBÉ, P. A., CARBONARA, A. O. & HEREMANS, J. F. (1965) The normal human intestinal mucosa as a major source of plasma cells containing γA-immunoglobulin. *Lab. Invest. 14*, 235

CRAIG, S. W. & CEBRA, J. J. (1971) Peyer's patches: an enriched source of precursors for IgA-producing immunocytes in the rabbit. *J. Exp. Med. 134*, 188

FERGUSON, A. & PARROTT, D. M. V. (1972) The effect of antigen deprivation on thymus-dependent and thymus-independent lymphocytes in the small intestine of the mouse. *Clin. Exp. Immunol. 12*, 477

FORD, W. L. (1975) Lymphocyte migration and immune responses. *Prog. Allergy 19*, 1

GOWANS, J. L. (1959) The recirculation of lymphocytes from blood to lymph in the rat. *J. Physiol. (Lond.) 146*, 54

GOWANS, J. L. & KNIGHT, E. J. (1964) The route of re-circulation of lymphocytes in the rat. *Proc. R. Soc. Lond. B Biol. Sci. 159*, 257

GRISCELLI, C., VASSALLI, P. & MCCLUSKEY, R. T. (1969) The distribution of large dividing lymph node cells in syngeneic recipient rats after intravenous injection. *J. Exp. Med. 130*, 1427

GUY-GRAND, D., GRISCELLI, C. & VASSALLI, P. (1974) The gut-associated lymphoid system: nature and properties of the large dividing cells. *Eur. J. Immunol. 4*, 435

HALL, J. G. & MORRIS, B. (1963) The lymph-borne cells of the immune response. *Q. J. Exp. Physiol. 48*, 235

HALL, J. G., PARRY, D. M. & SMITH, M. E. (1972) The distribution and differentiation of lymph-borne immunoblasts after intravenous injection into syngeneic recipients. *Cell Tissue Kinet. 5*, 269

HALSTEAD, T. E. & HALL, J. G. (1972) The homing of lymph-borne immunoblasts to the small gut of neonatal rats. *Transplantation 14*, 339

HAY, J. B., MURPHY, M. J., MORRIS, B. & BESSIS, M. C. (1972) Quantitative studies on the proliferation and differentiation of antibody-forming cells in lymph. *Am. J. Pathol. 66*, 1

HUSBAND, A. J. & LASCELLES, A. K. (1974) The origin of antibody in intestinal secretion of sheep. *Aust. J. Exp. Biol. Med. Sci. 52*, 791

JONES, P. P. & CEBRA, J. J. (1974) Restriction of gene expression in B lymphocytes and their progeny. III. Endogenous IgA and IgM on the membranes of different plasma cell precursors. *J. Exp. Med. 140*, 966

MANN, J. D. & HIGGINS, G. M. (1950) Lymphocytes in thoracic duct, intestinal and hepatic lymph. *Blood 5*, 177

MARKOWITZ, J., ARCHIBALD, J. & DOWNIE, H. G. (1964) in *Experimental Surgery*, p. 143, Williams & Wilkins, Baltimore

MASON, D. W. (1976) The class of surface immunoglobulin on cells carrying IgG memory in rat thoracic duct lymph: the size of the subpopulation mediating IgG memory. *J. Exp. Med. 143*, 1122

MCWILLIAMS, M., PHILLIPS-QUAGLIATA, J. M. & LAMM, M. E. (1975) Characteristics of mesenteric lymph node cells homing to gut-associated lymphoid tissue in syngeneic mice. *J. Immunol. 115*, 54

PARISH, C. R. & HAYWARD, J. A. (1974) The lymphocyte surface. II. Separation of Fc receptor, C'3 receptor and surface immunoglobulin-bearing lymphocytes. *Proc. R. Soc. Lond. B. Biol. Sci. 187*, 65

PARROTT, D. M. V. & FERGUSON, A. (1974) Selective migration of lymphocytes within the mouse small intestine. *Immunology 26*, 571

PIERCE, N. F. & GOWANS, J. L. (1975) Cellular kinetics of the intestinal immune response to cholera toxoid in rats. *J. Exp. Med. 142*, 1550

RUDZIK, O., PEREY, D. Y. E. & BIENENSTOCK, J. (1975a) Differential IgA repopulation after transfer of autologous and allogeneic rabbit Peyer's patch cells. *J. Immunol. 114*, 40

Rudzik, R., Clancy, R. L., Perey, D. Y. E., Day, R. P. & Bienenstock, J. (1975b) Repopulation with IgA-containing cells of bronchial and intestinal lamina propria after transfer of homologous Peyer's patch and bronchial lymphocytes. *J. Immunol. 114,* 1599

Williams, A. F. & Gowans, J. L. (1975) The presence of IgA on the surface of rat thoracic duct lymphocytes which contain internal IgA. *J. Exp. Med. 141,* 335

Discussion

Ahlstedt: To take up the question of antigen causing the cells to home to particular areas, in our studies with colostral cells, where we treated pregnant women with *Escherichia coli* O83 bacteria, antibody-producing cells were found in the colostrum for over three weeks, while the bacteria were very difficult to detect in faecal samples (Goldblum *et al.* 1975). It would seem unlikely that the antigen is transported from the gut up to the mammary gland and stays there for three weeks, making the cells there produce antibodies.

Gowans: So antibody-forming cells are entering the mammary gland and passing out into the colostrum continuously?

Ahlstedt: Yes, maybe, if the cells are not proliferating within the gland. This finding may also be peculiar to the mammary gland, since we cannot detect any secretory antibodies in saliva or urine, or any antibodies in serum. We haven't looked at the gut.

Brandtzaeg: I agree with Professor Gowans that secretory component apparently has no role in the homing of IgA cell precursors to the gut. We have looked at circulating human B lymphocytes and we detect no surface affinity for secretory component and no J chain on these cells (Brandtzaeg 1976).

Booth: Strober and his colleagues (1976) have described a single case recorded of secretory piece deficiency. There was a normal population of IgA cells in the lamina propria.

Brandtzaeg: As will be discussed in my paper (pp. 77–108), I doubt very much that that report shows a complete deficiency of the secretory component.

Professor Gowans referred to Hall's recent study (Hopkins & Hall 1976) and used this as an argument that the IgA cells in the lamina propria do not come from peripheral lymph nodes, but have an intestinal source. However, if your conclusions about the role of antigen in B cell trapping are correct, this mechanism may equally well apply to the immunocyte populations in spleen and peripheral lymph nodes in Hall's study. The intestinal lymphoid cells were naturally stimulated by the intestinal flora, whereas the cells in spleen and peripheral lymph nodes were primed by a subcutaneously deposited mixture of *Corynebacterium parvum, Brucella abortus* and *Salmonella typhi.*

I am not sure that this study proves that the blast cells homing to the gut come exclusively from intestinal sources.

Gowans: Hopkins & Hall (1976) have shown that radio-labelled blast cells from the intestinal lymph of sheep home preferentially to the small intestine whereas those from the efferent lymph of peripheral nodes elsewhere migrate mainly to the spleen. You are right to emphasize that the blasts in intestinal lymph were formed in response to normal gut antigens whereas the spleen-seeking blasts were a response to intentional stimulation with a mixed bacterial vaccine. So it could be argued that the latter were not given an opportunity to display gut-homing since the specific antigen was not present in the gut. It would be interesting to know whether these blasts entered the lamina propria and then left it again, but this appears unlikely since Hopkins and Hall say that 'they did not reappear in significant numbers in samples of either lymph or blood'.

Brandtzaeg: One should stimulate the peripheral lymph nodes with the gut flora, to do a clear-cut experiment.

Gowans: I agree.

Rosen: Can one interfere with the homing of IgA-forming cells by treating them with anti-IgA antibody, and is the homing population completely eliminated if one treats the thoracic duct suspension with anti-IgA and complement?

Cebra: That experiment using mesenteric lymph node cells has been done by McWilliams *et al.* (1976). Anti-IgA antibody plus complement ablates the small extra increment of cells that are found in mesenteric nodes and that lodge in gut rather than elsewhere. These sensitive cells probably account for at least some of the IgA precursors which populate gut lamina propria.

Gowans: This experiment is difficult to interpret because treatment with anti-IgA may opsonize the cells for phagocytosis by the liver and spleen.

Seligmann: Have you any information on the membrane-bound immunoglobulins of the large dividing cells in thoracic duct lymph which do not have intracytoplasmic IgA, and particularly have you information on IgD?

Gowans: I cannot give you a precise answer to your question but from estimates of the proportion of large lymphocytes with surface IgA (Williams & Gowans 1975) and of the proportion of blasts carrying surface Ig of all classes (Mason 1976*a*) I would guess that very few large lymphocytes in rat thoracic duct lymph possess membrane Ig other than IgA. About half do not bind anti-L chain reagents and are presumably T blasts.

We have no reagent for detecting IgD in rats (assuming it exists) but Mason (1976*b*) has concluded that the existence of B cells carrying IgD *exclusively* in rat thoracic duct lymph is very unlikely: the sum of the proportions of **B cells** with surface IgM, IgG and IgA is about equal to the proportion of all cells which bind anti-L chain antibodies. On the other hand, estimates of the amount of anti-Ig reagents bound to individual cells certainly leave room for cells carrying more than one class, for example IgM *plus* presumptive IgD.

I should emphasize that everything I have said applies to thoracic duct cells from rats which were not intentionally immunized: that is, to blast cells generated in gut lymphoid tissue in response to gut antigens. I would guess that blast cells generated in peripheral nodes elsewhere might carry predominantly IgM.

Booth: In loop experiments, a technical problem is that the loop atrophies after about a month and the segment distal to the anastomosis hypertrophies. What is your technique for counting the cells and how do you express the number—per length of tissue or per villus, or what?

Gowans: All the experiments were done within a week or so of preparing the loops and the problems you describe were not encountered.

On the second point, we express the density of antibody-forming cells as the number per centimetre of gut in histological sections cut at 4 μm. The unit length includes the whole thickness of the mucosa down to the muscular coat.

Parrott: In the primed rats with loops, have you put a non-cross-reacting antigen into the loops, or traumatized the second loop, to get the cells to go to that loop?

Gowans: No, we have not tried mechanical, chemical or other immunological stimuli in the second loop.

Porter: You highlighted the difference in the populations of lymphoid cells in the colon and small intestine; there is also a difference among the small intestinal lymphoid cells that was first shown by Crabbé & Heremans (1966). The duodenum, for example, showed a considerably higher lymphoid cell population than the jejunum or ileum. We have made a similar observation in relation to intestinal infection with *E. coli* in mono-contaminated germ-free pigs. The response of the gut shows ten times more cells in the duodenum than the jejunum and ileum, yet the antigen density, or the *E. coli* population, is almost inverse, in that it is higher at the lower end of the intestine. I have argued teleologically that this is a good way for the gut to defend itself, in that it is better to pour the antibody out at the upper end of the intestine than at the lower, but it goes against the antigen-trapping idea, and I favour some intrinsic factor which would tend to bind antibody-forming cells in the upper small intestine rather than to mediate at the site of challenge.

Pepys: Why does intraperitoneal antigen prime for subsequent gut challenge? Is it because antigens reach the gut or because non-gut blast cells home into the intestine?

Gowans: It is surprising that intraperitoneal priming prepares the gut for a secondary response (Pierce & Gowans 1975). I assume that memory cells created by intraperitoneal priming accumulate in Peyer's patches and are thus available for stimulation by the subsequent intra-intestinal challenge. Dr Pierce tells me that subcutaneous priming is much less effective, which is hard to explain. Antigen injected intraperitoneally is collected by the diaphragmatic lymphatics, a few of which join the thoracic duct in the chest; most, however, drain into the mediastinal lymph nodes. I suppose that it is possible that intraperitoneal antigen in complete Freund's adjuvant, which is extremely corrosive, may stimulate Peyer's patches directly by penetrating them from their peritoneal surface, but this has never been established. We need to know what happens to an antigen in CFA which is injected into the peritoneal cavity.

Pepys: We have data that may be relevant. We have been looking at the production of IgE antibody in mice after the intraperitoneal injection of 0.1 μg of ovalbumin on alum, with a priming dose at six weeks of age and a booster four weeks later. The mice make good IgE responses. When we killed them some weeks after the booster, we found IgE-containing lymphoid cells in the Peyer's patches, although antigen had not been given into the gut (W. D. Brighton, B. E. Hewitt & M. B. Pepys, unpublished work).

Secondly, on the question of whether lymphocytes are stimulated by antigen, or divide, in the lamina propria, Marsh (1975) has studied both the morphology and the tritiated thymidine incorporation of lymphocytes in the intestinal epithelium of mice. He found that at any one time about 5% are blasts of which many appear to be T cells, but some look like B cells.

Gowans: The simple scheme which I put forward envisages each DNA-synthesizing large lymphocyte in the lymph as giving rise to no more than two IgA-secreting cells in the lamina propria. This may well be an over-simplification. We need to know whether IgA-precursor cells which have not yet started proliferating in either the Peyer's patches or the lymph can enter the lamina propria and proliferate and differentiate locally; and whether large lymphocytes which are already in DNA synthesis in the lymph can undergo several further divisions after migration into the gut. The clustering of IgA plasma cells in some villi is certainly consistent with continued local proliferation, although equally consistent with accumulation due to specific attraction.

Bienenstock: You mentioned that it isn't known where some of the respiratory tract lymphoid cells go to. We have shown that lymphoid cells in the follicles of the respiratory tract go to the gut and will repopulate the spleen in a similar fashion to cells from Peyer's patches (Rudzik *et al.* 1975).

As far as intraperitoneal priming is concerned, antigen put into the peritoneal cavity certainly goes up into the mediastinal area and enters what is loosely described as the area draining the respiratory tract (Gerbrandy & Bienenstock 1976). I suggest that this may be a higher localization of potential IgA precursor cells than if the antigen is given either parenterally or orally. I wonder why, in the experiments done with Dr Pierce, oral priming is worse than intraperitoneal priming?

Pierce: I am not certain it is worse, because the conditions are not the same. We cannot prime the gut of rats with either a single intraperitoneal or intraduodenal injection of purified fluid toxoid. We obtain good priming when toxoid is injected intraperitoneally with Freund's complete adjuvant but we have not evaluated this combination given into the gut lumen.

Cebra: Complete Freund's adjuvant given intraperitoneally with antigen induces a high proportion of cooperating T cells. What is the relative importance of the priming, on the one hand to give cooperating T cells and on the other to affect the B cell compartment of the Peyer's patches? In experiments mentioned earlier (p. 26), if cooperating T cells were transferred together with Peyer's patch cells we found more IgA-forming PFC cells (plaque-forming cells) in the spleen, and at earlier times. The response that Professor Gowans observes may be only one part of the overall secondary IgA response, the earliest phase. Secondary IgA cells may mature in a few days following very few divisions and end up in the lamina propria. Those B cells which are able to mature so rapidly must be already committed to generating IgA plasma cells and also must surely have available a lot of cooperating T cells to facilitate rapid maturation with few cell divisions. Ordinarily, an adoptive transfer of unprimed cells requires seven or eight cell divisions before significant numbers of IgA plasma cells are seen. The rapidity of your response suggests both cooperation early with pre-existing T cells and that the B cells functioning in your system are already committed to generating IgA plasma cells (i.e., are secondary B cells). One wonders whether they have reached that secondary state by priming or whether natural gut stimulation has put a few cells in this state, which are susceptible to early maturation to IgA plasma cells. There may be a reservoir of other cells that can take part in later stages of the IgA response.

Pierce: In the rat intraperitoneal priming of the gut immune response does not require Freund's *complete* adjuvant; it is produced equally well by the incomplete adjuvant. This may diminish concern that the response depends on T cell stimulation primarily. It is *not* reproducible by intraperitoneal priming with an alum-precipitated toxoid, or by toxoid plus Freund's adjuvant given subcutaneously.

Second, we have observed apparent species differences in the responses of rats and dogs. In dogs we can prime the gut by the subcutaneous route *without* Freund's adjuvant, so the requirement for an oil adjuvant given intraperitoneally may apply to rats but not to the system in general.

Lachmann: You have discussed afferent and efferent homing, Professor Gowans, and you have evidence that the cells that come from the Peyer's patches are committed to make IgA, but how do they get there in the first place? They must presumably come from bone marrow; but how do the cells there that are committed to make IgA know to go to Peyer's patches?

Gowans: We have no idea. Peyer's patches are very odd structures. They possess no afferent lymphatics so they are not regional lymph nodes in the conventional sense. Presumably, antigen reaches them directly by passage through the overlying intestinal epithelium, or through defects in it. On the other hand, they are similar to lymph nodes in that both B and T lymphocytes recirculate through them and that, in cell transfer experiments, they can mount IgM and IgG adoptive antibody responses, at least to sheep erythrocytes. Their special feature is that, *in situ*, Peyer's patches generate cells that make IgA. We know that the precursor B cell in Peyer's patches is a non-dividing (small) lymphocyte (McWilliams *et al.* 1974) which carries IgA on its surface (Jones & Cebra 1974).

Now we come to Dr Lachmann's questions. If the marrow produces virgin sIgA (surface IgA) lymphocytes, then Peyer's patches may simply concentrate them by some unknown mechanism. On the other hand, all sIgA small lymphocytes may be memory cells in which there has been an antigen-driven switch from sIgM → sIgA and it is the facility to mediate this switch which is a particular property of Peyer's patches. A further possibility is that sIgA cells, whether virgin or memory, may undergo non-clonal expansion in Peyer's patches under the influence of locally active mitogens (? gut derived). All this is pure speculation, as I am sure Dr Lachmann will immediately recognize.

Cebra: One point directly pertinent to Dr Lachmann's question has to do with transfer of bone marrow cells into irradiated congenic BALB recipients. We can restore the peripheral lymphoid tissue, and then test the peripheral nodes, spleen and Peyer's patches. The bone marrow cells, which bear almost no surface IgA, are able, when they proliferate in the Peyer's patches, to generate cells among which are cells capable of mounting an IgA response. We believe that one unique feature of the Peyer's patches, aside from a possible selective effect on differentiation or development, is that divisions occur there without maturation. That seems to be the key to getting a cell line advanced towards, if not already committed to, generating IgA plasma cells.

Gowans: There is, as yet, no evidence for a B cell expansion of this kind in Peyer's patches, is there?

Cebra: There is extensive cell division there; moreover, from the results of the clonal precursor analysis using a variety of antigens, a pattern emerges. Antigens most likely to stimulate patch cells naturally and chronically reveal a population of antigen-sensitive precursors that generate large clones making IgA plus IgGl or IgA plus IgGl and IgM. Clonal precursor analysis with rarer antigens reveals antigen-sensitive cells which generate clones making only IgM or IgM plus IgGl. Some change in potential of patch cells appears to occur which is division-related.

Lachmann: Can we go any further towards resolving the question of whether there is a switch to IgA production by precursors that are not already fully committed to producing that isotype before they meet antigen? It makes a difference to explanations of the generation of IgA responses whether or not there are cells which make IgM and, after they meet antigen in the bowel, go on to make something else.

Cebra: Our data are consistent with the existence of B lymphocytes that can be precursors for IgA plasma cells and in addition have a broader isotype potential. Antigen-sensitive cells reactive with the DNP determinant generate clones making IgM plus IgA, IgGl plus IgA and IgA plus IgGl and IgM. A 'switch' must occur during the generation of a clone to explain how one cell gives rise to a thousand cells, some of which make one isotype and some another. Gearhart *et al.* (1975) showed that all the antibody made by such a clone to the phosphorylcholine determinant bears the same idiotype marker, which means that the same V genes are being expressed in connection with C_α, C_μ, and $C_{\gamma 1}$. A major question is how the patch environment, or antigen stimulation, influences the expression of the V gene together with a particular C gene. At that level, we are ignorant of what happens. Many geneticists concede that a translocation or gene rearrangement might occur, and that V and C genes are not a single gene to begin with. However, they consider it less likely that with successive divisions the V gene can move around. The alternative must be expansion (selective replication) of a particular V gene giving VC_α, VC_μ, $VC_{\gamma 1}$, etc. and thereafter gene regulation by conventional mechanisms. It is hard to see how antigen could affect gene rearrangement or gene expression, so I suggest that potentials to express various isotypes are in all the primary cells, that regulating components may be in their milieu, and that the number of divisions which a B cell undergoes influences which isotypes are expressed. Perhaps divisions can be stimulated in many ways—hormonally, or by mitogens; antigen might just induce the last division(s) before final maturation when a particular VC gene will be expressed. We don't know how antigen intervenes but I suggest that is by the facilitation of division rather than by acting on the genetic material itself.

Lachmann: So you would predict that any cell would go on to make IgA, if you stimulated it to divide intensively enough?

Cebra: It is possible that either it or its progeny might do that.

Pepys: Parkhouse and his collaborators have demonstrated in mice that the memory cells of some stable clones committed to IgG antibody formation have receptors of IgM class (Abney *et al.* 1976). The clonal cells were treated *in vitro* so as to 'cap' and 'strip' with various anti-mouse immunoglobulin antisera, before being transferred together with antigen and carrier-primed helper cells into irradiated recipients. Pretreatment with anti-μ or anti-Fab prevented the production of IgG antibody, while anti-γ and anti-putative mouse δ had no effect.

Cebra: If both classes are synthesized, there must be two V genes active in each cell and presumably those are identical.

Gowans: The recent work of D. W. Mason (1976*b*) should be quoted in connection with that just cited by Dr Pepys. Mason used the fluorescence activated cell sorter to identify the B lymphocytes which generated a secondary IgG anti-DNP response in rats. He found the precursors exclusively among a small population of cells bearing surface IgG. The IgM-positive cells, which constituted the majority of the primed population, contributed little or nothing to the response. I would guess that sIgG memory cells were derived, during priming, from sIgM precursors but this remains to be proved.

Lachmann: There is the work from Max Cooper's laboratory showing that all future antibody-forming cells go through a phase where they have IgM on their membranes, and that anti-μ antibody given in early life will destroy subsequent antibody production, even of IgG (Kincade *et al.* 1970). There must presumably be a time when the cells switch from transcribing the μ isotype to, say, the γ isotype. If there is enough messenger RNA left they can still be making IgM receptors although inside the cell the switch in the DNA being copied may have taken place and any new messenger will be for the γ chain.

Mayrhofer: To my knowledge, there has been no study of the class of immunoglobulin on differentiating cells in animals undergoing a primary immune response leading to production of IgA. Oral immunization with soluble proteins would be a difficult system to work with because prolonged feeding of antigen appears necessary in order to obtain a secretory antibody response. If a switch of class occurs during differentiation, it might easily be missed. Studies on the surface immunoglobulin of precursors of IgA plasma cells in normal animals are looking at on-going immune responses to normal gut antigens (Craig & Cebra 1975; Williams & Gowans 1975) and therefore do not necessarily bear on the precursors that respond with primary exposure to antigen. The cholera toxoid system (Pierce & Gowans 1975) gives a brisk IgA response, but requires parenteral priming, the effect of which may be to generate IgA memory cells. One possible reason for the lack of a brisk response to oral immunization might be the failure to engage sufficient antigen with the lymphoid tissue of the gut. It would seem worthwhile to try a live enterovirus as an antigen, as this might deliver a more powerful challenge of shorter duration. After such an infection, specific antibody-forming cells might be found in Peyer's patches or thoracic duct lymph showing evidence of class switching. Gowans & Williams (unpublished) for instance found one rat during the course of their study in which a significant minority of thoracic duct cells containing IgA bore IgM on their surfaces. This was unusual as, in most rats, IgA-containing cells have surface IgA (Williams & Gowans 1975). It could be that this animal was responding to an infective agent that it had not previously encountered at the time of study.

Seligmann: There have been two cases of Ig myeloma with IgG inside the cell and IgM with the same light chain on the cell membrane (Seligmann *et al.* 1973). Unfortunately, the idiotypes have not been studied.

Cebra: Operationally we always elicit a primary response in our experiments, in the adoptive transfer system, in the clonal precursor analysis and in the direct gut stimulation. But one question is what a real primary response is, and I am suggesting that environmental antigens impinging on the cells in the Peyer's patch could cause divisions to yield cells which immunologists would call secondary B lymphocytes, even though they had not been stimulated deliberately. Lipopolysaccharide or other mitogens might also stimulate cells in the Peyer's patches to arrive at such a secondary state where a cell might display IgM on its membrane but synthesize and secrete another isotype on maturation.

Davies: Dr Cebra, in your experiments in which you transferred Peyer's patch cells and compared them with transferred spleen cells, there were some added thymocytes, which did not seem to be essential. You certainly demonstrated that cells from the Peyer's patches can, under the given circumstances, be found in the lamina propria doing their thing. How long were they found? You implied a week or so. I would be interested in the performance of these cells in comparison with that of transferred bone marrow cells. One wonders whether the kinds of activity that you have demonstrated *can* take place, but perhaps don't?

Cebra: Transfer of congenic cells from the Peyer's patch, with or without thymocytes, to irradiated BALB/c mice, and then antigen stimulation, results in an IgA plaque-forming response in the spleen. The transfer also results in a repopulation of the lamina propria by about day 14. Almost all the IgA cells bear the donor marker. At about day 30 total IgA cells decline in the lamina propria. The mice gradually replace the donor cells with their own, presumably from bone marrow.

We have transferred marrow and after 6–8 weeks can recover cells from the peripheral lymph nodes, spleen or Peyer's patch displaying the usual potential of cells from these sources, but bearing the marrow donor's marker, so you can totally repopulate the lamina propria with marrow-derived cells. This repopulation takes 3–4 weeks.

Davies: That shows that bone marrow *can* do this, but does not tell one much about the state of differentiation of the cells in the bone marrow. You have recolonized Peyer's patches with bone marrow cells, although the implication is that bone marrow eventually outgrows Peyer's patch cells. Whatever kind of 'stemness' they have, their capacity for persistence, or proliferation, is relatively limited. Is there anything incompatible with the notion that one is dealing ontogenetically with the development of microenvironments within which the synthesis of a particular antibody will be propitiated, rather than a development of cells which will produce a particular kind of antibody?

Cebra: I have no evidence for this, but it is an attractive notion, although how the microenvironment could direct the course of differentiation and maturation is not clear. I prefer a version of 'microenvironment' that includes cells or factors that act on B lymphocytes and, during the course of division, favour the expression of IgA by some siblings in a clone but not other isotypes by progeny of the same clone. That kind of immunoregulation, together with stimuli of division, might be all that the Peyer's patch 'microenvironment' provides to generate more IgA precursors than appear elsewhere.

Davies: The idea of microenvironments has precedents in the haemopoietic system. It seems likely that certain kinds of haemopoietic stem cells develop along one of two or perhaps three pathways of development in the spleen, and this gives credence to the microenvironmental notion. One wonders whether it applies to lymphoid cells.

Cebra: Initially we thought that patch cells displayed a differentiative pathway of potential to express IgM → IgG1 → IgA while peripheral node cells showed a parallel but different pathway of IgM → IgG1 → IgG2. However, with some antigens we saw a pronounced potential for IgG2 expression by Peyer's patch cells, so a clear-cut separate and distinctive development of B cells in different microenvironments does not seem to occur.

Davies: Did you see them making IgG2 in the spleen, however?

Cebra: Yes, but they were derived from patch precursor cells on adoptive transfer, even though they expressed IgG2 in the spleen of the recipient.

Porter: In relation to the sequential development of Ig-forming cells in the lamina propria, it is some time after birth in the mammal before the IgA cell dominates, and so the role of the IgA cell in the ontogeny of secretory Ig responses should not be over-emphasized. The pig and cow are at least 20 weeks old before there are more IgA cells than IgM cells in the lamina propria. It is almost a year before one sees the adult pattern of about 80% of the cells in the lamina making IgA.

In relation to the sequential development, IgM as a secretory immunoglobulin must be taken seriously into account. One wonders what the consensus is about Cooper's sequence of IgM to IgG to IgA in the chicken, because although IgG cells appear in the lamina they form a very small proportion of the population at any age, in mammals.

Brandtzaeg: I agree that the Ig A system has been too much emphasized, and that we should think more about the development of IgM cells. In IgA-deficient patients, IgM cell precursors, and to a smaller extent IgG cell precursors, home to the gut and to other glandular sites, and the local plasma cell population develops to about the same size as the normal IgA cell population.

Seligmann: The question is whether there is a *direct* switch from M to A without going through G. There is some evidence in favour of this hypothesis (Cooper *et al.* 1976).

Porter: In the normal sequence of development within the first week of life there are at least ten times more IgM cells than IgA cells in any part of the intestine.

Brandtzaeg: My point was that the gland-associated development of IgM- (and IgG-)producing cells is greatly enhanced when there is a maturation defect in the IgA system.

Porter: So it appears as if there is *no* competence to switch.

White: Kincade & Cooper (1973) made the firm assertion that switches do not occur in peripheral tissues, based on the experimental finding that the switch did not occur in bursectomized birds, and we await confirmation or rejection of that. Of course, the bursectomy additionally eliminated another possible peripheral site of switching, namely the germinal centres. On the other hand, the experiments of Martin & Leslie (1974) favour a direct switch from IgM to IgA. Chickens were bursectomized at hatch and treated with anti-μ antiserum; there was a depletion of IgA and IgM but not IgG. At least some of the switching was thought to occur in the periphery.

Lachmann: Cooper's hypothesis goes further and says that the switch is not antigen-driven and happens before the cells see antigen. It is a coherent story and therefore a good one for testing with data!

References

ABNEY, E. R., KEELER, K. D., PARKHOUSE, R. M. E. & WILLCOX, H. N. A. (1976) Immunoglobulin M receptors on memory cells of immunoglobulin G antibody-forming cell clones. *Eur. J. Immunol.* 6, 443-450

BRANDTZAEG, P. (1976) Studies on J chain and binding site for secretory component in circulating human B cells. I. The surface membrane. *Clin. Exp. Immunol.* 25, 50-58

COOPER, M. D., KEARNEY, J. F., LAWTON, A. R., ABNEY, E. R., PARKHOUSE, R. M. E., PREUD'HOMME, J. L. & SELIGMANN, M. (1976) Generation of immunoglobulin class diversity in B cells: a discussion with emphasis on IgD development. *Ann. Immunol. (Paris)*, in press

CRABBÉ, P. A. & HEREMANS, J. F. (1966) The distribution of immunoglobulin-containing cells along the human gastrointestinal tract. *Gastroenterologia 51*, 305

CRAIG, S. W. & CEBRA, J. J. (1975) Rabbit Peyer's patches, appendix, and popliteal lymph node B lymphocytes: a comparative analysis of their membrane immunoglobulin components and plasma cell precursor potential. *J. Immunol.* 114, 492-502

GEARHART, P. J., SIGAL, N. Y. & KLINMAN, N. R. (1975) Heterogeneity of the BALB/c antiphosphorylcholine antibody response at the precursor cell level. *J. Exp. Med. 141*, 56-71

GERBRANDY, J. L. F. & BIENENSTOCK, J. (1976) Kinetics and localization of IgE tetanus antibody response in mice immunized by the intratracheal, intraperitoneal and subcutaneous routes. *Immunology*, in press

GOLDBLUM. R. M., AHLSTEDT, S., CARLSSON, B., HANSON, L. Å., JODAL, U., LIDIN-JANSON, G. & SOHL-ÅKERLUND, A. (1975) Antibody-forming cells in human colostrum after oral immunisation. *Nature (Lond.)* 257, 797-799

HOPKINS, J. & HALL, J. G. (1976) Selective entry of immunoblasts into gut from intestinal lymph. *Nature (Lond.)* 259, 308-309

JONES, P. P. & CEBRA, J. J. (1974) Restriction of gene expression in B lymphocytes and their progeny. III. Endogenous IgA and IgM on the membranes of different plasma cell precursors. *J. Exp. Med. 140*, 966

KINCADE, P. W. & COOPER, M. D. (1973) Immunoglobulin A: site and sequence of expression in developing chicks. *Science (Wash. D.C.) 179*, 398-400

KINCADE, P. W., LAWTON, A. R., BOCKMAN, D. E. & COOPER, M. D. (1970) Suppression of immunoglobulin G synthesis as a result of antibody mediated suppression of immunoglobulin M synthesis in chickens. *Proc. Natl. Acad. Sci. U.S.A. 67*, 1918

MCWILLIAMS, M., LAMM, M. E. & PHILLIPS-QUAGLIATA, J. M. (1974) Surface and intracellular markers of mouse mesenteric and peripheral lymph node and Peyer's patch cells. *J. Immunol. 113*, 1326-1333

MCWILLIAMS, M., PHILLIPS-QUAGLIATA, J. M. & LAMM, M. E. (1976) Origin of IgA-secreting plasma cells in the gut. *Fed. Proc. 35*, 351 (abstr. 817)

MARSH, M. N. (1975) Studies of intestinal lymphoid tissue. *Gut 16*, 665-682

MARTIN, L. N. & LESLIE, G. A. (1974) IgM-forming cells as the immediate precursor of IgA-producing cells during ontogeny of the immunoglobulin-producing system of the chicken. *J. Immunol. 113*, 120-126

MASON, D. W. (1976a) The requirement for C3 receptors on the precursors of 19S and 7S antibody-forming cells. *J. Exp. Med. 143*, 1111

MASON, D. W. (1976b) The class of surface immunoglobulin on cells carrying IgG memory in rat thoracic duct lymph: the size of the subpopulation mediating IgG memory. *J. Exp. Med. 143*, 1122

PIERCE, N. F. & GOWANS, J. L. (1975) Cellular kinetics of the intestinal immune response to cholera toxoid in rats. *J. Exp. Med. 142*, 1550-1563

RUDZIK, O., CLANCY, R. L., PEREY, D. Y. E., DAY, R. P. & BIENENSTOCK, J. (1975) Repopulation with IgA-containing cells of bronchial and intestinal lamina propria after transfer of homologous Peyer's patch and bronchial lymphocytes. *J. Immunol. 114*, 1599-1640

SELIGMANN, M., PREUD'HOMME, J. L. & BROUET, J. C. (1973) B and T cell markers in human proliferative blood diseases and primary immunodeficiencies, with special reference to membrane bound immunoglobulins. *Transplant. Rev. 16*, 85-113

STROBER, W., KRAKAUER, R., KLAEVEMAN, H. L., REYNOLDS, H. Y. & NELSON, D. L. (1976) Secretory component deficiency: a disorder of the IgA immune system. *N. Engl. J. Med. 294*, 351-356

WILLIAMS, A. F. & GOWANS, J. L. (1975) The presence of IgA on the surface of rat thoracic duct lymphocytes which contain internal IgA. *J. Exp. Med. 141*, 335-345

Significance of immune mechanisms in relation to enteric infections of the gastrointestinal tract in animals

P. PORTER, S. H. PARRY and W. D. ALLEN

Department of Immunology, Unilever Research Laboratory, Colworth House, Bedford

Abstract The impact of bacterial colonization on the alimentary tract in early life is reflected in gross changes in morphology. Subsequent health, if not survival, may largely be determined by a continuum of local intestinal immune mechanisms and it is essential for antibody development during the neonatal period to compensate adequately for declining passive maternal antibody. Consequent upon the development of the gut microflora the lamina becomes infiltrated with immunocytes in which the dominant immunoglobulins produced are IgM and IgA. Both immunoglobulins are transported across the epithelium by a process involving membrane-bound vesicles.

Germ-free and fistulated pigs and calves were shown to be able to respond to oral immunization with *Escherichia coli* O somatic antigens during the first week of life. Resistance to infection with enteropathogenic *E. coli* was significantly enhanced, along with other parameters of nutrition and performance. However, in the young chick, although the intestinal response to infection with *E. coli* was similar to that in the mammal, no response to *E. coli* O antigens could be determined on oral administration in germ-free or local intestinal applications in fistulated birds.

In the mammalian intestine secretory antibodies participate in the control of pathogenic *E. coli* by blocking adhesion to the mucosal epithelium, interfering with the elaboration of surface antigens, inhibiting toxins, and facilitating rapid elimination from the alimentary tract by agglutination and bacteriostasis. In consequence fewer enteropathogens are excreted into the environment, an important feature in modern intensive systems of animal production.

Animal species have evolved in intimate association with a complex microbial flora, and perhaps in consequence most living forms exhibit a strong dependence upon microbial activities. The alimentary tract provides an ideal environment for microbial colonization and the indigenous flora may play an indispensable role in regulating intestinal physiology and biochemistry and exert various morphogenetic effects on the host. The way in which the host tolerates the proliferation of certain microorganisms, and yet sets up mechanisms for rejection of others, remains to be determined. Colonization by a pathogen always has a traumatic effect on the morphology of the intestinal mucosa, interfering with the dynamics of epithelial cell renewal to the detriment of the function of the organ in nutrition (Kenworthy 1970). Under such circumstances the competence of intestinal immune mechanisms will govern the opportunity for rejection of the pathogen and subsequent survival of the host.

It is well known that *Escherichia coli* preponderates among those pathogens associated with enteric disease in domestic livestock. The animals most at risk are young ones, particularly those raised in modern intensive systems. We have studied the secretory immune mechanisms of the gut with particular reference to their role in effecting a balance in the host–pathogen relationship. In this context we have investigated oral immunization during the neonatal period, placing emphasis on nutritional performance and environment and not limiting the observations to the clinical manifestations of the problem.

MATERNAL IMMUNITY IN THE NEONATE

Most species have the ability to respond to a variety of antigenic stimuli during late fetal development. Indeed recent studies have shown that fetal lambs may be orally immunized by introducing antigens into the amniotic fluid (Husband & McDowell 1975). However, it is normal for passively acquired maternal immunoglobulins to compensate for the quantitative immunological deficiency of the neonate. The susceptibility of the neonate to enteric colibacillosis is readily evident in those species with chorioepithelial placentation. In such species, exemplified by pigs and calves, survival in the absence of colostrum will barely extend to 24 hours in a conventional environment. The quantitative weight of maternal immunity is evident from measurement of immunoglobulins which accumulate in the blood serum of the neonate. Thus the piglet in the first few hours of life will absorb colostral immunoglobulins through its gut wall amounting to approximately 3 g in total and the calf exceeds this by some 20-fold; even the chicken will take up some 60 mg from the yolk sac. What is of immediate consequence, however, is the class of antibody involved and its mode of antibacterial action in the intestinal mucosa and within the lumen.

A comparative study of immunoglobulin (Ig) classes in the pig, calf and chicken is of interest in this respect (Fig. 1), providing several different features of alimentary tract physiology and of the mode of operation of maternal immunity. The universal role of IgG is seen to operate in terms of its quantitative abundance in each species. The selective characteristics of the ruminant

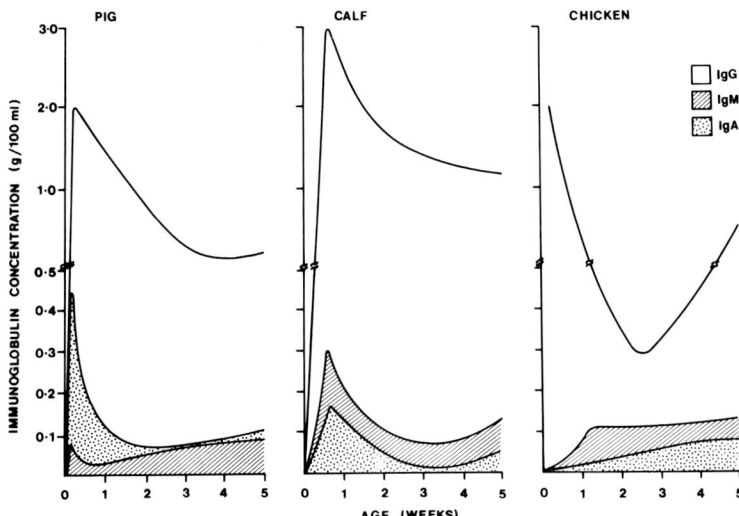

FIG. 1. Comparison of serum immunoglobulin (Ig) profiles of pig, calf, and chicken during the first few weeks of life.

allowing transport of IgG_1 into mammary secretions are well known and will not be dealt with here. In both pig and calf, IgM and IgA are transferred and play a significant role in antibacterial immunity. There is no transfer of IgM or IgA via the yolk sac in birds.

In mammals the lactational changes in the immunoglobulin profile of the dam in relation to neonatal requirement are of considerable interest. During the first few days of lactation the total concentration of immunoglobulin falls steeply in the milks of both pigs and cows. It is the rapid fall in IgG during this period which contributes most to the total decline, thus exercising a necessary economy in a maternal immunoglobulin which is transferred almost exclusively from the blood circulation by a transudative process across the mammary acinar epithelium.

In the pig, IgA emerges as the dominant immunoglobulin in the milk (Porter et al. 1970) whereas in the cow there is a uniformly low level of immunoglobulin secretion, which is a feature of ruminants in general. Secretory 11S IgA anti-*E. coli* antibodies in porcine colostrum and milk have been shown to operate entirely in the lumen without contributing significantly to antibody in the blood circulation of the neonatal piglet. The physiological patterns of milk antibody secretion, ingestion by the neonate and subsequent passage through the alimentary tract combine to provide a continuous bathing of the intestinal mucosa with maternal IgA antibody. Since the bovine mammary gland does not continue to secrete high levels of IgA throughout lactation (Butler *et al.* 1972), it is interesting to see how the calf compensates for this deficiency. It exhibits no intestinal selection in absorption of maternal immunoglobulins and temporarily high levels of 11S IgA occur in the blood circulation (Porter 1972). This IgA declines with a half-life of approximately two days, being lost into various external secretions, principally those of the gut. This process continues for a period of approximately 10 days, providing the basis of a short-term barrier to infection.

In this context the recent observations on the appearance of IgA and IgM in the amniotic fluid of embryonating eggs and the intestinal tract of chick embryos are of interest (Rose *et al.* 1974). It is suggested that the maternal IgA and IgM present in oviduct secretions are acquired by the egg as it passes down the oviduct where the white is laid down. These appear in the embryonic gut via swallowed amniotic fluid, giving some analogy to the situation that exists in the newborn mammal.

DEVELOPMENT OF INTESTINAL SECRETORY IMMUNITY IN THE NEONATE

There are very few lymphoid cells in the intestinal lamina propria of the newborn mammal and lymphoid follicles are poorly defined. In the germ-free state the lymphoid cell population of the lamina propria remains at a negligible level and the lamina becomes infiltrated with lymphocytes and plasma cells in response to the development of a gut microflora. Sequential studies on pigs have shown that during the first days of life, IgM cells outnumber those containing IgA or IgG (Fig. 2) and during this period IgM is the principal immunoglobulin secreted across the crypt epithelium (Allen & Porter 1973*a,b*). Immunoelectron microscopical studies suggest that the mechanism of transport of both immunoglobulins is essentially the same. Vesicles containing either IgM or IgA were found in the apical cytoplasm of crypt epithelial cells, suggesting that the immunoglobulin is transported across the epithelium by a process of reverse pinocytosis (Allen *et al.* 1973, 1976).

The relationship between the cellular component of the secretory immune system and the antigenic load in the lumen of the gut may be considered to be one of dynamic equilibrium. Thus the greater the load the higher the level of cellular activity required to counter it. The major antigenic stimulus derives from the enteric flora and it is interesting to note that lipopolysaccharide from Gram-negative organisms appears free in the lumen and is not only a B cell mitogen but also an antigen which promotes preferential synthesis of IgM.

During the early stages of its development an animal is likely to experience challenges by new antigens more frequently than later on. The establishment of

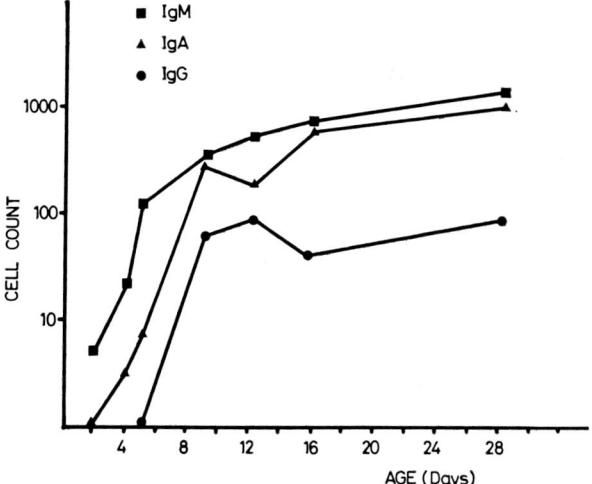

FIG. 2. Sequential development of immunoglobulin-producing cells in the lamina propria of the duodenum in the young pig.

the gut microflora together with a wide range of dietary antigens all contribute to this challenge. As the animal matures, the microflora becomes stabilized and the number of previously unencountered dietary components diminishes to a low level, and the cellular component of the lamina is better able to equilibrate with the luminal environment. Thus it is suggested that local antigenic challenge results in an initial proliferation of IgM-producing cells, to be followed by a possibly greater proliferation of IgA cells. Similarly, at any stage of maturity this development process is likely to occur in response to any previously unexperienced antigen. It is interesting that Crandall et al. (1967) showed a relative increase in the numbers of IgM-containing cells in the intestinal mucosa of adult rabbits soon after infection with Trichinella. Furthermore, in studies of infants with enteric colibacillosis, IgM antibodies formed an important part of the early response, especially in the youngest children of four or five months of age (McNeish et al. 1975).

The pattern of development of immunoglobulin-producing cells in response to antigens from the intestinal lumen can be gauged to advantage in the germ-free animal. In the germ-free pig IgM was demonstrated to play a dominant role in the early phases of the intestinal response to pathogenic E. coli. Furthermore, repeated administration of sterile preparations of bacterial antigens resulted in a response similar in terms of cell numbers to that produced by infection with the live organism in a comparable period.

In the young chick, however, no response to E. coli O antigens could be determined on either local application in fistulated birds or oral immunization in germ-free birds. This was surprising since the characteristics of the intestinal response to infection with *E. coli* are very similar to those in the mammal, implicating IgM-and IgA-producing cells in the tissues and antibody associated with these immunoglobulin classes in the secretions (Parry *et al.* 1977).

ORAL IMMUNIZATION IN PROPHYLACTIC CONTROL OF POST-WEANING ENTERIC INFECTION

The decline and termination of the protective function of maternal immunoglobulin is of signal importance in the complex of predisposing factors in the pathogenesis of post-weaning enteric syndromes. Immune mechanisms only play a significant role in inhibiting microbial proliferation after weaning provided that the intestinal mucosa is alerted to the production and secretion of antibodies long before the organisms achieve pathogenic proportions in the lumen. Thus if intestinal immunity is to have any potential at all, the young animal must be immunized early in life in order for a mucosal blockage to be established against the proliferation of enteropathogens consequent upon weaning. Only a limited number of serotypes are normally associated with diarrhoea syndromes of young farm livestock (Sojka 1971), so suitable prospects for vaccination exist.

The first criterion to establish in support of this rationale was that effective synthesis and secretion of anti-*E. coli* antibodies would occur in response to an antigenic stimulus to the intestinal mucosa of the neonate even in the presence of maternal antibodies. Studies were made in a litter of pigs in which intestinal fistulae were prepared at four days of age; four animals were maintained on the sow and four animals were reared separately and fed on cow's milk. One animal in each group was retained as a control and heat-inactivated *E. coli* were administered to the others. The characteristics of the secretory antibody response were very similar in all six animals, independent of whether the animals were maintained on maternal milk or a reconstituted cow's milk substitute lacking antibody (Fig. 3). Studies in the young calf provided essentially similar data; intestinal secretion of antibodies was registered in colostrum-fed animals in response to the oral administration of bacterial antigens at five days of age. Thus a useful relationship between passive maternal antibody and active intestinal antibody could be established in neonatal life. Since health and performance in young animals could be attributed to the establishment of this continuum, the stage was set to examine the efficacy of the local intestinal immune response in terms of the young animal's resistance to enteric infection.

Imbalance in the host–pathogen relationship will be shown in a range of

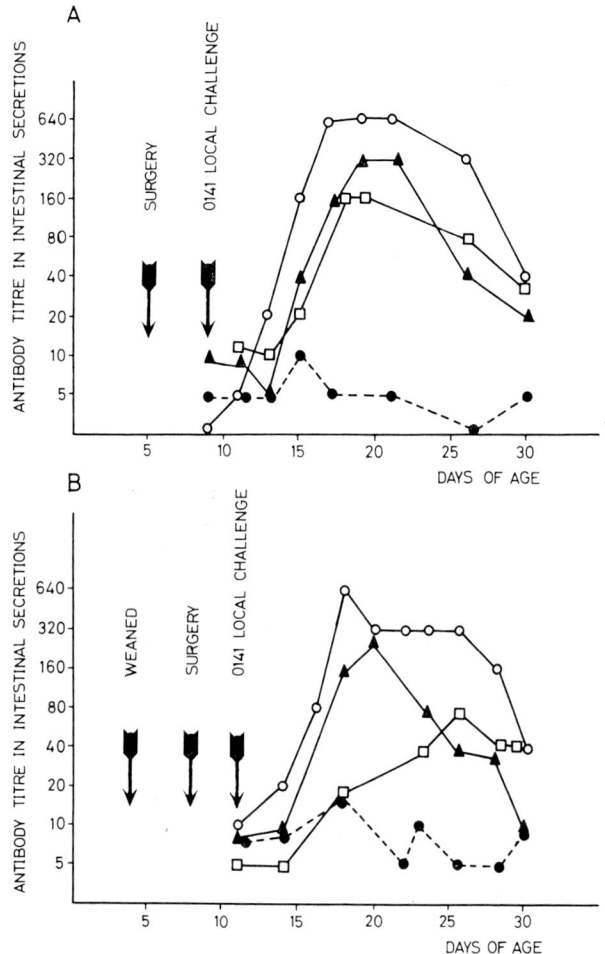

FIG. 3. Local intestinal antibody secretion after administration of heat-inactivated *E. coli* O141 to baby pigs.
(A) Animals maintained on the sow.
(B) Animals weaned at four days of age and raised on reconstituted spray-dried cow's milk.
●, control animals. ○, ▲ and ■, animals locally challenged with heat-inactivated *E. coli* O141.

responses creating a decline in performance, leading finally to overt disease and death. Young farm animals are growing rapidly during this stage of development and we have taken the view that maintenance of intestinal integrity and function against a bacterial challenge should be apparent in terms of animal performance. Thus, whereas the traditional approach to investigations of *E. coli*-associated enteric syndromes has been towards clinical manifestations of the problem, we have also placed emphasis on the overall nutritional and physiological status of the animal during a vital period of its life.

The requirement for antigens to be administered in repeated doses was met by including them in the diet, thus saving the labour of individual dosing. *E. coli* antigens were added at levels which ensured that on average animals consumed at least 10 times the minimum required dose.

In pilot trials with pigs, orally immunized animals showed a reduction in the natural excretion of pathogenic *E. coli* compared with controls. Significant benefits in weight gain were recorded along with improvements in food conversion, and the incidence of diarrhoea and requirement for medication were reduced (Porter *et al.* 1974*a*). Trials in calves provided much the same data. When calves are reared in units under continuous occupation, health and performance deteriorate in successive batches of animals associated with the bacterial loading of the environment created by previous occupants (Roy *et al.* 1955). It is interesting to note that in such a trial carried out over a period of 12 months involving 16 batches of calves, the overall deterioration in performance shown in control groups was practically abolished by oral immunization.

IMMUNE MECHANISMS OF HOST RESISTANCE TO ENTEROPATHOGENIC E. COLI AFTER ORAL IMMUNIZATION

Enteropathogenic *E. coli* may represent a substantial component of the intestinal microflora without manifestation of clinical symptoms. The enteric syndrome is usually associated with the establishment of enteropathogens in the anterior regions of the small intestine, a view supported by the observation that the tissues become progressively less responsive to the effects of *E. coli* enterotoxins after the first few feet, comprising the duodenum and upper jejunum. Thus attachment to the intestinal wall is considered to be an important prerequisite of an enteropathogen, enabling it to counter the flushing effects of peristalsis. Furthermore the toxic mechanisms will be optimized by the close proximity of the bacteria with the epithelial cells (Smith & Linggood 1971).

The commonest mechanism of adhesion identified in the Enterobacteriaceae is associated with the presence of filamentous surface antigens. A common K antigen, K88, occurs in porcine enteropathogenic strains and this, unlike other K antigens, is a protein component forming fine filaments on the surface of the bacterium. The antigen is the product of an episomal gene which can be transferred (Ørskov & Ørskov 1966) and elimination of the genetic elements

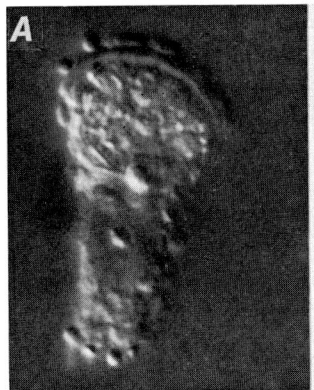 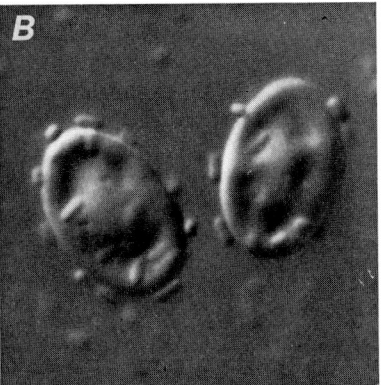

Fig. 4. Adhesion of pathogenic E. coli [O8; K87(B), K88ab(L)] to cell membranes shown by interference contrast microscopy.
(A) Intestinal epithelial cell from duodenum of newborn piglet ($\times$ 600).
(B) Chicken erythrocyte ($\times$ 600).

responsible for its synthesis results in loss of virulence (Smith & Linggood 1971).

Calf and lamb enteropathogenic strains also possess a common K antigen, designated K99, and this too is controlled by a transmissible plasmid (Smith & Linggood 1972). These antigens appear to display specific characteristics of attachment to host intestinal epithelium. Thus K88 determines virulence in the pig and K99 in the calf or lamb and not *vice versa*. This implies the presence of a specific receptor in the epithelial membrane of each species for the bacterial protein determinant. In this context it is of interest that *E. coli* possessing these antigens also agglutinate and adhere to the erythrocytes of certain species (Fig. 4). The erythrocyte and its membrane are a more suitable subject for investigation than the enterocyte and furthermore a simple haemagglutination technique provides a useful method for quantifying the bacterial K antigen.

We have used the chicken erythrocyte to facilitate our investigations of the K88 virulence determinant for the pig; by specific inhibition techniques we have correlated the agglutination of erythrocytes with adhesion to enterocytes. Additionally, both properties can be inhibited by antibodies raised against the purified K antigen. The presence of a possible membrane receptor in enterocytes and erythrocytes is demonstrated indirectly by treating the cells with K88 antigen and subsequently localizing the antigen with fluorescent antibody.

The role of virulence determinants in protective immunization has been examined in relation to porcine neonatal enteritis by Rutter & Jones (1973). Sows were immunized with a crude preparation of K88 antigen and passive protection in the suckling neonate was suitably demonstrated by oral challenge with enteropathogenic *E. coli*. Parenteral immunization of the sow results in transfer of antibody, mainly by transudative processes, and the antibody class yielded by the immunization protocol used in this study is invariably IgG. An active local antibody response to bacterial adhesion determinants would be expected to enhance the resistance of a young animal to intestinal colonization with enteropathogenic serotypes of *E. coli*, but so far these protein K antigens have not been used successfully as an oral immunogen.

There are, however, indirect means of eliminating the properties of bacterial adhesion. Agglutination may assist in creating bacterial aggregates which may successfully be eliminated by peristalsis, but of greater potential significance is our recent observation that piglets orally immunized with O antigens, and then infected with K88-containing enteropathogens, subsequently excrete only K88-negative *E. coli*. We failed to infect control pigs with cultures prepared from the excreted serotype, whereas the original enteropathogen was demonstrated to be virulent and excreted without modification in the control animals. Furthermore, in an *in vitro* model system in which K88-positive *E. coli* were passaged through media containing antibodies to O antigens, the K88 plasmid was progressively lost so that the level of antigen which was produced in culture declined rapidly over a series of passages. Thus modification of the antigenic composition of enteropathogens occurs in the presence of antibody *in vivo* and *in vitro*. The practical benefits of oral immunoprophylaxis therefore go beyond the immediate characteristics of host resistance, and a very significant advantage to the environment will accrue in terms of a limitation on the excretion of serotypes with virulence determinants, thereby reducing the risk to other animals.

The ability to produce enterotoxin is a prime requirement for enteropathogenicity and this too has been identified with the presence of a transmissible plasmid (Smith & Halls 1968). Enterotoxins of *Vibrio cholerae* and *E. coli* have several similarities and their main function is the creation of a prolonged disturbance of fluid and electrolyte balance. If we take the view that *E. coli* enterotoxins are poorly antigenic, it might be most appropriate to make an indirect approach to the problem via antibacterial mechanisms. Thus, if the bacterium is eliminated, the enterotoxic problem does not arise. In this respect it is significant that Smith & Linggood (1971) had concluded from studies of post-weaning diarrhoea in pigs that the protective function of immunity may be principally associated with bactericidal as opposed to anti-enterotoxic mechanisms.

This concept of indirect protection against enterotoxigenicity was tested in orally immunized pigs in which the main effect of mucosal antibodies was considered to be bacterial agglutination and stasis (Porter *et al.* 1974*b*).

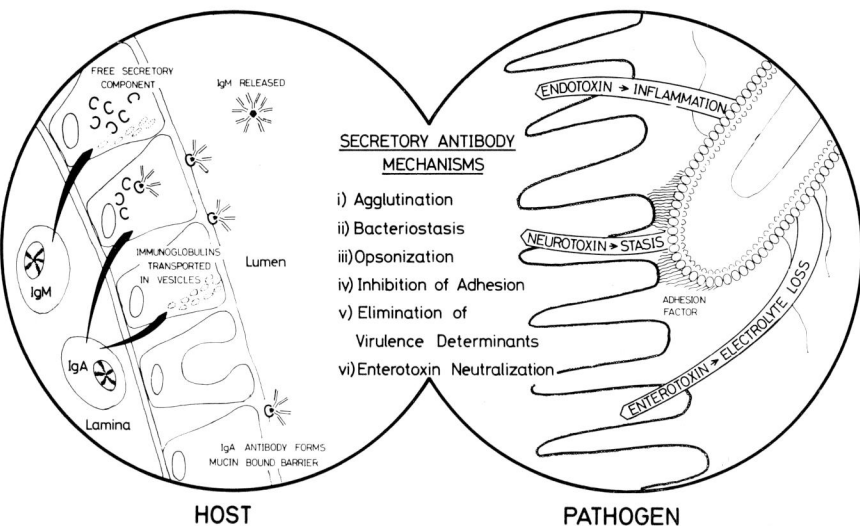

FIG. 5. Schematic representation of host–pathogen interaction in the intestine, showing mechanisms of secretion of antibody (*left*) and virulence characteristics of enteropathogenic *E. coli* (*right*). Defined characteristics of interference with microbial pathogenicity by secretory antibody are listed.

Bacterial proliferation in response to infection during the critical two-week period after weaning was substantially reduced by oral immunization with heat-inactivated antigens, and in consequence so was the severity and duration of diarrhoea. Furthermore, in recent studies orally immunized piglets were used in ligated gut tests to look for an inhibition of the enterotoxigenicity of live pathogens (Balger *et al.* 1975). Such animals were demonstrated to resist approximately 1000 times greater doses of *E. coli* than control animals and the effect was attributed to bacteriostasis. However, perhaps of greater significance are the recent observations of Linggood (1976) using the ligated gut model with cell-free isolates of *E. coli* enterotoxin. In these studies enterotoxin neutralization was observed in orally immunized animals and in addition the activity could be passively transferred with intestinal secretions. Thus enterotoxin inhibition can be mediated directly by mucosal antibodies, without necessarily invoking indirect antibacterial mechanisms.

The variety of ways in which secretory antibodies may mediate in local interference with microbial pathogenicity are summarized in Fig. 5. Most of these mechanisms will be required for solid immune defence.

Finally, in considering the mechanisms of synthesis and secretion of immunoglobulins and their presentation as a local antibody barrier on the intestinal epithelium, it is relevant also to consider the distribution of immunoglobulin-producing cells within the lamina propria. If we return to the observation of Smith & Linggood (1971), that in order to cause disease the bacteria needed to proliferate in the upper region of the small intestine, it is significant that immunocytes are more numerous here than anywhere else in the gut. A further link in quantitative terms is apparent when one considers that it is this region of the intestine which is most susceptible to the effects of enterotoxin (Smith & Halls 1967). Thus immune cell function predominates in the most vulnerable area of the gut rather than in the region which carries the greatest microbial population. Probably this characteristic of intestinal function will contribute to the control of the pathogenic component of the intestinal flora not only locally, but generally, by virtue of the release of antibody which will ultimately traverse the length of the alimentary tract in the digesta. In this context, our observation on the effects of low levels of secretory antibody causing loss of virulence determinants in cultures of enteropathogens will be relevant. Thus, in terms of the balance of the host–pathogen relationship, the environmental implications of the excretion of fewer organisms with lower virulence will definitely benefit the host.

References

ALLEN, W. D. & PORTER, P. (1973a) Localisation by immunofluorescence of secretory component and IgA in intestinal mucosa of the young pig. *Immunology 24*, 365-501

ALLEN, W. D. & PORTER, P. (1973b) The relative distribution of IgM and IgA cells in intestinal mucosa and lymphoid tissue of the young pig and their significance in ontogenesis of secretory immunity. *Immunology 24*, 493-501

ALLEN, W. D., SMITH, C. G. & PORTER, P. (1973) Localisation of intracellular immunoglobulin A in porcine intestinal mucosa using enzyme-labelled antibody. *Immunology 25*, 55-70

ALLEN, W. D., SMITH, C. G. & PORTER, P. (1976) Evidence for the secretory transport mechanism of intestinal immunoglobulin. The ultrastructural distribution of IgM. *Immunology 30*, 449-457

BALGER, G., CHORHERR, S., SICKEL, E. & GUBEN, D. (1975) Orale, aktine Immunisierung neugeborener Ferkel gegen *E. coli:* Wirksamkeitsnachweis in Darmligaturtest. *Zentralbl. Veterinaermed. 22*, 488-498

BUTLER, J. E., MAXWELL, C. G., PIERCE, C. J., HYLTON, M. B., ASOFSKY, R. & KIDDY, C. A. (1972) Studies on the relative synthesis and distribution of IgA and IgG1 in various tissues and body fluids of the cow. *J. Immunol. 109*, 38-46

CRANDALL, R. B., CEBRA, J. J. & CRANDALL, C. A. (1967) The relative proportions of IgG, IgA and IgM cells in rabbit tissues during experimental trichinosis. *Immunology 12*, 147-156

HUSBAND, A. J. & McDOWELL, G. H. (1975) Local and systemic immune responses following oral immunization of foetal lambs. *Immunology 29*, 1019-1028

KENWORTHY, R. (1970) Effect of *Escherichia coli* on germ-free and gnotobiotic pigs. 1. Light and electron microscopy of the small intestine. *J. Comp. Pathol. 80*, 53-63

LINGGOOD, M. A. (1976) Some observations on plasmid controlled characters that affect the virulence of porcine strains of *Escherichia coli*. PhD Thesis, University of London

MCNEISH, A. S., EVANS, N., GAZE, H. & ROGERS, K. B. (1975) The agglutinating antibody response in the duodenum in infants with enteropathic *E. coli* gastroenteritis. *Gut 16*, 727-731

ØRSKOV, I. & ØRSKOV, F. (1966) Episome carried surface antigen K88 of *E. coli*. I. Transmission of the determinant of the K88 antigen and the influence of chromosomal markers. *J. Bacteriol. 95*, 69-75

PARRY, S. H., ALLEN, W. D. & PORTER, P. (1977) Intestinal immune response to *Escherichia coli* antigens in the germ-free chicken. *Immunology*, in press

PORTER, P. (1972) Immunoglobulins in bovine mammary sections: quantitative changes in early lactation and absorption by the neonatal calf. *Immunology 23*, 225-237

PORTER, P., NOAKES, D. E. & ALLEN, W. D. (1970) Secretory IgA and antibodies to *E. coli* in porcine colostrum and milk and their significance in the alimentary tract of the young pig. *Immunology 18*, 245-257

PORTER, P., KENWORTHY, R. & ALLEN, W. D. (1974a) Effect of oral immunisation with *E. coli* antigens on post weaning enteric infection in the young pig. *Vet. Rec. 95*, 99-104

PORTER, P., KENWORTHY, R., NOAKES, D. E. & ALLEN, W. D. (1974b) Intestinal antibody secretion in the young pig in response to oral immunisation with *E. coli*. *Immunology 27*, 841-853

ROY, J. B. H., PALMER, J., SHILLAM, K. W. G., INGRAM, P. L. & WOOD, P. C. (1955) The nutritive value of colostrum for the calf. 10. Relationships between the period of time that a calf house has been occupied and the incidence of scouring and mortality in young calves. *Br. J. Nutr. 9*, 11-20

ROSE, M. E., ORLANS, E. & BUTTRESS, N. (1974) Immunoglobulin classes in the hen's egg: their segregation in yolk and white. *Eur. J. Immunol. 4*, 521-523

RUTTER, J. M. & JONES, G. W. (1973) Protection against enteric disease caused by *E. coli*—a model for vaccination with a virulence determinant. *Nature (Lond.) 242*, 531-533

SMITH, H. W. & HALLS, S. (1967) Observations by the ligated intestinal segment and oral inoculation methods on *E. coli* infections in pigs, calves, lambs and rabbits. *J. Pathol. Bacteriol. 93*, 499-529

SMITH, H. W. & HALLS, S. (1968) The transmissible nature of the genetic factor in *E. coli* that controls enterotoxin production. *J. Gen. Microbiol. 52*, 319-334

SMITH, H. W. & LINGGOOD, M. A. (1971) Observations on the pathogenic properties of the K88, Hly, and Ent plasmids of *E. coli* with particular reference to porcine diarrhoea. *J. Med. Microbiol. 4*, 467-486

SMITH, H. W. & LINGGOOD, M. A. (1972) Further observations on *E. coli* enterotoxins with particular regard to those produced by atypical piglet strains and by calf and lamb strains. *J. Med. Microbiol. 5*, 243-250

SOJKA, W. (1971) Enteric diseases in newborn piglets, calves and lambs due to *E. coli* infection. *Vet. Bull. 41*, 509-522

Discussion

Pierce: You suggested that it is necessary to continue to feed the antigen in order to sustain protection, as measured by the presence of coproantibody. In dogs immunized by one of several means that induce a local immune response to cholera toxoid, we obtained protection against live vibrio challenge which far outlasted the presence of preformed antibodies in gut washings (Pierce

1976). Have you considered that it may not be necessary to continually feed the antigen, or to have pre-existing secreted antibody in the gut, to protect the animals?

Porter: We have not examined this particular aspect. The mechanisms we have concentrated on would probably require the continuous secretion of antibody; for example, the loss of the virulence determinant, or inhibition of the adhesion determinant, and bacteriostasis, would all be mediated by secreted antibody.

Pierce: Perhaps antibody-mediated mechanisms can be effective even in the absence of pre-formed secretory antibody—for example, by a rapid secondary response after re-exposure of a primed animal.

Porter: Have you evidence of a rapid secondary response of this type?

Pierce: Only in terms of protection against experimental cholera in dogs, which has an incubation period of 12–16 hours. We have shown that significant protection against oral challenge with live *Vibrio cholerae* lasts at least eight months after effective local immunization with cholera toxoid (Pierce 1976).

Porter: There is a difference between the level of antibody secretion, and the antibody which would be present in the intestinal epithelium. There will be continuing antibody in the intestinal wall that is not revealed by the crude measurement of antibody in the secretion from the gut loop. However, I do not think that protection will go on for months.

Lehner: Dr Pierce's question touched on the problem of whether there is a memory in the secretory antibody (IgA) system, and some of the evidence you showed, Dr Porter, suggests that there wasn't; the antibodies did not appear early, the response was not greater in magnitude, and it didn't last longer. Can you enlighten us about the existence of an IgA memory system?

Porter: Professor Parrott has published work on bovine serum albumin (BSA) which indicated tolerance. We were studying a response that will not involve T cell help, since we use the O endotoxin. We use this antigen because it is very stable, is not degraded in mammalian intestine to any extent, and mediates important anti-bacterial mechanisms. We wouldn't have expected that the O antigen would mediate an anti-enterotoxic effect, and Balger's work suggests that it was a bacteriostatic mechanism rather than an anti-enterotoxic one (Balger *et al.* 1975), yet we are getting enterotoxin antigens surviving and producing antibodies that can be transferred between species.

The other important point is the mediation against the adhesion-virulence determinant. We can produce the virulence determinant very easily and can measure it, but we are not yet able to immunize by feeding this protein. In Professor Parrott's work with BSA there was little activity in terms of secreted antibody and yet there was tolerance, after oral feeding of antigen.

Parrott: We fed large amounts of protein antigen (BSA) and got partial tolerance (Thomas & Parrott 1974). There was also a small amount of systemic antibody but there were no IgA-secreting cells in the lamina propria; but there was no antibody production after challenge with BSA in Freund's complete adjuvant, so presumably no production of memory.

Brandtzaeg: In relation to a possible secondary response, Richard Newcomb repeatedly immunized his own nose with serum albumin from *Alligator mississippiensis*, and found after prolonged immunization an apparent feedback on the secretory IgA response as measured in the secretion (Newcomb & Sutoris 1974). It may be misleading just to look at the secretions, however. For example, if gland-associated secondary immune responses also lead to a gradual switch from production of dimeric IgA to an increased proportion of monomeric IgA and perhaps also IgG, these immunoglobulins will not appear in the secretions. A secondary response may thus be masked because of lack of secretory properties of the antibodies produced. This possibility should be considered in evaluating mucosal secondary immune responses.

Mayrhofer: Another factor is that if IgA has a role in preventing antigen absorption by the gut, then any possibility of producing a secondary response by gut challenge with an antigen is reduced for as long as secretory antibody to that antigen persists. This could make it difficult to demonstrate memory in the IgA system of the intact animal. An adoptive transfer of immune lymphocytes into a non-immune animal may be necessary in order to show it.

André: We found that a repeat intragastric administration of sheep red blood cells resulted in a spleen response with plaque-forming cells which belonged predominantly to the IgA class. This spleen response was in all points similar to the primary response and in no way suggestive of immunological memory when the animals were given their second immunization after a three-month rest period. In contrast, when the intragastric immunization was resumed two weeks after the priming period, no response was obtained (André *et al.* 1973). It is known that local immunization of the gut impairs its capacity to absorb the corresponding antigen (André *et al.* 1974). But we have also established that intragastric immunization caused an immunological hyporesponsiveness to parenteral challenge and that one is therefore dealing with tolerance and not with failure to absorb antigen from the gut (André *et al.* 1975).

Porter: We get different results with bacterial antigens. We get a booster response, not tolerance, by oral immunization. If we orally immunize with the *E. coli* antigens and follow with a single parenteral administration of the same heat-killed antigen, there is a booster response providing an IgM antibody in serum. We haven't looked at the secretions because we wanted to exploit this response in terms of colostral immunity, timing the IgM response to coincide with formation of colostrum, to get a high IgM antibody titre into the suckling neonate (this is John Chidlow's work). This is distinct from the tolerance observations made by Professor Parrott.

Lachmann: Is it significant that you are using on the one hand a T-dependent and on the other a T-independent antigen? The classical demonstration of tolerance following oral immunization is the Sulzberger & Chase phenomenon, where it is to delayed hypersensitivity that feeding hapten renders the animal tolerant (Sulzberger 1929; Chase 1963).

Porter: Yes. We are using a T-independent antigen. This is the difference from Dr Parrott's work.

White: You said that if you continuously administered the antigens of *E. coli* to pigs you found a response in terms of cell numbers that was like that generated by infection with gut pathogen; thus in the monocontaminated and in the orally immunized germ-free animal the cell responses were similar. In the chicken, whereas we obtained a similar cell response in the monocontaminated bird to that generated in the pig, the oral administration of *E. coli* O antigens produced no cell response. Is that related to adherence of the antigen to the intestinal wall? Does it adhere in the pig and not in the chicken?

Porter: I don't think so, but we haven't looked at this question specifically. We have examined the survival of the antigen along the alimentary tract of the chick; we fed iodine-labelled *E. coli* O2 antigen, which is pathogenic for the chick. It survives into the caecum. There is much degradation, since iodine-labelled fragments are absorbed into the blood and excreted in the urine. We wondered whether there is a lack of absorption of the antigen, or perhaps adherence of the antigen, or survival of antigen, in the region of the bursa. Furthermore, the distribution of Peyer's patches along the intestine of the pig gives a greater opportunity for immune stimulation than does the simple presentation of the antigen to the bursa in the chicken.

White: You said that antibody does not interfere with the immunization process. Does that depend on the specificity of the antibody?

Porter: No. We were using an immunization schedule that reproduced what we envisaged would exist in the sucking pig, in preparation for events at weaning, because the young animal normally then goes through an *E. coli* proliferation lasting two weeks. A survey by Svendsen *et al.* (1974) found 82% morbidity associated with *E. coli* pathogens at weaning. We envisage preparing the young animal and its intestinal immune system to take over from the protection continuously mediated by maternal IgA antibody in its intestine during the suckling period. The sow provides antibody to the gut lumen of the young animal throughout suckling and that presumably could interfere with any antigenic stimulus, given orally. The experiment I described (p. 60) showed that the maternal antibody did *not* interfere.

White: Was it antibody against the K antigen?

Porter: No, it was antibody against the O antigen, which was interfering with the production of the adherence factor.

Booth: One obvious feature of the gut mucosa is the mucus layer but whenever we look at preparations, by electron microscopy or any other method, we never see it. This applies to all techniques of fixation for electron microscopy. You have made scanning electron micrographs simply showing an impregnated surface of the membrane.

Porter: Those electron micrographs illustrate adherence. In an animal that had died because of *E. coli* infection, or is in the worst phases of infection, the anterior small intestine is completely coated with millions of organisms, whereas in an animal excreting the same pathogen and not showing clinical symptoms, the anterior small intestine can be free. So whether the animal shows clinical symptoms is determined by the upper region of the small intestine.

Booth: The question is whether the organisms adhere in the small intestine. It has been proved for the mouth.

Porter: Yes. The bacterium must gain access to the upper small intestine and adhere where it has close association with the epithelial cell and the capability to multiply and secrete its toxin, because *E. coli* is non-invasive and the effect is mediated by toxin. The interesting point is that the antibodies are mediating not against adhesion but against the ability of the pathogen to produce the adhesion factor.

Gowans: Has the ability of virulent bacteria to adhere to the intestinal epithelium any connection with the ability of the organisms to prevent mucus secretion? Mucus does not appear on your list of possible mechanisms, presumably because it is not an immunological mechanism, but one would like to know whether it is important.

Lachmann: In fact it is not altogether non-immunological. Eggert (1976) in Professor Coombs' laboratory has evidence of IgA complexes with mucin that mediate antibacterial reactions in saliva.

Porter: We have interesting observations in relation to the reaction of the K88 antigen which go some way towards answering this question. If we prepare extracts of this antigen from a virulent organism and treat sections of gut with it, and then with a fluorescent antiglobulin, or do the same with chicken erythrocytes, we see receptor domains for that antigen.

Booth: The background of my question was an observation of Tabagchali (1970) using electron microscopy and non-pathogenic *E. coli* in man, showing the bacteria beautifully wrapped up in mucus, which is very puzzling.

Porter: We can agglutinate bacteria *in vitro* with anti-O antibody and do not prevent adhesion, so the agglutinate still adheres by available determinants to the gut epithelial cells.

Bienenstock: Bloch & Walker studied antigen uptake in the rat ligated everted gut sac. If the rats are pre-immunized or there are immune complexes in the bathing medium, the goblet cells eject mucus (K. J. Bloch & A. Walker, personal communication 1976). It would be interesting to look at the relationship of immune complexes to that.

Cebra: You seem to be suggesting, Dr Porter, that IgM could pass into the gut lumen but that IgA could adhere to the mucosal surface of the cells. Perhaps there is an interaction between the Fc region of IgA and the cell surface, or perhaps an Fc–mucin interaction. Have you any observations on the relative adhesion of serum as against secretory IgA to the surface of cells? We had wondered if the passage of IgA across undifferentiated crypt cells might lead to the sequential addition of monosaccharides, leading to a mucin-like oligosaccharide and resulting in a cell surface interaction directly or via a mucin binding. Have you done comparative studies?

Porter: No, nothing in that realm, but would you not think that the secretory component mediates this binding effect with mucin?

Cebra: I am open-minded on this. But just how different are the two isotypes, IgM and IgA, with respect to mucin binding which in turn may lead to cell adhesion?

Porter: We obtained intestinal secretions from Thiry-Vella loops in calves. By the time we put the secretions into the fridge to cool, the mucin had clotted and when we compared the supernatant and the clot, the binding of IgA and IgM was very different. Only IgM went into the supernatant, whereas IgA was bound into the mucin gel.

Lachmann: What is the evidence of opsonization by virtue of IgA antibodies?

Porter: Rowley made the initial observations on this (Wernet *et al.* 1971) but I believe he has subsequently retracted this thesis.

Soothill: Unfortunately Dr Breu was unable to reproduce this phenomenon while working in our laboratory.

Porter: There is other work that has shown this. Girard & de Kalbermatten (1970) made similar observations using intestinal antibodies. One should remember also that intestinal antibody function is not solely mediated by IgA; I have emphasized the role of IgM (Fig. 5, p. 65). This may also exert a potent antibacterial effect in gut immunity.

Lachmann: IgGl in serum at least is a perfectly good opsonizing and complement-fixing antibody.

Porter: There is interesting work by Bellamy (1973) in relation to the appearance of neutrophils in the intestinal lumen, which seems to be antibody-mediated. Bellamy looked in the calf at the transudation of neutrophils into Thiry-Vella loops in response to the local administration of BSA and also *E. coli* antigens. This seemed to be antibody-mediated rather than T cell-mediated, so there may be a basis for opsonization within the gut lumen.

Lehner: On the same basis, has anyone shown Fc receptors for IgA?

Pepys: There is evidence that IgG and IgA from the plasma bind in the cold to human peripheral blood lymphocytes and monocytes; the immunoglobulins can be removed by washing the cells at 37 °C instead of 4 °C, or by a low pH shock (Kumagai *et al.* 1975; Lobo *et al.* 1975). It has not been established that this binding, particularly of IgA, takes place via receptors for Fc.

Lehner: Is there any evidence for the IgA Fc receptor on polymorphs or macrophages by rosetting or by using aggregated IgA and anti-IgA conjugate?

Pepys: The work of Kumagai *et al.* (1975) demonstrated the following. A proportion of human peripheral blood lymphocytes and monocytes, prepared by Ficoll-Hypaque separation and washed at 4 °C, can be stained with fluorescent anti-IgA antibodies. If the cells are washed at 37 °C before fluorescent staining, very few stain with anti-IgA. Reincubation at 4 °C of the warm-washed cells with a source of IgA restores the staining with anti-IgA.

Lachmann: It has been shown that IgA will not inhibit K cell cytotoxicity (Wislöff *et al.* 1974).

Rosen: There is an interesting situation in man where the early feeding to the newborn of poliovirus results in the prompt cessation of poliovirus secretion and in no immunity. This occurs when the mother has a reasonable titre of antibody to poliovirus. The reason is that the human newborn has Fab fragments in the intestine which are washed out at about 48 hours after birth. Fab fragments can even be found in newborn infants with oesophageal atresia. Fab has about 10 times less viral-neutralizing capacity than intact γ-globulin. Nonetheless, these Fab fragments are effective in neutralizing poliovirus.

Bienenstock: Chickens are interesting in that they have very few, but large, Peyer's patches; there are only two in the whole gastrointestinal tract, exclusive of the bursa. It might be worth exploring some of the questions we discussed earlier using the chicken, because this species has many IgA cells with relatively few Peyer's patches.

Porter: Most characteristics of the secretory immune system in the chicken have an analogy to the mammal; there is an analogue, if not a homologue, to the secretory component, and there is the same sort of response to bacterial infections, yet antigen given orally fails to mediate responses seen in mammals.

Bienenstock: One reason may be that the bird doesn't have the Peyer's patches and therefore lacks the lymphoid tissue necessary for the response.

Parrott: Perhaps you should sit chickens in a bath of antigen, so that it can get to the bursa—the converse of oral immunization!

White: This has been done with HSA. The antigen is cloacally drunk by the chicken; there is not much immediate antibody formation, but there is sensitization to subsequent systemic challenge and you lay down the mechanism for antibody production, the antigen going via the cloaca into the bursa.

References

ANDRÉ, C., BAZIN, H. & HEREMANS, J. F. (1973) Influence of repeated administration of antigen by the oral route on specific antibody-producing cells in the mouse spleen. *Digestion 9*, 166-175

ANDRÉ, C., LAMBERT, R., BAZIN, H. & HEREMANS, J. F. (1974) Interference of oral immunization with the intestinal absorption of heterologous albumin. *Eur. J. Immunol. 4*, 701-704

ANDRÉ, C., HEREMANS, J. F., VAERMAN, J. P. & CAMBIASO, C. L. (1975) A mechanism for the induction of immunological tolerance by antigen feeding: antigen–antibody complexes. *J. Exp. Med. 142*, 1509-1519

BALGER, G., CHORHERR, S., SICKEL, E. & GUBEN, D. (1975) Orale, aktine Immunisierung neugeborener Ferkel gegen *E. coli:* Wirksamkeitsnachweis in Darmligaturtest. *Zentralbl. Veterinaermed. 22*, 488-498

BELLAMY, J. E. C. (1973) Neutrophil emigration into the lumen of the porcine small intestine. PhD. Thesis, University of Saskatchewan, Canada

CHASE, M. W. (1963) Tolerance towards chemical allergens, in *La tolerance acquise et la tolerance naturelle à l'égard de substances antigéniques définés* (Bossard, A., ed.), pp. 139-160, CNRS, Paris

EGGERT, M. (1976) The nature of human salivary agglutinins and aggregating factors. Ph.D. Dissertation, University of Cambridge

GIRARD, J. P. & DE KALBERMATTEN, A. (1970) Antibody activity in human duodenal fluid. *Eur. J. Clin. Invest. 1*, 188-195

KUMAGAI, K., ABO, T., SEKIZAWA, T. & SASAKI, M. (1975) Studies of surface immunoglobulin on human B lymphocytes. I. Dissociation of cell-bound immunoglobulin with acid pH or at 37°C. *J. Immunol. 115*, 982-987

LOBO, P. I., WESTERVELT, F. B. & HORWITZ, D. A. (1975) Identification of two populations of immunoglobulin-bearing lymphocytes in man. *J. Immunol. 114*, 116-119

NEWCOMB, R. W. & SUTORIS, C. A. (1974) Comparative studies on human and rabbit exocrine IgA antibodies to an albumin. *Immunochemistry 11*, 623-632

PIERCE, N. F. (1976) Intestinal immunization with soluble bacterial antigens: the example of cholera toxoid, in *Acute Diarrhoea in Childhood (Ciba Found. Symp. 42)*, pp. 129-143, Elsevier/Excerpta Medica/North-Holland, Amsterdam

SULZBERGER, M. B. (1929) Hypersensitiveness to neoarsphenamine in guinea pigs. 1. Experiments in prevention and desensitization. *Arch. Dermatol. Syphilol. 20*, 669

SVENDSEN, J., LARSON, J. L., BILLE, M. & NIELSEN, M. C. (1974) Post weaning *E. coli* diarrhoea in pigs. *3rd Int. Pig Soc. Vet. Congress*, Lyons, D7

TABAGCHALI, S. (1970) The pathophysiological role of small intestinal bacterial flora. *Scand. J. Gastroenterol. 5*, Suppl. 6, 139-163

THOMAS, H. C. & PARROTT, D. M. V. (1974) The induction of tolerance to soluble protein antigen by oral administration. *Immunology 27*, 631

WERNET, P., BREU, H., KNOP, J. & ROWLEY, D. (1971) Antibacterial action of specific IgA and transport of IgM, IgA and IgG from serum into the small intestine. *J. Infect. Dis.* *124*, 223-229

WISLÖFF, F., MICHAELSEN, T. E. & FROLAND, S. S. (1974) Inhibition of antibody-dependent human lymphocyte-mediated cytotoxicity by immunoglobulin classes, IgG subclasses, and IgG fragments. *Scand. J. Immunol. 3*, 29-36

Intestinal secretion of IgA and IgM: a hypothetical model

PER BRANDTZAEG and KÅRE BAKLIEN

Department of Microbiology, Dental Faculty; Immunohistochemical Laboratory, Institute of Pathology and Medical Department A, University Hospital, Rikshospitalet, Oslo

Abstract The secretory component (SC) has recently been found to be associated with IgM in external secretions, although in a less stable complex than secretory IgA. Moreover, SC combines spontaneously *in vitro* with both IgA and IgM. A prerequisite is that the immunoglobulins contain the J chain, which is present only in dimers and polymers. This polypeptide is essential for the formation of an SC-binding site which appears already at the cytoplasmic level in IgA- and IgM-producing immunocytes. Locally formed J-chain-containing immunoglobulins are therefore readily available for complexing with SC present in the membranes of columnar secretory epithelial cells of glandular sites. This complexing initiates pinocytosis and external transport. Immunohistochemically the gland cells are shown to contain SC, IgA and IgM in identical locations, except that SC alone appears in the Golgi zone. Locally formed IgA and IgM antibodies are thus efficiently transferred to the mucosal surface where they exert an immunological exclusion of antigens. Conversely, IgG antibodies, which are not actively drained away from the lamina propria, may rather become engaged in complement activation and cell-mediated cytotoxicity with potentially deleterious effects on the tissue. Secondary to severe inflammatory reactions, secretory epithelium may show decreased production of SC; the selective external transport of SC-stabilized secretory IgA and IgM is thus jeopardized, and a vicious circle may be set up in the mucosa.

Because of its quantitative dominance and unique association with an epithelial secretory component (SC), IgA is considered as the most important immune factor in human exocrine secretions (for reviews, see Tomasi & Grey 1972; Hanson & Brandtzaeg 1973; Heremans 1974). Nevertheless, some individuals appear completely healthy despite a selective lack of IgA, at least in countries with good hygiene. It has been speculated that this may depend on a compensatory local immune mechanism expressed by enhanced local synthesis and secretion of IgM, known to occur in IgA deficiency (Heremans & Crabbé 1967);

Brandtzaeg et al. 1968; Eidelman & Davis 1968; Brandtzaeg 1971a). The observation that locally produced IgM may exhibit anti-virus activity in IgA-deficient individuals (Ogra et al. 1974) supports a possible contribution of this immunoglobulin to mucosal defence mechanisms. On the basis of our quantifications of immunoglobulins in pure glandular secretions we proposed several years ago that IgM should be considered as a secretory immunoglobulin with epithelial transport properties similar to secretory IgA (Brandtzaeg 1968). Indeed, subsequent studies of reptiles and amphibians suggested that IgM probably served the function of protecting mucosal surfaces before the evolution of IgA (Portis & Coe 1975). Recent immunochemical studies of IgM present in human secretions have moreover demonstrated that the 19S pentamers contain SC, which is retained in 60–70% of the molecules after purification (Brandtzaeg 1975c). Compared with secretory IgA, the quaternary structure of secretory IgM is less stabilized, since SC shows reactive I determinants after incorporation and depends on an excess of free component for permanent association with the remaining 30–40% of IgM in the secretions.

A MODEL FOR THE GLANDULAR TRANSPORT OF IgA AND IgM

It was speculated in several early studies that SC may facilitate the entry of extracellular IgA into glandular epithelial cells (Tomasi et al. 1965; South et al. 1966; O'Daly et al. 1971). SC was therefore originally called 'transport piece' (South et al. 1966). This suggestion was prompted by the fact that SC was complexed with secretory IgA, but there was no obvious explanation for its postulated transport function.

We proposed originally that a common glandular transport mechanism operates for IgA and IgM independently of SC, perhaps involving unique characteristics ('transfer sites') in the Fc portions of these two immunoglobulin classes and a corresponding epithelial receptor of unknown nature (Brandtzaeg 1968; Brandtzaeg et al. 1970). This view was mainly influenced by our early failure to demonstrate a regular association between SC and secretory IgM (Brandtzaeg et al. 1968; Brandtzaeg 1971a). An epithelial receptor specific for IgG1 has recently been demonstrated in bovine mammary glands, which preferentially transmits this immunoglobulin unchanged from serum during the colostrum-forming period (Kemler et al. 1975).

Subsequent observations, however, have made it increasingly likely that the epithelial membrane receptor specific for IgA and IgM is identical with SC. We have therefore recently proposed a common glandular transport model for these two immunoglobulins including five critical steps as depicted in Fig. 1: (1) J chains are produced and incorporated into IgA dimers or larger polymers

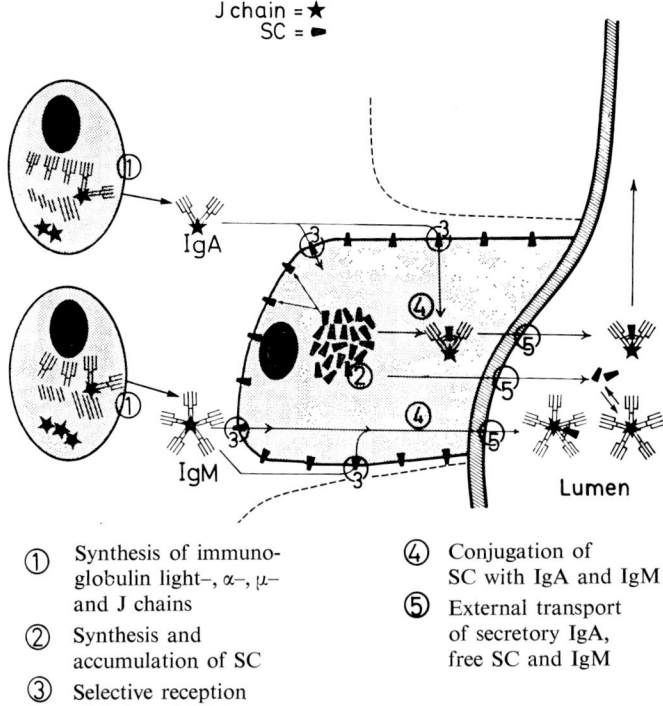

①	Synthesis of immuno-globulin light-, α-, μ- and J chains	④	Conjugation of SC with IgA and IgM
②	Synthesis and accumulation of SC	⑤	External transport of secretory IgA, free SC and IgM
③	Selective reception of IgA and IgM		

FIG. 1. Schematic representation of gland-associated synthesis and selective external transport of dimeric IgA and pentameric IgM. It is proposed that SC acts as a specific receptor for these two immunoglobulins, and that Ig–SC complexes are formed and become mobilized in the plasma membrane of secretory epithelial cells. The completed secretory immunoglobulins finally reach the gland lumen via the cytoplasm outside the Golgi region. While conjugation of IgA with SC is efficient and gives rise to stable complexes, this is so for only 60–70% of the IgM; the rest of the secreted IgM contains SC in an association that is unstable and depends on excess of free SC in the fluid. The five schematic steps are discussed in the text. (Modified from Brandtzaeg 1974d.)

and into IgM pentamers in gland-associated immunocytes; (2) SC is produced by secretory epithelial cells, concentrated in the Golgi zone, and made available for the general secretory process as well as for plasma-membrane incorporation; (3) structural characteristics induced by the J chains in polymeric IgA and pentameric IgM constitute a specific SC-binding site; the polymers will therefore after release from the immunocytes readily become bound to epithelial cells by non-covalent interactions, which apparently depend on the I-determinant-bearing part of the membrane-associated SC (Brandtzaeg 1975a); (4) the Ig–SC complexes are then taken up by the epithelial cell by adsorptive pinocytosis and subjected to stabilizing conjugation by disulphide exchange (enzymically catalysed?); such exchange reactions depend on the immunoglobulin class as well as on an excess of free SC (Brandtzaeg 1974a); (5) finally, the completed secretory polymers are extruded into the gland lumen along general secretory pathways (Kagnoff et al. 1973). The possibility also exists that some of the Ig–SC complexes floating in the cell membrane may reach the gland lumen without entering the cytoplasm.

In man the covalent conjugation of IgA with SC is efficient and gives rise to polymers which are very stable in the exocrine fluids. SC is thus disulphide-bonded in 75–80% of human secretory 11S IgA (Brandtzaeg 1974a), and only about 10% of the IgA dimers separated from human colostrum lack SC (Mestecky et al. 1970). As discussed in the introduction, a permanent association between SC and secretory IgM is more dependent on an excess of free SC (Brandtzaeg 1975c). The ratio of free to bound SC varies in different secretions (Brandtzaeg 1973b) and also depends on the fluid flow rate (Brandtzaeg 1971d). In normal human saliva and colostrum the amount of free SC may approach that of the bound component (Brandtzaeg 1973b). In pig colostrum, on the other hand, there are only traces of free SC and 60% of the dimeric IgA lacks SC after purification (Bourne 1974). A stabilization of Ig–SC complexes, as regularly seen for human secretory IgA, may hence be explained by surplus SC production and unique possibilities for disulphide-exchange reactions. The fact that there is no other known situation where a receptor becomes permanently attached to the transported molecule (Lamm 1976) is therefore no valid argument against a receptor function of SC. The phylogenetic selection of the secretory IgA system may indeed have its basis in the unique stability conferred on dimeric IgA by covalently bound SC (Lindh 1974), since the less stabilized secretory IgM apparently has a shorter functional survival time, at least in the gastrointestinal secretions (Haneberg 1974 a,b).

The proposed model for selective epithelial immunoglobulin reception and transmission is compatible with the fluid mosaic structure suggested for cell membranes (Singer & Nicolson 1972). However, it must be stressed from the outset that our transport model is based mainly on test tube experiments with purified proteins and on the immunofluorescence of dead tissue. Nevertheless, it should be possible in the near future to test several of the proposed steps by kinetic studies on living cells.

IMMUNOCHEMICAL AND PHYSICOCHEMICAL OBSERVATIONS SUPPORTING THE MODEL

1. Quantitation and characterization of human immunoglobulins

The concentration ratio of IgG:IgA in pure glandular secretions, such as

TABLE 1

Average immunoglobulin concentrations (mg/100 ml) in serum and some exocrine secretions

Sample	Immunoglobulin class			Ratio	
	IgG	IgA	IgM	IgG:IgA	IgG:IgM
Serum[a]	1230	328	132	3.8	9.3
Colostrum[a]	10	1234	61	0.008	0.16
Parotid secretion[a]	0.036	3.95	0.043	0.009	0.84
Whole saliva[a]	1.44	19.40	0.20	0.07	6.86
Duodenal secretion[b]	10.4	31.3	20.7	0.33	0.50
Jejunal secretion[c]	34.0	27.6	N.D.[d]	1.23	N.D.
Colonic secretion[c]	86.0	82.7	N.D.	1.04	N.D.

[a] From Brandtzaeg et al. (1970).
[b] From Girard & de Kalbermatten (1970).
[c] From Bull et al. (1971).
[d] N.D., not determined.

colostrum and parotid saliva, is 400–500 times lower than the same ratio in normal serum (Table 1). This suggests that the exocrine glands actively or selectively transmit IgA. The same reasoning applies to the glandular transfer of IgM, although the reduction of the IgG:IgM ratio is less marked (10–60 times) and varies between different secretions (Table 1). Fluids collected from surfaces of mucous membranes contain relatively more IgG, indicating that the external transmission of this immunoglobulin mainly depends on extraglandular passive diffusion. Such 'leakage' is enhanced by inflammatory processes (Brandtzaeg et al. 1970). Comparisons of the parotid transmission of immunoglobulins in patients with G myeloma or macroglobulinaemia have further attested to the selectivity inherent in the glandular transport of IgA and IgM (Brandtzaeg 1971a). Moreover, parotid IgA and IgM show similar secretory dynamics on gustatory stimulation of the gland (Brandtzaeg 1971d).

Since secretory IgM is chiefly a 19S pentamer (Brandtzaeg 1971a, 1975c), its immunoglobulin moiety may be derived from serum. Conversely, the IgA pattern in pure glandular secretions is quite different from that in serum, comprising a major J-chain-containing 11S dimer fraction (Tomasi et al. 1965; Halpern & Koshland 1970), two minor (heavier than 11S) polymer populations, and only 10–13% monomeric 7S IgA (Brandtzaeg et al. 1970). About 80–90% of human serum IgA normally consists of monomers devoid of J chain (see Vaerman 1973); most secretory IgA must therefore originate in gland-associated immunocytes which produce both IgA and J chain (see later section, p. 87).

The predominance of IgA in external secretions could hence depend on preferential local synthesis alone rather than on selective external transmission. Nevertheless, glandular transfer selectivity for IgA and IgM is firmly substantiated by immunohistochemical observations (see later, p. 89). Since pure glandular fluids contain about ten times more monomeric IgA than IgG (Brandtzaeg et al. 1970), transfer selectivity might seem to be more easily explained by an Fc characteristic of IgA and IgM (Brandtzaeg 1968) than by a J-chain-induced SC-binding site (Fig. 1, p. 79). However, a relative enrichment of 7S IgA compared with IgG may well be accounted for by a combination of passive external transmission and degradation. Intercellular diffusion through the epithelium probably includes monomeric IgA derived both from serum and from the abundant local IgA-producing immunocytes, which release a mixture of monomers and dimers (see later, p. 87). As discussed above for IgM, dimers of IgA are probably unstable before covalent conjugation with SC, and may in part be converted to monomers by intraepithelial and intraluminal degradation. Some breakdown of SC-conjugated dimers is also likely, and may explain why a fraction of the monomeric IgA present in colostrum is apparently associated with SC (Mestecky et al. 1970).

A preferential glandular transfer of IgA dimers compared with monomers is supported by analyses of monoclonal IgA components appearing in the saliva of patients with multiple myeloma (Coelho et al. 1974), and intravenously injected monomeric IgA does not seem to be selectively secreted (for review, see Heremans 1974; Lamm 1976). One possible exception was reported after the infusion of large quantities of plasma into two hypogammaglobulinaemic patients (South et al. 1966). However, it could not be excluded that the traces of IgA transmitted to the saliva were polymers.

A varying fraction (10–20%) of IgA in normal serum is composed of dimers and larger polymers (see Vaerman 1973). This fraction is small in view of the abundant polymer-producing IgA cells found in bone marrow (Rádl et al. 1974) and especially in the digestive tract (Brandtzaeg 1973a, 1974c). The fraction of polymeric IgA in lymph from the thoracic duct is not significantly raised (Tomasi & Grey 1972), perhaps because locally produced IgA polymers are rapidly transmitted to the gut lumen. Moreover, Rádl et al. (1975) showed that most IgA polymers present in normal human serum lack the J chain. Since there is a dynamic equilibrium between proteins in serum and interstitial fluid, this observation supports the idea that an efficient clearing mechanism selective for J-chain-containing IgA operates in glandular regions. Only about 20% of serum IgM (molecular weight about 1 000 000) is distributed extravascularly (Waldmann & Strober 1969); a J-chain-dependent clearing mechanism would therefore *a priori* be less efficient for IgM than for serum-derived dimeric IgA (molecular weight about 320 000). It should also be considered that the two molecular species are competing for the same epithelial receptor if this indeed is SC. The proposed transport model could easily explain the lack of external transmission of intravenously injected secretory 11S IgA (Stiehm *et al.* 1966; Butler *et al.* 1967) since the SC-binding site of these polymers is occupied.

2. *In vitro combination of SC with IgA and IgM*

The discovery of SC as a regular subunit of human secretory IgA (Tomasi *et al.* 1965) stimulated a series of attempts to show specific affinity between SC and IgA. Tomasi & Bienenstock (1968) first reported that reduced and alkylated SC added to whole serum combined fairly specifically with IgA. Hanson *et al.* (1969) mixed native free SC with purified IgA and obtained a low yield of poorly stabilized complexes. We likewise found that the affinity of native free SC was relatively specific for serum IgA, although there was some evidence of SC-IgM association (Brandtzaeg 1971*c*). Thompson (1970) had previously reported that small amounts of SC-IgM complexes might occur in sera of IgA-deficient individuals, and also found that IgM in the duodenal juice of one such patient to some extent was associated with SC.

The first indication that a particular conformation is necessary for an efficient binding of free SC came from studies of rabbit secretory IgA; when the polymer had been separated from its bound SC it became highly active in recombination with free SC (Lawton *et al.* 1970*b*; O'Daly & Cebra 1971). Mach (1970) and Rádl *et al.* (1971) independently demonstrated the importance of the IgA-dimer conformation by studying the combination between human myeloma proteins and free SC isolated from colostrum. Complexing with IgM was also noted in these studies, but only polymers larger than 19S pentamers seemed to be active (Rádl *et al.* 1971). In a subsequent study we were unable to confirm the latter finding (Brandtzaeg 1974*a*). By contrast, we showed that SC is able to combine with 19S IgM as readily as with dimeric IgA (Fig. 2*a,c*), and that specific complex formation depends on non-covalent interactions (Brandtzaeg 1974 *a,b*). This would be a prerequisite for a receptor function of membrane-associated SC. Our observations have been verified by Weicker & Underdown (1975).

When Mach published his results in 1970 the J chain had just been detected in polymeric IgA and IgM (for review, see Inman & Mestecky 1974; Koshland 1975); in an addendum to his paper he therefore postulated a role for this polypeptide in the SC-binding process. We obtained the first evidence to

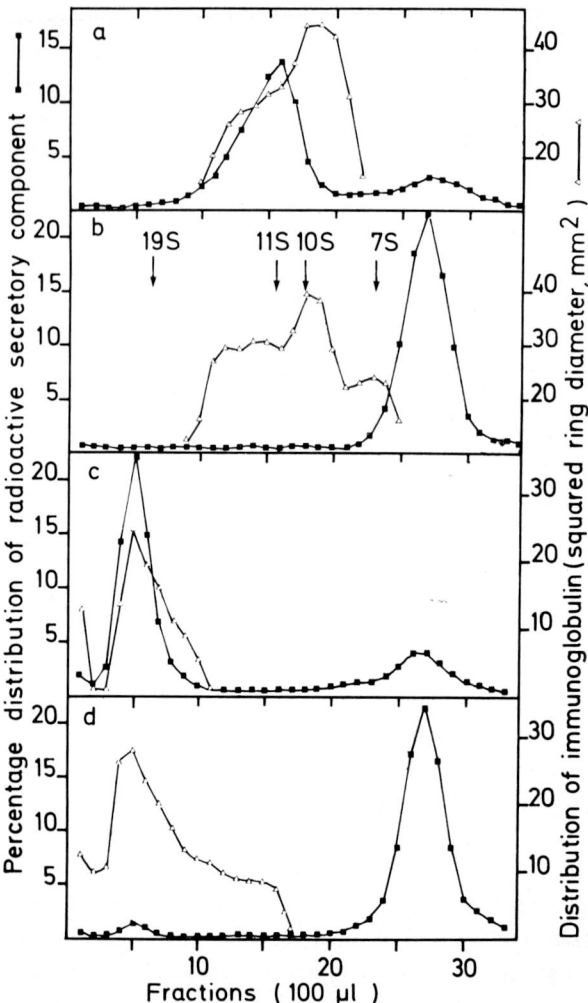

FIG. 2. Ultracentrifugation analyses (42 000 r.p.m., 20 h, 10–35% linear sucrose gradients) of immunoglobulin polymers after incubation with radioactive SC (2.5 μg). The immunoglobulin distribution was determined by testing each fraction in single radial immunodiffusion; SC distribution was shown by scintillation counting. Bottom of gradients is to the left. The positions of four marker proteins are indicated (vertical arrows) as reference for S values. Samples: (a) 100 μg of J-chain-containing polyclonal IgA polymers (mainly 10S dimers); (b) 100 μg of J-chain-deficient monoclonal IgA polymers; (c) 50 μg of J-chain-containing monoclonal IgM 19S pentamers; and (d) 110 μg of J-chain-deficient monoclonal IgM polymers.

support such a function of the J chain when we found that an IgM polymer lacking it failed to bind SC *in vitro* (Eskeland & Brandtzaeg 1974). In a subsequent study we quantified immunochemically the reductive release of J chain in twenty-four IgA preparations (Brandtzaeg 1976b). Five polymeric fractions that contained only 0.2–0.8 mg J chain per 100 mg protein showed an SC-binding capacity of 6–12% compared with 69–82% for polymers containing more than 4.0 mg J chain per 100 mg (Fig. 2). Monomeric IgA without contaminating J-chain-positive polymers did not bind SC. The report of Jerry *et al.* (1972) has caused some confusion in this respect. They found that in the presence of a large excess of SC obtained from reduced secretory IgA, covalent complexing took place with monomeric IgA of the subclass α_2 and genetic variant Am_2 (+). These findings must be clearly distinguished from our results which are based on non-covalent interactions with small amounts of native free SC.

We have thus demonstrated that the J chain is mandatory for a spontaneous association of SC with IgA and IgM, but the mechanism of its function in this binding process is still unknown. One possibility is that the SC-binding site is located in the Fc region of the Ig polymers, the conformation of which may depend on J-chain incorporation. Direct non-covalent interactions between SC and the J chains may be another explanation, although the purified polypeptide only marginally blocks the binding of SC to dimeric IgA and 19S IgM (Brandtzaeg 1975d). Antibody to J chain, on the other hand, efficiently blocks the SC-binding site of these polymers (Brandtzaeg 1975d). Such experiments are difficult to interpret, but the results are compatible with the hypothesis that polymer-incorporated J chains have acquired a configuration conducive to specific interactions with SC.

Contrary to the present view (see Koshland 1975), our recent studies of human J chain have indicated that it occurs as a dimer in IgA and as a trimer or two dimers in IgM (Brandtzaeg 1975b). IgM should hence show stronger SC affinity than IgA if this property is determined by the J chain. Indeed, the binding of SC to IgM is less inhibited by high salt concentrations (Brandtzaeg 1974a), and on a molar basis pentameric IgM has five to thirty times better affinity for SC than dimeric or trimeric IgA in competitive tests (P. Brandtzaeg, unpublished data). It is tempting to speculate that these observations reflect the 'bonus effect' of a higher molar J-chain content in IgM. Thus, if our glandular transport model is correct, the relative amount of bound J chain may have biological consequences by enhancing the epithelial reception and transmission of IgM, whose local synthesis normally is inferior to that of dimeric IgA (see below, p. 86).

IMMUNOHISTOCHEMICAL OBSERVATIONS SUPPORTING THE MODEL

1. Characterization of intestinal immunocyte populations

The reliability of immunohistochemical observations depends on the quality of the fluorochrome conjugates as well as on the tissue-processing technique (for review, see Brandtzaeg & Baklien 1976). Our aim is complete retention of diffusible immunoglobulins in one piece of the biopsy specimen (see Fig. 11 *a-c*, p. 100) and extensive removal of these components from another with preservation of immunocytes and facilitated characterization of their cytoplasmic content (see Fig. 11*e-h*, p. 100). The former piece is fixed directly in cold alcohol, whereas the latter is first extracted by washing in isotonic buffered saline (Brandtzaeg 1974*d*).

TABLE 2

Immunoglobulin-containing cells in normal adult intestinal mucosa

	Cell numbers expressed as mean, observed range, and average % contribution		
	IgA cells	IgM cells	IgG cells
Jejunum	104(60-163) 81%	21(8-36) 17%	3.2(1-8) 2.6%
Ileum	37(21-61) 83%	5(1.5-10) 11%	2.5(0.3-6) 5%
Large bowel	129(28-237) 90%	8(1-27) 6%	6(2-14) 4.2%

Table modified from Brandtzaeg & Baklien (1976). Data based on a 'mucosal tissue unit' constituting a 6-μm-thick and 500-μm-wide block of tissue including the mucosa at full height from the muscularis mucosae.

A marked preponderance of IgA-producing cells is found at all levels of the human intestinal tract (Table 2). We have calculated that almost 10^{10} such immunocytes normally occur per metre of small bowel. The share of IgM-producing cells varies between 6% and 17%, being highest proximally, and IgG cells are normally even fewer. The immunocytes are not homogeneously distributed throughout the various mucosal layers. In the normal large bowel about 60% occur in the luminal 200-μm zone, with decreasing numbers towards the muscularis mucosae. In the small bowel about 70% occur in the 200-μm zone around the base of the villi. Marked alterations are seen associated with bowel disease. Thus, in coeliac disease an increase takes place for all immunocyte classes, in relative terms most prominent for IgG and IgM cells.

In ulcerative colitis and Crohn's disease the IgG cell response is very dramatic (for review, see Brandtzaeg & Baklien 1976).

Gland-associated IgA immunocytes were initially thought to produce monomers which subsequently polymerized by complexing with SC (Fig. 10a,b, p. 97). Random combination of the polymer subunits was supported by the apparent occurrence in human colostrum of hybrid 11S IgA isoagglutinins containing both κ and λ light chains (Costea et al. 1968). But molecules hybrid with regard to allotypic markers could not be detected in rabbit colostral 11S IgA (Lawton & Mage 1969). Also, studies of suspended rabbit appendix immunocytes indicated a direct release of dimeric IgA (Cohen & Kern 1969). Our finding of J chains with partially buried antigenic determinants in human intestinal IgA cells is likewise indicative of dimer production (Brandtzaeg 1976a). Moreover, SC-affinity tests on tissue sections (Brandtzaeg 1973a) show that the J-chain-containing IgA and IgM immunocytes (Fig. 3) can bind SC to their cytoplasm *in vitro* (Brandtzaeg 1974c). This non-covalent affinity characteristic (Brandtzaeg 1974a) demonstrates that the polymer subunits to a substantial extent are 'correctly' aligned already at the cytoplasmic level. Thus, when these immunoglobulins are released into the extracellular fluid, they are readily available for spontaneous complexing with membrane-associated SC of columnar epithelial cells.

The intestinal IgA immunocytes are heterogeneous with regard to cytoplasmic SC affinity (Brandtzaeg 1973a) and J-chain content (Fig. 3a-c). This indicates that the cells produce varying proportions of monomers and polymers. According to our glandular transport model most of the monomers should be drained away by the vessels and thus contribute to the pool of serum IgA.

Very little conclusive information is available about the origin of the intestinal immunocytes, but they apparently develop from blast cells seeded into the mucosa (for review, see Brandtzaeg & Baklien 1976; Lamm 1976). Most of these blasts probably express J-chain synthesis, since this seems to be turned on early in the immune response (Brandtzaeg & Berdal 1975; Brandtzaeg 1976a). We have therefore proposed that circulating J-chain-containing blasts regardless of immunoglobulin class may contribute to the predominant gland-associated population of dimer-producing IgA immunocytes (Fig. 4). In individuals with selective IgA deficiency there is a block in the final B cell differentiation; according to the maturation scheme (Fig. 4), IgM- and IgG-producing cells should then accumulate adjacent to the glands, which agrees with immunohistochemical observations (Brandtzaeg et al. 1968; Savilahti 1973).

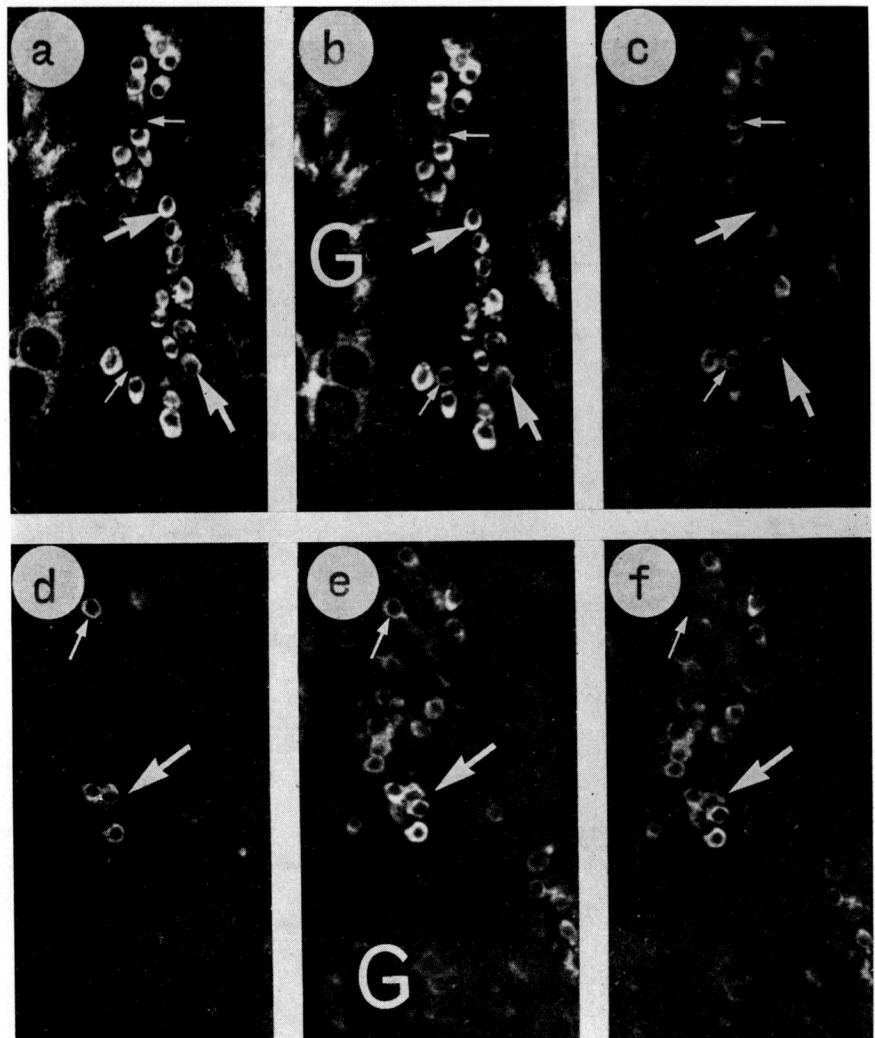

FIG. 3. Immunohistochemical demonstration of J chain in human intestinal IgA and IgM immunocytes. Sections of a saline-extracted specimen of normal rectal mucosa were preincubated for 60 min in 6M-urea, pH 3.2, to expose concealed J-chain determinants.
(*a-c*) Double tracing of 'green' IgA and 'red' J chain shown by selective filtration of green (*a*) and red (*c*) fluorescence and double exposure (*b*) in the same field. Most IgA immunocytes are J-chain-positive, although of varying intensity; a few are negative (*large arrows*). Two J-chain-positive cells are of another immunoglobulin class (*small arrows*).
(*d-f*) Double tracing of 'green' IgM and 'red' J chain shown by selective filtration of green (*d*) and red (*f*) fluorescence and double exposure (*e*) in the same field. Three IgM immunocytes are J-chain-positive (*large arrow*), whereas one is negative (*small arrow*). Some J chain is revealed in the gland cells (*G*). Magnification: × 340.

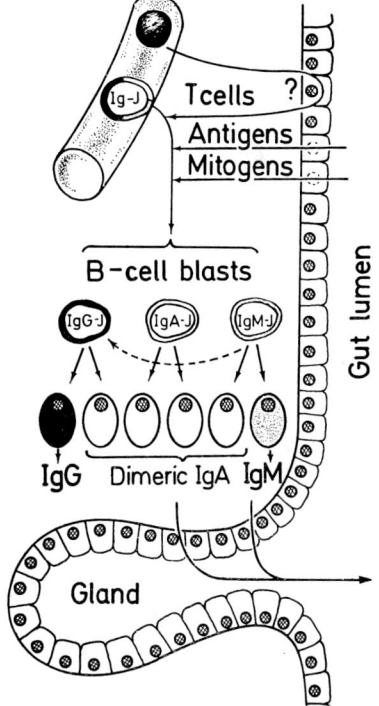

FIG. 4. Hypothetical scheme for the maintenance of a normal gland-associated immunocyte population. Circulating J-chain-positive B cell blasts of IgG, IgA, or IgM class become continuously seeded into the lamina propria, where further clonal differentiation is induced by a 'second signal' mediated by helper T cells or directly by antigens or mitogens. During this differentiation most cells end up as IgA dimer producers due to switching of class expression in the precursors. The direction of differentiation may be from IgM to IgG to IgA or directly from IgM to IgA. If an insufficient amount of J chain is synthesized by mature IgA cells, a mixture of dimeric and monomeric IgA will be produced (not indicated in figure). Monomeric IgA will, like IgG, not be transported externally by gland cells. (From Brandtzaeg & Baklien 1976.)

2. Interstitial and epithelial distribution of immunoglobulins and SC

In sections of directly fixed mucosal specimens the connective tissue ground substance exhibits diffuse fluorescence for IgG, particularly intense in the basement membrane zones along epithelia and vessel walls (Figs. 5a and 6a). The epithelium is virtually devoid of cytoplasmic IgG, but there may be an irregular faint fluorescence related to interstices in the glands and especially in the epithelium facing the gut lumen, indicating intercellular diffusion. Some IgG is also occasionally seen in goblet cells (Fig. 6a). An influence of the biopsy procedure on the epithelial IgG distribution cannot be excluded.

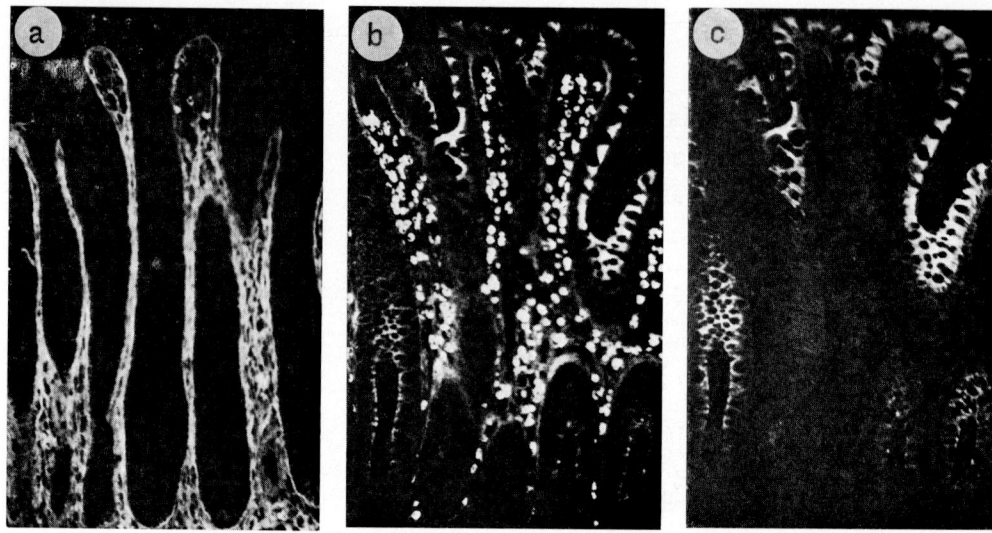

FIG. 5. Immunohistochemical localization of immunoglobulins and SC in normal rectal mucosa fixed directly in alcohol to retain diffusible protein components. Comparable fields shown after single tracing of 'red' IgG in one section (a) and double tracing of 'red' IgA (b) and 'green' SC (c) in the adjacent section. Note that IgG predominates in connective tissue ground substance and basement membranes but is hardly detectable in epithelium. IgA is located in numerous immunocytes, but only small amounts are seen extracellularly in this specimen. In the epithelium IgA is especially prominent apically in the columnar cells of the crypts, whereas little is present in surface epithelium (at the top). SC shows an overall distribution in epithelium similar to that of IgA. Magnification: × 100.

In most normal specimens the lamina propria contains much less extracellular IgA than IgG, despite extensive local synthesis of the former (Fig. 5b). This is compatible with an efficient external transport of the locally produced dimeric IgA. However, in connection with an intensified mucosal immune response, the specific background staining is very bright and obscures many of the IgA immunocytes (Figs. 6c and 11c). The crypt epithelium shows staining for IgA in the cytoplasm and in relation to interstices. The intracellular fluorescence is bright in the apical part of the columnar cells near the crypt openings, especially in the large bowel. Much less IgA is present in the surface epithelium (Fig. 5b) and hardly any occurs in the epithelium covering the villi of the small intestine (Fig. 6c).

The ground substance shows relatively little IgM staining, except for basement membrane zones and vessel walls. The epithelial distribution mimics that of IgA, but the fluorescence intensity is normally weaker (Fig. 6b). IgM is most readily demonstrated in colonic and rectal glands (Fig. 7b), as noted before

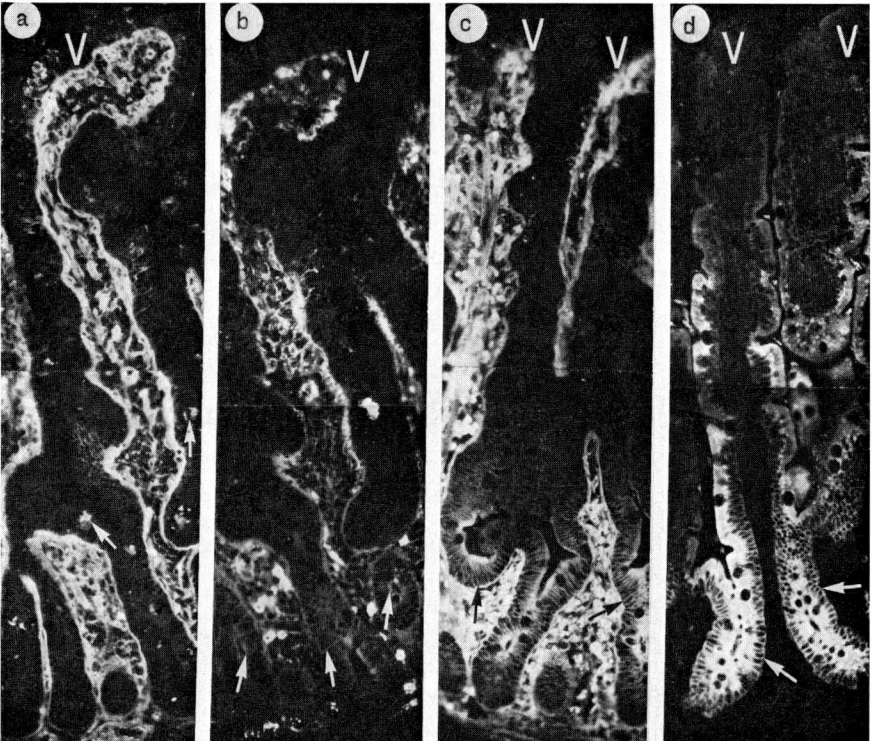

FIG. 6. Immunohistochemical localization of immunoglobulins and SC in morphologically normal duodenal mucosa from a patient with *Giardia lamblia* infestation. The specimen was fixed directly in alcohol to retain diffusible proteins. Single tracing with rhodamine conjugates in four serial sections: (a) IgG; (b) IgM; (c) IgA; and (d) SC. Lamina propria is rich in extracellular IgG, but also contains unusually large amounts of extracellular IgA, probably because of extensive local production by numerous IgA immunocytes which are difficult to discern against the bright background. Smaller amounts of extracellular IgM are present and some IgM immunocytes can be seen. Columnar crypt cells contain cytoplasmic SC and there is also distinct staining related to their basal and lateral borders (*arrows* in d). The SC concentration is gradually diminished in epithelium covering the villi (V). Mucinous content of goblet cells is unstained. Epithelial distribution of IgA parallels that of SC with distinct staining related to lateral borders of crypt cells (*arrows* in c) as well as apically in their cytoplasm. Similar but much weaker epithelial staining is seen for IgM (*arrows* in b). Cytoplasmic IgG fluorescence is absent from columnar crypt cells, but some striated staining is seen related to epithelial interstices. Some goblet cells contain IgG (*arrows* in a). Magnification: × 50.

in normal (Chen 1971) and especially in IgA-deficient individuals with enhanced local synthesis of IgM (Heremans & Crabbé 1967; Savilahti 1973). Paired staining with contrasting colours reveals no difference in the epithelial distribution of IgA and IgM in colonic glands (Brandtzaeg 1975c).

There is reason to believe that most of the 'intercellular' staining for IgA and IgM in crypt epithelium may be interpreted as cell-membrane fluorescence. Firstly, if passive diffusion from the lamina propria was the only explanation, the concentration of IgG between the epithelial cells should greatly exceed that of IgA and especially that of IgM. A possible molecular filtration in the basement membrane should moreover favour IgG. Secondly, all epithelial IgG can be removed by washing the tissue specimens, whereas IgA and IgM may still be found related to the borders of epithelial cells (Fig. 11*e-h*, p. 100). This indicates that IgA and IgM are adsorbed to the cell membranes, as proposed before (Brandtzaeg 1974*e*). The presence of IgA in crypt cell membranes has likewise been suggested at the ultrastructural level (Brown *et al.* 1975).

Many conflicting reports have appeared about the cellular origin of SC. Rossen *et al.* (1968) proposed that it is a plasma cell product, and Tourville *et al.* (1969) claimed that the goblet cell is the major intestinal source of SC. Other workers have refuted these findings (Munster 1972; Søltoft & Söeberg 1972; Poger & Lamm 1974). Our studies (Brandtzaeg 1973*b*, 1974*d*) have demonstrated SC in the columnar crypt cells of the large bowel and generally also in the surface lining cells (Fig. 5*c*). In the small bowel it is present in the columnar cells of the glands, decreasing in concentration in the epithelium covering the villi and rarely reaching their tips (Fig. 6*d*). Regardless of the tissue-processing technique, we have been unable to demonstrate SC associated with the mucinous content of goblet cells. At the ultrastructural level SC has been detected on the lateral membranes of both goblet and columnar crypt cells (Brown *et al.* 1975). Poger & Lamm (1974) failed to demonstrate SC corresponding to cell membranes by immunofluorescence, but we see specific staining related to the intercellular and basal borders of glandular cells, especially with highly sensitive rhodamine conjugates (Figs. 6*d* and 7*d*). This

Fig. 7. Immunohistochemical localization of immunoglobulins and SC in a directly alcohol-fixed autopsy specimen from the colon of a 32-week-old boy with intractable diarrhoea and marasmus. There was a maturation defect in his B cell system until the age of 5 months, when marked synthesis of IgM and IgG began. From that age immunocytes appeared in his bowel mucosa with a predominance of IgM-producing cells. Single tracing with rhodamine conjugates is shown in serial sections: (*a*) IgG; (*b*) IgM (corresponding fields); (*c*) IgA; and (*d*) SC (corresponding fields). Lamina propria contains large amounts of extracellular IgG and IgM, whereas IgA is localized to immunocytes. In the crypt epithelium IgM is located in the cytoplasm of columnar cells and along their lateral borders (*arrows* in *b*). Some striated staining is seen for IgG. IgA is present only in crypt cells situated adjacent to small groups of IgA immunocytes. SC is ubiquitously present in the cytoplasm of columnar epithelial cells and along their lateral and basal borders (*small arrows* in *d*). *Large arrows* point to similar locations in (*c*) and (*d*). Magnification: × 90.

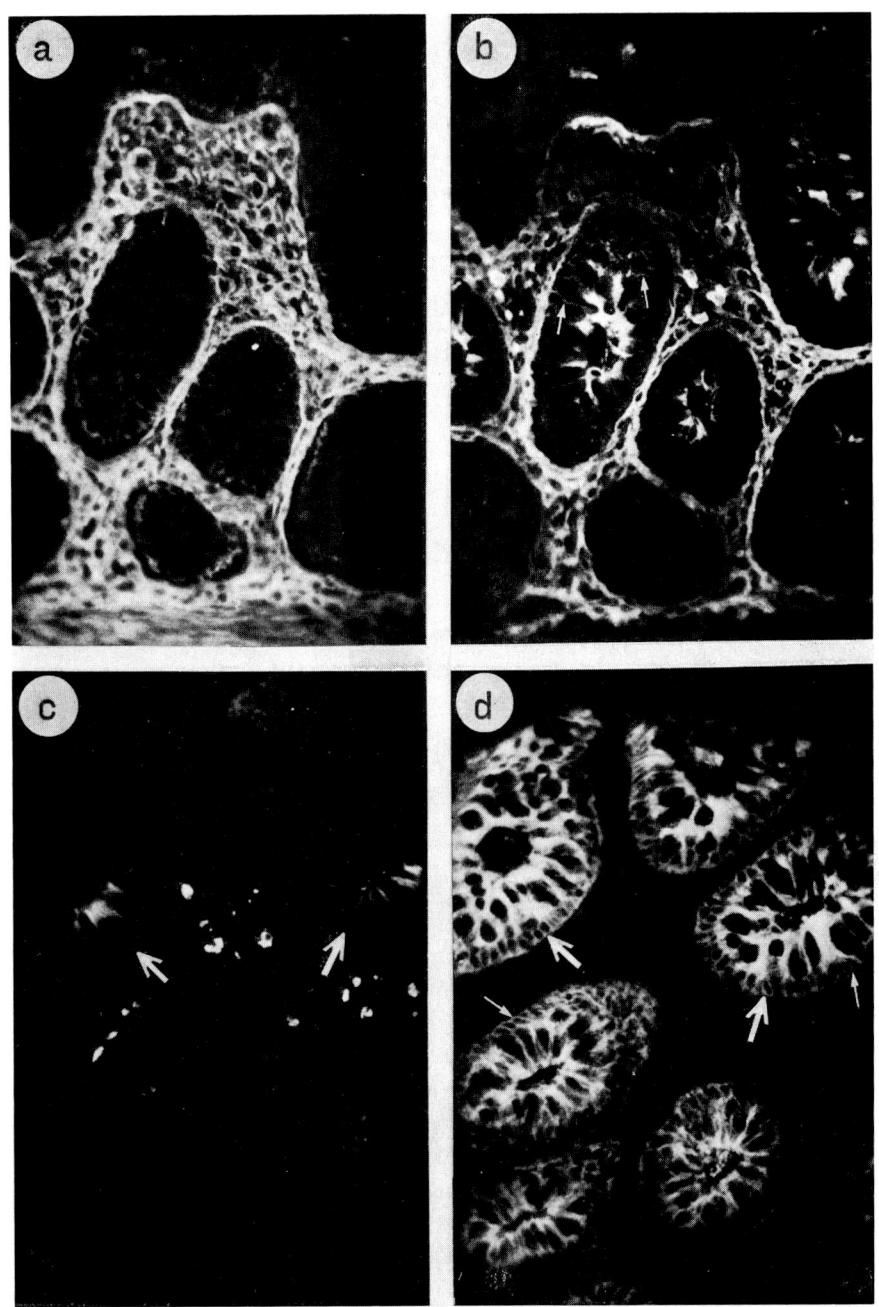

Fig. 7

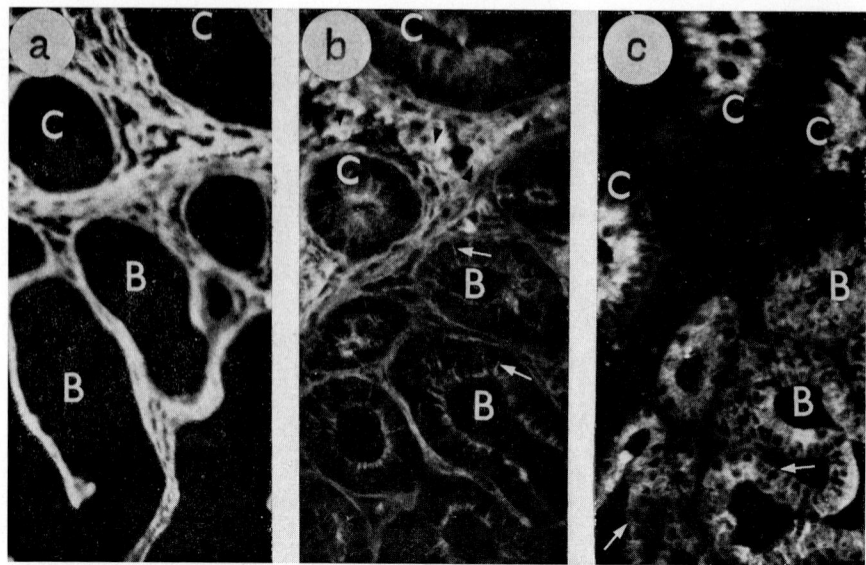

FIG. 8. Immunohistochemical localization of immunoglobulins and SC in a directly alcohol-fixed specimen of duodenal mucosa from an adult with coeliac disease. The bottom of two or three crypts (C) and some Brunner's glands (B) are shown. Single tracing with rhodamine conjugates in serial sections: (a) IgG; (b) IgA; and (c) SC. Note differences between crypts and tubules of Brunner's glands with regard to IgA and SC distribution. Distinct localization of IgA and SC is seen related to the borders of tubule cells (*arrows* in *b* and *c*), whereas IgA in apical cytoplasm and accumulations of SC in Golgi zone are typical for columnar crypt cells. Stroma of Brunner's glands contains IgA, but there are no IgA immunocytes, in contrast to the mucosal lamina propria which is crowded by such cells (*arrowheads* in *b*). Note abundance of IgG in connective tissue, but absence of IgG staining in epithelium (*a*). Magnification: × 200.

feature may well represent membrane-associated SC. Indeed, Huang et al. (1976) recently succeeded in establishing long-term cultures of colon carcinoma cells bearing SC which regenerated after removal by trypsinization. These findings lend strong support to the proposed receptor function of SC.

The congruent distribution of SC, IgA and IgM in epithelium showing immunoglobulin transport further suggests that SC is involved in this process (Figs. 5b,c and 6b-d). When the local synthesis of IgA is limited to a few immunocytes, the immunohistochemical appearance indicates that IgA passes directly into the adjacent SC-containing epithelial cells (Fig. 7c). O'Daly et al. (1971) made similar observations in rabbits, using allotypic markers to trace the local immunoglobulin products after B cell transfer experiments. Conversely, when there is a pronounced IgA synthesis in the gut the immunoglobulin may apparently diffuse over a considerable distance before it is taken up by the epithelial cells. This is exemplified in Fig. 8, which shows unusually prominent IgA transport by a group of SC-producing Brunner's glands devoid of IgA immunocytes. However, the interstitial fluid surrounding the tubules contains appreciable amounts of IgA, probably derived from the mucosal lamina propria which in this patient with coeliac disease is very rich in IgA-producing cells.

Compared with the crypt epithelium, the staining for SC and IgA is intense in relation to the borders of the epithelial cells in these Brunner's glands (Fig. 8b,c). This may indicate that relatively more SC–IgA complexes accumulate in the gland cell membranes and perhaps reach the lumen without entering the cytoplasm, as has previously been suggested for respiratory and salivary glands (Brandtzaeg 1974e). That the striated staining does not represent intercellular IgA is indicated by the lack of IgG in the epithelial interstices of the tubules (Fig. 8a).

Although the epithelial distributions of SC and IgA are in general very similar, the detailed staining patterns of crypts revealed by double tracing are not completely congruent (Brandtzaeg 1974d,e). A common feature is the fluorescence apparently related to the cell membranes, as discussed above. Intracellularly, both SC and IgA are present in the apical portion of the cytoplasm, but SC alone is distinctly concentrated in a granular pattern corresponding to the Golgi zone (Fig. 9). Ultrastructural studies of rabbit mammary glands lend support to these observations, since SC but no IgA could be found in the Golgi elements of the epithelial cells, whereas both components were present in more apically located vesicles (Kraehenbuhl *et al.* 1975). Moreover, the antigenic properties of SC present in human colonic crypt cells indicate that it exists in a free form in the Golgi zone and in a bound form apically in the cytoplasm (Brandtzaeg 1974e; Poger & Lamm 1974).

OTHER PROPOSED MODELS FOR THE GLANDULAR TRANSPORT OF IgA

There is now general agreement that secretory IgA represents the synthetic product of two cell types. Since free SC is concentrated in the Golgi zone of serous secretory epithelial cells (Fig. 9), it seems unquestionable that it is produced by these cells. The synthesis of SC may be regarded as independent of IgA and IgM because it appears to be normal in hypogammaglobulinaemic individuals (see Brandtzaeg & Baklien 1976) and occurs in the fetus before the initiation of immunoglobulin production (Ogra *et al.* 1972). However, there may be as yet undefined interrelations between SC and immunocytes. Thus, Hassall's corpuscles synthesize SC (Tomasi & Yurchak 1972) and the maturation of IgA-producing cells is clearly thymus-dependent (for review, see Lamm

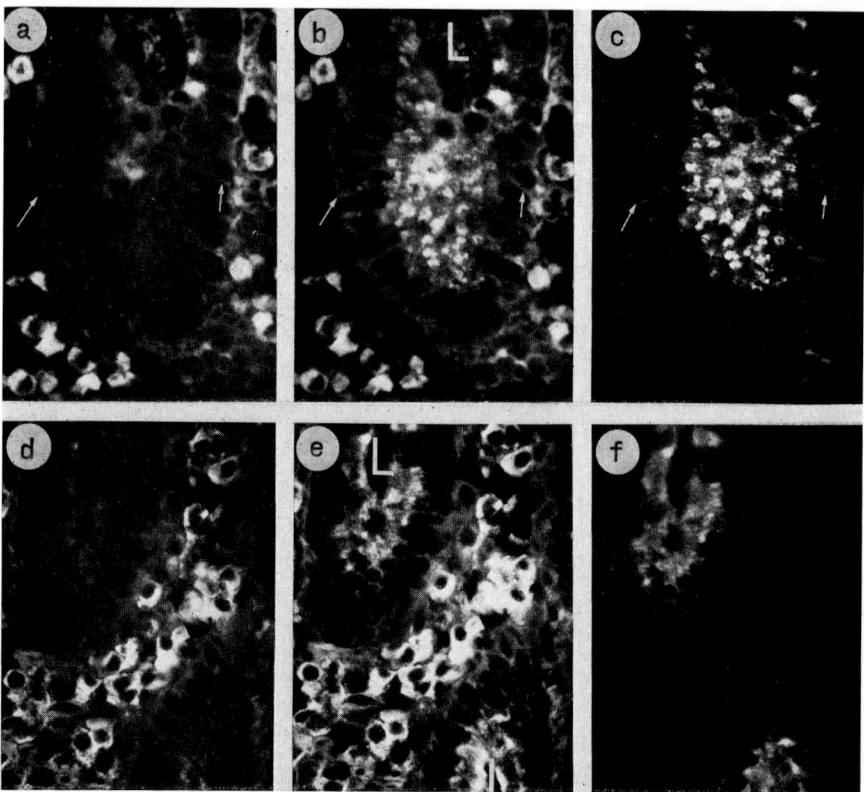

Fig. 9. Double tracing of IgA and SC in directly alcohol-fixed intestinal specimens: (*a-c*) Oblique section through crypt in colon mucosa from a patient with ulcerative colitis. (*d-e*) Section through two hypertrophied crypts in duodenal mucosa from an adult with coeliac disease. (*a*) Selective red filtration for IgA; (*c*) selective green filtration for SC; and (*b*) double exposure in same field. Many columnar cells in the colon crypt have been cut through the Golgi zone where granular accumulations of SC (*c*) and absence of IgA (*a*) are distinctly shown. Both IgA and SC occur in the apical part of the cytoplasm close to the lumen (*L*) of the gland, and also related to lateral and basal borders of columnar cells (*arrows*). Mucinous content of goblet cells is unstained. (*d*) Selective green filtration for IgA; (*f*) selective red filtration for SC; and (*e*) double exposure in same field. The duodenal specimen contains numerous IgA immunocytes and considerable amounts of extracellular IgA in lamina propria. Epithelial distribution of SC and IgA is similar to that seen in the colon crypt, but SC is not so distinctly concentrated in the Golgi zone. Magnification: × 510.

1976). Lawton *et al.* (1970*a*) obtained some evidence from tissue culture experiments with rabbit mammary glands of an influence of IgA on the synthesis of SC. Moreover, it is claimed that some unidentified cells in lymphoid organs such as bone marrow, spleen and lymph nodes are able to produce SC (Lai A Fat *et al.* 1974).

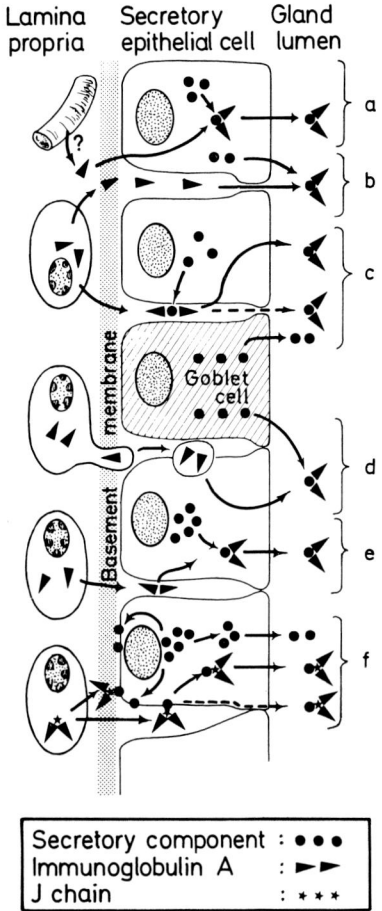

FIG. 10. Schematic representation of glandular transport of secretory IgA as proposed by various research groups. The six models depicted are discussed in the text.

In the first model proposed for the glandular secretion of IgA (Tomasi *et al.* 1965; South *et al.* 1966) it was envisioned that the SC-producing epithelial cell mediated the immunoglobulin transport, and that the union of two IgA monomers took place by intracellular complexing with SC (Fig. 10*a*). The IgA monomers were thought to be produced by local plasma cells, but a contribution from serum was not excluded. It was not clear whether the epithelial transport was active, or whether it depended on high concentrations of locally formed IgA. This model was recently supported by Shiner & Ballard (1973) using commercial immunofluorescent antibodies to 7S IgA, 11S IgA and

SC. However, their results are questionable since the reagents obviously did not discriminate between monomeric and dimeric IgA, nor between free and bound SC.

Heremans & Crabbé (1967) challenged the view that IgA follows an intracellular route through the epithelium. They felt that the apical IgA fluorescence seen in intestinal glands should be ascribed to adsorbed mucus rather than to cytoplasmic IgA. On the other hand, they stressed the localization of IgA in epithelial interstices and proposed that most intestinal IgA diffuses between the epithelial cells into the gut lumen where complexing with SC takes place (Fig. 10b).

A direct passage of IgA into the lumen would be restricted by the apical tight junctions between the epithelial cells. Tomasi and co-workers (Tourville et al. 1969; Tourville & Tomasi 1969; Franklin et al. 1973) have therefore maintained the view that IgA combines with SC in the epithelial interstices; most of the complexes then enter the glandular cell and are subsequently extruded into the lumen (Fig. 10c). This model raises many questions. Why should the basement membrane selectively allow IgA (and IgM) to diffuse into the epithelial interstices? Why is SC usually undetectable in sera of hypogammaglobulinaemic individuals (Brandtzaeg 1971b) if it is regularly secreted into the intercellular spaces? Why do the secretory IgA molecules go into the epithelial cell? These authors (Tourville et al. 1969; Tourville & Tomasi 1969) have moreover claimed that the mucous-type glandular cell is especially active in the production of SC, but it is not clear how this fits into their transport model.

Allen et al. (1973) tried to follow the intestinal secretion of IgA in pigs at the ultrastructural level. They suggested that pseudopodia from plasma cells adjacent to the glands are sloughed off as vesicles which cross the basement membrane into the epithelial interstices and thereafter enter the columnar cells (Fig. 10d). In this way IgA could be protected during the entire external transfer. After release into the gut lumen IgA combines with SC, which also according to the latter authors is derived mainly from goblet cells. The ultrastructural localization of IgA and SC in human intestinal epithelium does not agree with these findings (Brown et al. 1975), and the proposed model cannot explain the transport of IgA by glands lying at a considerable distance from the IgA-producing cells (Fig. 8, p. 94).

The recent immunohistochemical study of Poger & Lamm (1974) agrees to some extent with our findings. Firstly, the serous secretory epithelial cell is identified as the major source of SC. Secondly, when IgA is transported through this cell, free SC is present in the Golgi zone, whereas the bound component occurs in the apical part of the cytoplasm. Since no indication of membrane-associated SC was obtained, their observations were interpreted (Lamm 1976) to suggest that the assembly of secretory IgA takes place inside the epithelial cell after the fusion of pinocytotic and SC-containing Golgi vesicles (Fig. 10e).

If the epithelial uptake of IgA occurred as a 'fluid' or 'bulk' pinocytosis, the latter model would not easily explain the selectivity in the transport. One possibility mentioned by Lamm (1976) is that SC protects IgA against degradation by intracellular enzymes, whereas IgG and other proteins included in the pinocytotic vesicle are degraded. Even fragments of IgG should retain some antigenicity, however, and the complete lack of cytoplasmic IgG staining in glandular epithelia (see previous section, p. 89) speaks against an entry of this protein into intact secretory cells. Thus, a selection of IgA most likely takes place at the epithelial cell membrane by means of a receptor. According to our transport model this receptor is specific for J-chain-containing IgA and IgM (Fig. 1, p. 79). Receptor–substrate complexes formed on the cell surface are either taken up by adsorptive pinocytosis or may float in the membrane and reach the gland lumen without entering the cytoplasm (broken arrow in Fig. 10f). Which route is preferred may depend on the cellular distribution of SC, which apparently varies among different glands (Fig. 8). Although there is no formal proof demonstrating the identity of the epithelial receptor with SC, circumstantial evidence is accumulating to support our view. Heremans (1974) in his recent review also favoured a similar model for the transport of IgA.

Some authors argue against a participation of SC in glandular immunoglobulin transport (Weicker & Underdown 1975) by referring to the lack of *in vivo* (Newcomb & Ishizaka 1970) and *in vitro* association between SC and IgE (P. Brandtzaeg, unpublished data). This argument is not valid, however, since the previous assumption of selectivity in the secretion of IgE comparable to that of IgA does not hold true (Nakajima *et al.* 1975); a relative enrichment of IgE in some exocrine fluids compared with serum apparently depends on local synthesis combined with passive diffusion through epithelial interstices. The function of SC has further been confused by the recent suggestion that it may act as a γ-glutamyltransferase; a possible involvement of this enzyme activity in the glandular transport or function of secretory IgA has been discussed (Binkley & Wiesemann 1975). However, we have distinctly separated the γ-glutamyltransferase activity of colostrum from SC and secretory IgA (P. Brandtzaeg & A. Winsnes, unpublished data). In our opinion, therefore, the only established activity of SC is to complex spontaneously with J-chain-containing IgA and IgM by specific non-covalent interactions. This property is certainly compatible with its proposed receptor function.

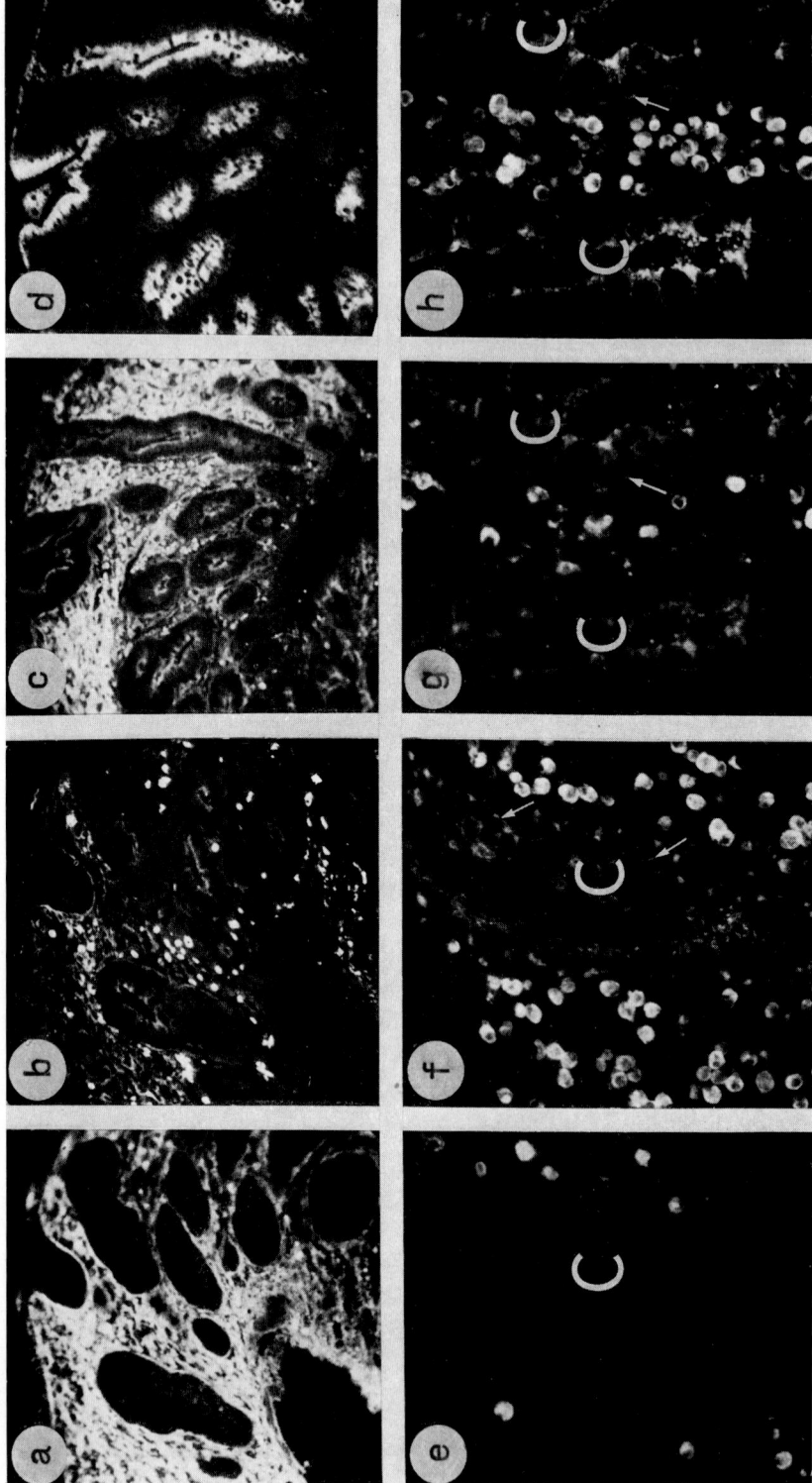

Fig. 11

GLANDULAR IMMUNOGLOBULIN TRANSPORT IN DISEASE

A defect in glandular immunoglobulin transport has not been convincingly shown to be a primary cause of intestinal disease. The SC pattern of duodenal and jejunal mucosa from patients with coeliac disease (Fig. 11d) mimics that of the normal colon, and signs of intracellular IgA and IgM transport are seen along the entire hypertrophied crypts (Fig. 11b,c). We do not agree with Shiner & Ballard (1973) who claimed that there is a marked 'backflow' of secretory IgA into the lamina propria in this disease. In our hands the usual epithelial distribution of SC and IgA is found (Fig. 9d-f). The same holds true for normal-appearing glandular epithelium in ulcerative colitis and Crohn's disease, where SC may be present to the very brink of the ulceration (Fig. 12a-c). However, pathological epithelium may contain reduced amounts of SC, and there seems to be a parallel decrease (Fig. 12d,e) and sometimes complete lack (Fig. 12f,g) of intracellular IgA and IgM transport. Green & Fox (1975) and Das et al. (1975) have likewise reported altered SC distribution in Crohn's disease and idiopathic proctitis. These findings must be ascribed to localized secondary events, and no significant overall reduction of SC synthesis is shown when mucosal specimens from various intestinal diseases are cultured in vitro (McClelland et al. 1976).

A few reports have recently appeared indicating deficient SC synthesis as the primary cause of disease. A 52-year-old male (Krakauer et al. 1975) and a 15-year-old boy (Strober et al. 1976) with severe diarrhoea were found to have normal levels of serum immunoglobulins including IgA, but secretory IgA and SC were virtually undetectable in saliva and intestinal fluid. Moreover, the intestinal mucosa of the latter patient showed only negligible IgA production

---

←

FIG. 11. Immunohistochemical localization of immunoglobulins and SC in directly fixed (a-d) and saline-extracted (e-h) specimens of jejunal mucosa from an adult with coeliac disease. Single tracing with rhodamine conjugates in serial sections: (a) IgG; (b) IgM; (c) IgA; and (d) SC. The extracellular concentration of IgG is high as usual, but in coeliac disease with intensified local immune responses large amounts of extracellular IgA are also present in lamina propria and obscure the visualization of numerous IgA immunocytes. Extracellular IgM is less abundant, and most IgM cells can be discerned. Hypertrophied crypts produce SC along their entire length, and also cells lining the surface show some SC staining. The epithelial distribution of IgA parallels that of SC. Small amounts of cytoplasmic IgM can likewise be seen in the crypt epithelium, whereas faint IgG staining seems to be restricted to epithelial interstices. Double tracing of: (e) 'red' IgG and (f) 'green' IgA (same field); and of: (g) 'red' IgM and (h) 'green' IgA (same field). Extracellular immunoglobulins have been removed from lamina propria by the extraction procedure, and immunocytes of all classes are clearly revealed against the dark background. IgG has also been completely removed from lateral and basal borders of crypt cells (C), whereas some IgA and IgM seems to be retained along the epithelial cell membranes (arrows). Magnification: (a-d) × 80; (e-h) × 190.

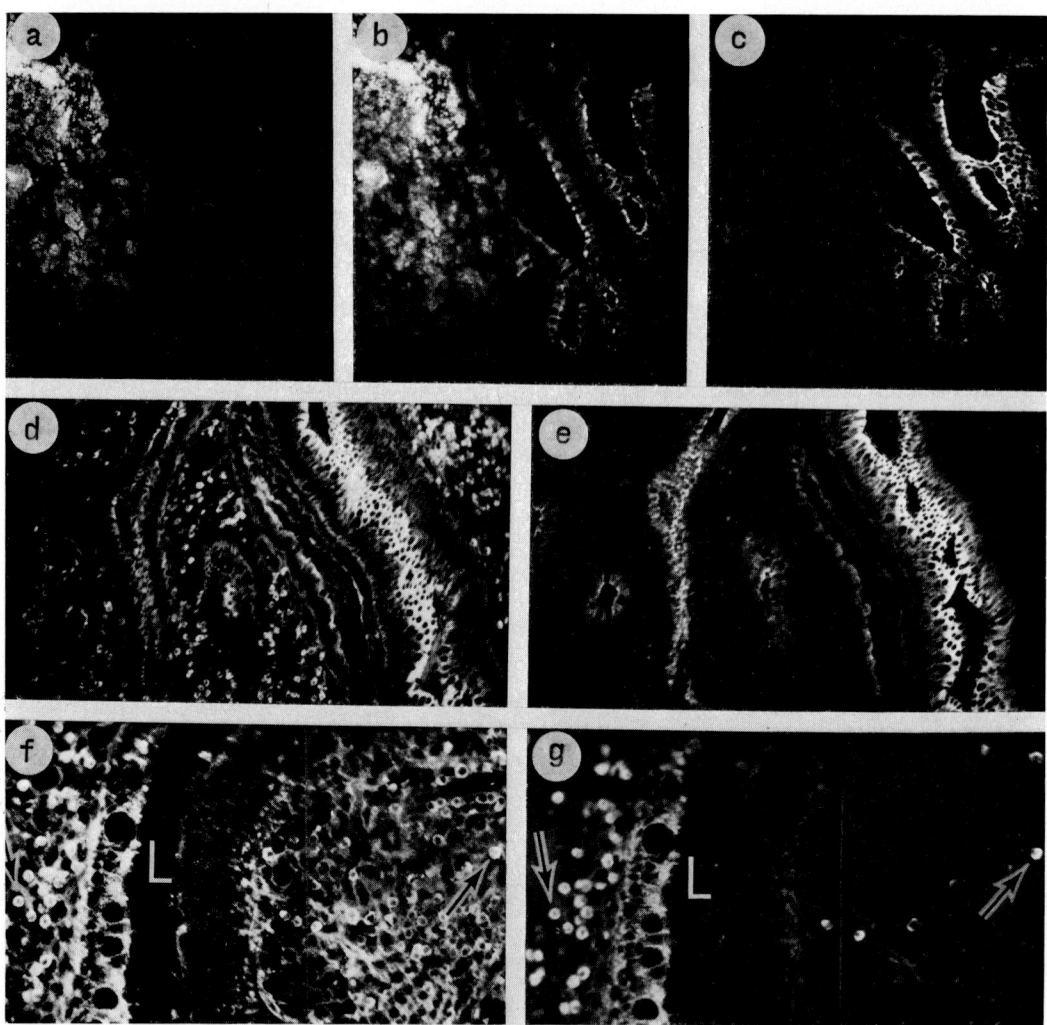

FIG. 12. Immunohistochemical localization of epithelial IgA and SC in inflammatory bowel disease. (a-c) Double tracing of 'green' lactoferrin and 'red' SC in rectal mucosa of patient with ulcerative colitis shown by selective filtration of green (a) and red (c) fluorescence and double exposure (b) in same field. Note that there is a normal distribution of SC almost to the brink of the ulceration, which appears as an accumulation of lactoferrin-containing neutrophilic granulocytes. (d, e) Tracing of IgA (d) and SC (e) in comparable fields from neighbouring sections of large bowel mucosa of a patient with Crohn's disease of colon. The pathological epithelium shows highly varying content of SC, and there are parallel variations in the epithelial distribution of IgA. (f, g) Double tracing of 'green' IgA and 'red' IgG in saline-extracted specimen from the colon of a patient with ulcerative colitis shown by double exposure (f) and selective filtration of green fluorescence (g) in same field. Examples of identical positions in the two pictures are indicated by arrows. Note that the crypt epithelium to the left of the lumen (L) apparently shows a normal distribution of IgA in columnar cells, whereas there is no intracellular immunoglobulin in the pathological epithelium facing the dense IgG-cell infiltrate to the right. Magnification: (a-e) × 100; (f, g) × 240.

in tissue culture. A common feature was a 20-fold increase of the IgM concentration in jejunal aspirates, indicating normal epithelial transport combined with enhanced local synthesis. A maturation defect of B cell blasts being seeded into the mucosa might explain the fact that intestinal IgA production apparently was replaced by IgM. According to our proposed glandular transport model, however, IgM should not be transmitted to the gut lumen without the participation of SC. Lack of SC synthesis in the two patients was not directly shown by immunohistochemistry or tissue culture techniques, neither was any attempt made to demonstrate SC bound to IgM in the intestinal fluid. Critical definition of these important points in such rare patients would be invaluable for the understanding of mucosal immunity.

A primary defect in SC-synthesizing capacity has been proposed as a possible cause of the sudden-infant-death syndrome (Ogra et al. 1975). Decreased amounts of SC were found in mucosal tissue extracts and sections from most of eight patients studied. The authors speculated that this deficiency might have jeopardized the respiratory mucosal defence. However, it was not excluded that a defect in SC production could be secondary to a recent virus infection of the epithelium. Williams et al. (1976) detected SC in submandibular gland extracts from all of ten such patients. A primary SC deficiency therefore seems unlikely as a general aetiological factor in this syndrome.

BIOLOGICAL IMPLICATIONS OF SELECTIVE GLANDULAR IMMUNOGLOBULIN TRANSPORT

It may be conceived that a normal immunological homeostasis is maintained in the intestinal mucosa through a critical balance between the various immunoglobulin classes. Polymeric IgA and IgM act as a first line of defence by immunological antigen exclusion at the mucosal surface. Antigens by-passing this exclusion mechanism may meet corresponding antibodies of all the three major immunoglobulin classes in the lamina propria. IgM and IgG are able to activate complement and IgG may participate in antibody-dependent cell-mediated cytotoxicity, but adverse reactions are normally most likely moderated within the mucosa by blocking antibody activities of IgA, which lacks phlogistic properties.

The initial phase of an intestinal immune response is characterized by increased synthesis and external transport of IgM and IgA. When noxious influences are counterbalanced by such a response, only moderate and reversible alterations of the local immunological homeostasis take place. An example is probably seen in coeliac disease; a pronounced mucosal IgM and IgA response develops but also a disproportionately increased local formation of

IgG, which indeed may be responsible for a considerable fraction of the gluten antibodies (Brandtzaeg & Baklien 1976). Since IgG is not actively transferred to the body exterior, antibodies of this class are of little value in the immunological exclusion of antigens and may rather have adverse effects within the mucosa.

Persistent and excessive stimulation of the intestinal B cell system leads to a pronounced local overproduction of IgG, as seen in ulcerative colitis and Crohn's disease (see Brandtzaeg & Baklien 1976), and the immunological homeostasis is severely altered. Antigens gain increased access to the lamina propria through epithelial breaks and because of defective external transport of SC-stabilized secretory IgA and IgM by injured epithelium. The IgG-cell response will be maintained and intensified by a continuous exposure of the interior of the body to a massive antigen load.

ACKNOWLEDGEMENTS

The studies of the authors have been supported by The Norwegian Research Council for Science and the Humanities, Anders Jahres Fond, and Helga Sembs Fond.

References

ALLEN, W. D., SMITH, C. G. & PORTER, P. (1973) Localization of intracellular immunoglobulin A in porcine intestinal mucosa using enzyme-labelled antibody. *Immunology 25*, 55-70

BINKLEY, F. & WIESEMANN, M. L. (1975) Glutathione and gamma glutamyl transferase in secretory processes. *Life Sci. 17*, 1359-1361

BOURNE, F. J. (1974) Structural features of pig IgA. *Immunol. Commun. 3(2)*, 157-173

BRANDTZAEG, P. (1968) Glandular secretion of immunoglobulins. *Acta Pathol. Microbiol. Scand. 74*, 624

BRANDTZAEG, P. (1971a) Human secretory immunoglobulins. II. Salivary secretions from individuals with selectively excessive or defective synthesis of serum immunoglobulins. *Clin. Exp. Immunol. 8*, 69-85

BRANDTZAEG, P. (1971b) Human secretory immunoglobulins. V. Occurrence of secretory piece in human serum. *J. Immunol. 106*, 318-323

BRANDTZAEG, P. (1971c) Human secretory immunoglobulins. VI. Association of free secretory piece with serum IgA *in vitro*. *Immunology 29*, 323-332

BRANDTZAEG, P. (1971d) Human secretory immunoglobulins. VII. Concentrations of parotid IgA and other secretory proteins in relation to the rate of flow and duration of secretory stimulus. *Arch. Oral Biol. 16*, 1295-1310

BRANDTZAEG, P. (1973a) Two types of IgA immunocytes in man. *Nature New Biol. 243*, 142-143

BRANDTZAEG, P. (1973b) Structure, synthesis and external transfer of mucosal immunoglobulins. *Ann. Immunol. (Inst. Pasteur) 124C*, 417-438

BRANDTZAEG, P. (1974a) Characteristics of SC-Ig complexes formed *in vitro*, in The Immunoglobulin A System (Mestecky, J. & Lawton, A. R., eds.) (*Adv. Exp. Med. Biol. 45*), pp. 87-97, Plenum Press, New York

BRANDTZAEG, P. (1974b) Human secretory component. II. Physicochemical characterization of free secretory component purified from colostrum. *Scand. J. Immunol. 3*, 707-716

BRANDTZAEG, P. (1974c) Presence of J chain in human immunocytes containing various immunoglobulin classes. *Nature (Lond.)* 252, 418-420

BRANDTZAEG, P. (1974d) Mucosal and glandular distribution of immunoglobulin components. Immunohistochemistry with a cold ethanol fixation technique. *Immunology* 26, 1101-1114

BRANDTZAEG, P. (1974e) Mucosal and glandular distribution of immunoglobulin components. Differential localization of free and bound SC in secretory epithelial cells. *J. Immunol.* 112, 1553-1559

BRANDTZAEG, P. (1975a) Human secretory component. IV. Aggregation and fragmentation of free secretory component. *Immunochemistry* 12, 877-881

BRANDTZAEG, P. (1975b) Immunochemical studies on free and bound J chain of human IgA and IgM. *Scand. J. Immunol.* 4, 439-450

BRANDTZAEG, P. (1975c) Human secretory immunoglobulin M. An immunochemical and immunohistochemical study. *Immunology* 29, 559-570

BRANDTZAEG, P. (1975d) Blocking effect of J chain and J-chain antibody on the binding of secretory component to human IgA and IgM. *Scand. J. Immunol.* 4, 837-842

BRANDTZAEG, P. (1976a) Studies on J chain and binding site for secretory component in circulating human B cells. II. The cytoplasm. *Clin. Exp. Immunol.* 25, 59-66

BRANDTZAEG, P. (1976b) Complex formation between secretory component and human immunoglobulins related to their content of J chain. *Scand. J. Immunol.* 5, 411-419

BRANDTZAEG, P. & BAKLIEN, K. (1976) Immunohistochemical studies of the formation and epithelial transport of immunoglobulins in normal and diseased human intestinal mucosa. *Scand. J. Gastroenterol.* 11, Suppl. 36, 1-45

BRANDTZAEG, P. & BERDAL, P. (1975) Presence of J chain in human IgG immunocytes related to the early phase of clonal expansion? *Scand. J. Immunol.* 4, 748-749

BRANDTZAEG, P., FJELLANGER, I. & GJERULDSEN, S. T. (1968) Immunoglobulin M: local synthesis and selective secretion in patients with immunoglobulin A deficiency. *Science (Wash. D.C.)* 160, 789-791

BRANDTZAEG, P., FJELLANGER, I. & GJERULDSEN, S. T. (1970) Human secretory immunoglobulins. I. Salivary secretions from individuals with normal or low levels of serum immunoglobulins. *Scand. J. Haematol.* Suppl. 12, 1-83

BROWN, W. R., ISOBE, Y. & NAKANE, P. K. (1975) Ultrastructural localization of IgA and secretory component (SC) in human intestinal mucosa by immunoperoxidase techniques. *Gastroenterology* 68, A-12/869

BULL, D. M., BIENENSTOCK, J. & TOMASI, T. B. (1971) Studies on human intestinal immunoglobulin A. *Gastroenterology*, 60, 370-380

BUTLER, W. T., ROSSEN, R. D. & WALDMANN, T. A. (1967) The mechanism of appearance of immunoglobulin A in nasal secretions in man. *J. Clin. Invest.* 46, 1883-1893

CHEN, S.-T. (1971) Cellular sites of immunoglobulins. II. The relative proportions of mucosal cells containing IgG, IgA, and IgM, and light polypeptide chains of kappa and lambda immunoglobulin in human appendices. *Acta Pathol. Jap.* 21, 67-83

COELHO, I. M., PEREIRA, M. T. & VIRELLA, G. (1974) Analytical study of salivary immunoglobulins in multiple myeloma. *Clin. Exp. Immunol.* 17, 417-426

COHEN, H. J. & KERN, M. (1969) Synthesis and secretion of γ-globulin by lymph node cells. VI. Characteristics of the structure of immunoglobulin A and its pattern of secretion by appendix cell suspensions. *Biochim. Biophys. Acta* 188, 255-264

COSTEA, N., YAKULIS, V., SCHMALE, J. & HELLE, P. (1968) Light chain determinants of exocrine isoagglutinins. *J. Immunol.* 101, 1248-1252

DAS, K. M., ERBER, W. & RUBINSTEIN, A. (1975) Immunological studies in patients with idiopathic proctitis: changes in systemic immune reactions, secretory component and immunoglobulins in histologically involved and uninvolved colonic mucosa. *Gastroenterology* 68, A-23/880

EIDELMAN, S. & DAVIS, S. D. (1968) Immunoglobulin content of intestinal mucosal plasma cells in ataxia telangiectasia. *Lancet* 1, 884-886

ESKELAND, T. & BRANDTZAEG, P. (1974) Does J chain mediate the combination of 19S IgM and dimeric IgA with the secretory component rather than being necessary for their polymerization? *Immunochemistry 11*, 161-163

FRANKLIN, R. M., KENYON, K. R. & TOMASI, T. B. (1973) Immunologic studies of human lacrimal gland: localization of immunoglobulins, secretory component and lactoferrin. *J. Immunol. 110*, 984-992

GIRARD, J. P. & DE KALBERMATTEN, A. (1970) Antibody activity in human duodenal fluid. *Eur. J. Clin. Invest. 1*, 188-195

GREEN, F. H. Y. & FOX, H. (1975) The distribution of mucosal antibodies in the bowel of patients with Crohn's disease. *Gut 16*, 125-131

HALPERN, M. S. & KOSHLAND, M. R. (1970) Novel subunit in secretory IgA. *Nature (Lond.) 228*, 1276-1278

HANEBERG, B. (1974a) Human fecal agglutinins to rabbit erythrocytes. *Scand. J. Immunol. 3*, 71-76

HANEBERG, B. (1974b) Immunoglobulins in feces from infants fed human or bovine milk. *Scand. J. Immunol. 3*, 191-197

HANSON, L. Å. & BRANDTZAEG, P. (1973) Secretory antibody systems, in *Immunologic Disorders in Infants and Children* (Stiehm, E. R. & Fulginiti, V. A., eds.), pp. 107-126, Saunders, Philadelphia

HANSON, L. Å., HOLMGREN, J., JODAL, U., JOHANNSSON, B. G. & LØNNROTH, F. (1969) On secretory IgA. *Scand. J. Clin. Lab. Invest.* Suppl. 110, 86-89

HEREMANS, J. F. (1974) Immunoglobulin A, in *The Antigens*, vol. 2 (Sela, M., ed.), pp. 365-522, Academic Press, London

HEREMANS, J. F. & CRABBÉ, P. A. (1967) Immunohistochemical studies on exocrine IgA, in *Gammaglobulins* (Killander, J., ed.), pp. 129-139, Almqvist & Wiksell, Uppsala

HUANG, S. W., FOGH, J. & HONG, R. (1976) Synthesis of secretory component by colon cancer cells. *Scand. J. Immunol. 5*, 263-268

INMAN, F. P. & MESTECKY, J. (1974) The J chain of polymeric immunoglobulins. *Contemporary Topics in Mol. Immunol. 3*, 111-141

JERRY, L. M., KUNKEL, H. G. & ADAMS, L. (1972) Stabilization of dissociable IgA_2 proteins by secretory component. *J. Immunol. 109*, 275-283

KAGNOFF, M. F., SERFILIPPI, D. & DONALDSON, R. M. (1973) In vitro kinetics of intestinal secretory IgA secretion. *J. Immunol. 110*, 297-300

KEMLER, R., MOSSMAN, H., STROHMAIER, K., KICKHÖFEN, B. & HAMMER, D. K. (1975) In vitro studies on the selective binding of IgG from different species to tissue sections of the bovine mammary gland. *Eur. J. Immunol. 5*, 603-608

KOSHLAND, M. E. (1975) Structure and function of the J chain. *Adv. Immunol. 20*, 41-69

KRAEHENBUHL, J. P., RACINE, L. & GALARDY, R. E. (1975) Localization of secretory IgA, secretory component, and α heavy chain in the mammary gland of lactating rabbits by immunoelectron microscopy. *Ann. N.Y. Acad. Sci. 254*, 190-202

KRAKAUER, R., ZINNERMAN, H. H. & HONG, R. (1975) Deficiency of secretory IgA and intestinal malabsorption. *Am. J. Gastroenterol. 64*, 319-323

LAI A FAT, R. F. M., MCCLELLAND, D. B. L. & VAN FURTH, R. (1974) The synthesis of secretory component by lymphoid tissues in vitro. *J. Immunol. 113*, 1199-1203

LAMM, M. E. (1976) Cellular aspects of immunoglobulin A. *Adv. Immunol. 22*, 223-290

LAWTON, A. R. & MAGE, R. G. (1969) The synthesis of secretory IgA in the rabbit. I. Evidence for synthesis as an 11S dimer. *J. Immunol. 102*, 693-697

LAWTON, A. R., ASOFSKY, R. & MAGE, R. G. (1970a) Synthesis of secretory IgA in the rabbit. II. Production of alpha, light and T chains by *in vitro* cultures of mammary tissue. *J. Immunol. 104*, 388-396

LAWTON, A. R., ASOFSKY, R. & MAGE, R. G. (1970b) Synthesis of secretory IgA in the rabbit. III. Interaction of colostral IgA fragments with T chain. *J. Immunol. 104*, 397-408

LINDH, E. (1974) Increased resistance of immunoglobulin A dimers to proteolytic degradation after binding of secretory component. *J. Immunol. 114*, 284-286

MACH, J.-P. (1970) *In vitro* combination of human and bovine free secretory component with IgA of various species. *Nature (Lond.) 228*, 1278-1282

MCCLELLAND, D. B. L., SHEARMAN, D. J. C., LAI A FAT, R. F. M. & VAN FURTH, R. (1976) *In vitro* synthesis of immunoglobulins, secretory component, complement and lysozyme by human gastrointestinal tissues. II. Pathological tissues. *Clin. Exp. Immunol. 23*, 20-27

MESTECKY, J., KRAUS, F. W. & VOIGHT, S. A. (1970) Proportion of human colostral immunoglobulin A molecules containing the secretory determinant. *Immunology 18*, 237-243

MUNSTER, P. J. J. VAN (1972) De secretoire component. Een immunochemisch onderzoek. Isolatie, eigenschappen, uitscheiding in secreta en localisatie in jejunumbiopten. [The secretory component. An immunochemical investigation. Isolation, properties, excretion in secretions and localization in jejunal biopsy samples.] Thesis, University of Nijmegen

NAKAJIMA, S., GILLESPIE, D. N. & GLEICH, G. J. (1975) Differences between IgA and IgE as secretory proteins. *Clin. Exp. Immunol. 21*, 306-317

NEWCOMB, R. W. & ISHIZAKA, K. (1970) Physicochemical and antigenic studies on human γE in respiratory fluid. *J. Immunol. 105*, 85-89

O'DALY, J. A. & CEBRA, J. J. (1971) Rabbit secretory IgA. II. Free secretory component from colostrum and its specific association with IgA. *J. Immunol. 107*, 449-455

O'DALY, J. A., CRAIG, S. W. & CEBRA, J. J. (1971) Localization of b markers, α-chain and SC of sIgA in epithelial cells lining Lieberkühn crypts. *J. Immunol. 166*, 286-288

OGRA, S. S., OGRA, P. L., LIPPES, J. & TOMASI, T. B. (1972) Immunohistochemical localization of immunoglobulins, secretory component and lactoferrin in the developing human fetus. *Proc. Soc. Exp. Biol. Med. 139*, 570-574

OGRA, P. L., COPPOLA, P. R., MACGILLIVRAY, M. H. & DZIERBA, J. L. (1974) Mechanism of mucosal immunity to viral infections in γA immunoglobulin-deficiency syndromes. *Proc. Soc. Exp. Biol. (N. Y.) 145*, 811-816

OGRA, P. L., OGRA, S. S. & COPPOLA, P. R. (1975) Secretory component and sudden-infant-death syndrome. *Lancet 2*, 387-390

POGER, M. E. & LAMM, M. E. (1974) Localization of free and bound secretory component in human intestinal epithelial cells. A model for the assembly of secretory IgA. *J. Exp. Med. 139*, 629-642

PORTIS, J. L. & COE, J. E. (1975) IgM the secretory immunoglobulin of reptiles and amphibians. *Nature (Lond.) 258*, 547-548

RÁDL, J., KLEIN, F., VAN DEN BERG, P., DE BRUYN, A. M. & HIJMANS, W. (1971) Binding of secretory piece to polymeric IgA and IgM paraproteins *in vitro*. *Immunology 20*, 843-852

RÁDL, J., SCHUIT, H. R. E., MESTECKY, J. & HIJMANS, W. (1974) The origin of monomeric and polymeric forms of IgA in man, in *The Immunoglobulin A System* (Mestecky, J. & Lawton, A. R., eds.) (*Adv. Exp. Med. Biol. 45*), pp. 57-68, Plenum Press, NewYork

RÁDL, J., SWART, A. C. W. & MESTECKY, J. (1975) The nature of polymeric serum IgA in man. *Proc. Soc. Exp. Med. 150*, 482-484

ROSSEN, R. D., MORGAN, C., HSU, K. C., BUTLER, W. T. & ROSE, H. M. (1968) Localization of 11S external secretory IgA by immunofluorescence in tissues lining the oral and respiratory passages in man. *J. Immunol. 100*, 706-717

SAVILAHTI, E. (1973) IgA deficiency in children. Immunoglobulin-containing cells in the intestinal mucosa, immunoglobulins in secretions and serum IgA levels. *Clin. Exp. Immunol. 13*, 395-406

SHINER, R. J. & BALLARD, J. (1973) Mucosal secretory IgA and secretory piece in adult coeliac disease. *Gut 14*, 778-783

SINGER, S. J. & NICOLSON, G. L. (1972) The fluid mosaic model of the structure of cell membranes. *Science (Wash. D.C.) 175*, 720-731

SÖLTOFT, J. & SÖEBERG, B. (1972) Immunoglobulin-containing cells in the small intestine in viral hepatitis. *Acta Pathol. Microbiol. Scand. B 80*, 379-387

SOUTH, M. A., COOPER, M. D., WOLLHEIM, F. A., HONG, R. & GOOD, R. A. (1966) The IgA system. I. Studies of the transport and immunochemistry of IgA in the saliva. *J. Exp. Med. 123*, 615-627

STIEHM, E., VAERMAN, J. P. & FUDENBERG, H. H. (1966) Plasma infusions in immunologic deficiency states: metabolic and therapeutic studies. *Blood 28*, 918-937

STROBER, W., KRAKAUER, R., KLAEVEMAN, H. L., REYNOLDS, H. Y. & NELSON, D. L. (1976) Secretory component deficiency. A disorder of the IgA immune system. *N. Engl. J. Med. 294*, 351-356

THOMPSON, R. A. (1970) Secretory piece linked to IgM in individuals deficient in IgA. *Nature (Lond.) 226*, 946-948

TOMASI, T. B. & BIENENSTOCK, J. (1968) Secretory immunoglobulins. *Adv. Immunol. 9*, 1-96

TOMASI, T. B. & GREY, H. M. (1972) Structure and function of immunoglobulin A. *Prog. Allergy 16*, 81-213

TOMASI, T. B. & YURCHAK, A. M. (1972) The synthesis of secretory component by the human thymus. *J. Immunol. 108*, 1132-1135

TOMASI, T. B., TAN, E. M., SOLOMON, A. & PRENDERGAST, R. A. (1965) Characteristics of an immune system common to certain external secretions. *J. Exp. Med. 121*, 101-124

TOURVILLE, D. R. & TOMASI, T. B. (1969) Selective transport of γA. *Proc. Soc. Exp. Biol. Med. 132*, 473-477

TOURVILLE, D. R., ADLER, R. H., BIENENSTOCK, J. & TOMASI, T. B. (1969) The human secretory immunoglobulin system: immunohistological localization of γA, secretory 'piece', and lactoferrin in normal tissues. *J. Exp. Med. 129*, 411-429

VAERMAN, J. P. (1973) Comparative immunochemistry of IgA. *Res. Immunochem. Immunobiol. 3*, 91-183

WALDMANN, T. A. & STROBER, W. (1969) Metabolism of immunoglobulins. *Prog. Allergy 13*, 1-110

WEICKER, J. & UNDERDOWN, B. J. (1975) A study on the association of human secretory component with IgA and IgM proteins. *J. Immunol. 114*, 1337-1344

WILLIAMS, A. L., HOSKING, C. S. & WAKEFIELD, E. (1976) Secretory component and sudden infant death. *Lancet 1*, 485-486

Discussion

Cebra: You suggested that secretory component may be a membrane component of the epithelial cells and be found on their basal borders. Have you any idea about the selectivity of secretory component as a receptor explaining differences in the concentrations of exported Ig? If you compare IgM with IgA1 and IgA2, are the changes in proportions outside in gut lumen explained by a difference in specificity?

Brandtzaeg: So far there is no evidence for any difference between IgA1 and IgA2 dimers in SC binding properties. There is one study indicating binding of SC to monomeric IgA2 of the genetic variant Am_2 (+), but that experiment was done with a large excess of SC obtained from colostral IgA by reduction (Jerry *et al.* 1972). The situation was therefore not comparable to the specific, non-covalent interaction I have discussed.

Cebra: Have you looked at the relative proportions of IgA2 and IgA1 cells in the lamina propria? There is a difference in the proportion of the two isotypes in the secretions and in the circulation, and one wonders what the basis for the difference is.

Brandtzaeg: This information is based on one publication (Grey *et al.* 1968) which has not been confirmed, and there are as yet no published cellular studies.

André: You gave evidence of some IgG cells synthesizing J chains. Do these cells bind secretory component?

Brandtzaeg: The IgG producers containing J chain do not bind SC, neither do J-chain-positive IgD cells. The SC-binding site depends on the incorporation of J chain into IgA or IgM polymers. Apparently J chain is unable to combine with IgG and IgD.

Gowans: How firm is the evidence that there is a J-chain specific binding site for secretory component?

Brandtzaeg: The evidence is two-fold. Firstly, you need the presence of J chain in the IgM or IgA polymers in order to obtain SC binding. Secondly, you can block the binding site by means of antibody to J chain. The latter experiment is difficult to interpret, however, because of the possibility of non-specific steric hindrance.

Lachmann: When you say you need the J chain, have you taken *polymeric* forms of IgM and IgA that are free of J chain and shown they have not bound secretory piece?

Brandtzaeg: Yes; that was shown in Fig. 2. SC likewise binds only to the cytoplasm of J-chain-producing IgA and IgM cells when tested on tissue sections.

Cebra: According to Hanly *et al.* (1973), there may well be a requirement for J chain but there seems also to be a second requirement, for the hinge region of the Fc fragment. They can prepare Fc dimer from IgA2 molecules which fails to bind SC. One can infer that perhaps one requires the J chain but also a part of the heavy chain around the hinge.

Brandtzaeg: I agree completely, because J chain isolated from polymeric IgA does not block the binding reaction to any great extent. Also cells containing native free J chain (we call it 'free' when it is in an IgG or IgD plasma cell) do not bind secretory component, so free J chain apparently has very low affinity for the secretory component. The Fc portion of Ig polymers is thus essential for the SC-binding site. Why it is important is not known. Is it because of the conformation of the heavy chains or because of the configuration of the bound J chains? Our results favour the latter possibility.

Vaerman: It has also been proved by Mach (1970) that dimeric IgA which was re-formed from reduced IgA and from which J chain had been removed could not bind.

Gowans: Where precisely do you think the membrane-bound secretory component is located? You illustrated a striated pattern which you suggested might indicate a distribution along the sides of the epithelial cells. However, another picture showed basement membrane staining. Do you think the receptors are arranged on the basement membrane, or on the epithelial cells?

Brandtzaeg: I think they are on the plasma membrane, and this is supported by the work of Huang *et al.* (1976).

Gowans: Has this ever been demonstrated on suspensions of intestinal epithelial cells? The epithelium can be readily dissociated into a cell suspension.

Brandtzaeg: We have not been able to produce such cell suspensions with the capacity to make SC, which would be required for proving the point.

Cebra: Some beautiful studies were made by Kraehenbuhl *et al.* (1973) using microperoxidase-labelled Fab anti-secretory component. He used normal sections and looked at the epithelial cells, and found a staining of the whole cell membrane going round into the intercellular space before the tight junction. This distribution of SC is very much like the one that Rodewald (1975) finds for Fc receptors on the absorptive epithelium in the neonatal rat.

Brandtzaeg: As I mentioned (p. 95), Kraehenbuhl *et al.* (1975) also showed that SC but not IgA is present in the Golgi complex in rabbit mammary gland cells. The same sort of findings as you mention have been made by Brown *et al.* (1975) showing a plasma membrane localization of IgA plus SC, in human gut sections examined electron microscopically.

Gowans: Can you really tell that it is on the surface in sections?

Cebra: This technique uses thick sections which are 'marinated' in the Fab-microperoxidase and then cut into ultra-thin sections.

Brandtzaeg: I agree that the final proof of a model such as I have been suggesting must be obtained on cells in suspension. The first step in this direction is the studies reported by Huang *et al.* (1976). I hope that they will do further experiments on cultivated colon cancer cells.

Evans: With the Sainte-Marie technique you could lose up to 50% of antigenic activity of IgG, especially if it is at an extracellular site. Scott (1976) found that with jejunal biopsies which had been washed for up to two days in phosphate-buffered saline and then sectioned as frozen sections, IgG was often still present in the stroma.

Brandtzaeg: It depends on the technique and on the type of tissue. The dimensions of the tissue piece in one direction must not exceed 2–3 mm if one is to get rid of the diffusible proteins. But our slides show a satisfactory absence of background staining for IgG.

Evans: This might be denaturation. Have you tried it with frozen sections?

Brandtzaeg: Why is it not denatured in the plasma cells, then?

Evans: It may be much easier to denature material at an extracellular site.

Brandtzaeg: I have doubts about frozen sections in relation to the specificity of extracellular staining.

Evans: The specificity control I used was the same as one usually uses in such studies, namely absorption and blocking studies.

Brandtzaeg: I cannot answer your question but I doubt that one will have pronounced denaturation at 4 °C in our washing process, and the alcohol procedure is the same as for the directly fixed material. The fact that diffuse background staining is present, despite a 48-hour washing of tissue pieces that were too big, speaks against extracellular denaturation of Ig.

Vaerman: I was struck by the lack of IgG staining between the epithelial cells. Andersen *et al.* (1963) claimed that the gut was an important site of IgG catabolism. This suggests that some IgG reaches the gut lumen. I am surprised then to find no IgG staining, especially in view of the high concentration of IgG in the extracellular fluid. This implies that if there is some IgG there, it is very quickly removed from the spaces between the epithelial cells by an unknown mechanism.

Brandtzaeg: Our directly fixed material indicates that there is some intercellular staining of IgG in the crypts, and especially in all types of surface epithelium, like the tips of the villi and the surface of the colon. It depends on the type of epithelium: in the Brunner's glands and salivary glands the epithelium seems to be very tightly packed, because there we hardly see any IgG staining, while it is easily seen in columnar surface epithelia. Normally IgG is not present in the cytoplasm of epithelial cells.

Ferguson: You touched on the technical problems of fluorescence staining related to extracellular fluid. Do you think that when there is extravascular staining with anti-immunoglobulin and anti-complement conjugates (on the basement membrane or elsewhere), this can be taken to imply the presence of immune complexes? I am thinking in the context of mucosal appearances in coeliac disease, Crohn's disease and ulcerative colitis.

Brandtzaeg: We find extravascular immunoglobulins of all classes and also extravascular complement factors (Baklien & Brandtzaeg 1974), but whether they are present in complexes, I do not know. One can't tell from tissue sections.

Porter: Allen and I showed that IgA was transported in vesicles (Allen *et al.* 1973). This particular vesiculation takes place outside the epithelial cell. We showed the vesicles within the intercellular channels. Our model includes the pushing of a pseudopodium from the plasma cell into the intercellular space. Would you feel that in the transport of this vesicle, secretory component is necessary?

Brandtzaeg: Let me first ask you whether you still feel that there are vesiculations from the plasma cell going into the interstices.

Porter: We have seen these inside and outside the epithelial cell, within the intercellular channel.

Brandtzaeg: How then is IgA transported considerable distances from plasma cells to epithelium, if it depends on such vesicles?

Porter: I agree that free IgA may be transported by transudation on to the secretory component. My question is whether you feel that the secretory component would be a necessary receptor in terms of transporting that vesicle.

Brandtzaeg: I have no idea about these vesicles because I am not working at the ultrastructural level, but in the study of Brown *et al.* (1975) such vesicles were not found.

Lachmann: Can one conclude that there seems to be some difference of opinion on whether secretory piece, either bound on cell membranes or free in solution, acts as a receptor for IgA? We have been told that secretory piece occurs on the membranes of epithelial cells and picks up material, presumably either directly from a plasma cell, or from solution. But on the other hand there seems to be no good evidence that secretory piece is an important receptor for localizing IgA-forming cells in the lamina propria. If the secretory piece is not the receptor responsible, is the IgA itself the identifying molecule? There would seem to be no convincing evidence for this either.

References

ANDERSEN, S. B., GLENERT, J. & WALLEVIK, K. (1963) Gamma globulin turnover and intestinal degradation of gamma globulin in the dog. *J. Clin. Invest.* 42, 1873-1881

ALLEN, W. D., SMITH, C. G. & PORTER, P. (1973) Localization of intracellular immunoglobulin A in porcine intestinal mucosa using enzyme-labelled antibody. *Immunology* 25, 55-70

BAKLIEN, K. & BRANDTZAEG, P. (1974) Immunohistochemical localization of complement in intestinal mucosa. *Lancet* 2, 1087-1088

BROWN, W. R., ISOBE, Y. & NAKANE, P. K. (1975) Ultrastructural localization of IgA and secretory component (SC) in human intestinal mucosa by immunoperoxidase techniques. *Gastroenterology* 68, A-12/869

GREY, H. M., ABEL, C. A., YOUNT, W. J. & KUNKEL, H. G. (1968) A subclass of human γA-globulins (γA$_2$) which lacks the disulfide bonds linking heavy and light chains. *J. Exp. Med.* 128, 1223-1236

HANLY, C. W., LICHTER, E. A., DRAY, S. & KNIGHT, K. L. (1973) Rabbit immunoglobulin A allotypic specificities. Localization to two papain fragments Fab$_{2a}$ and Fc$_{2a}$, of secretory immunoglobulin A. *Biochemistry* 12, 733-741

HUANG, S. W., FOGH, J. & HONG, R. (1976) Synthesis of secretory component by colon cancer cells. *Scand. J. Immunol.* 5, 263-268

JERRY, L. M., KUNKEL, H. G. & ADAMS, L. (1972) Stabilization of dissociable IgA$_2$ proteins by secretory component. *J. Immunol.* 109, 275-283

KRAEHENBUHL, J. P., GALARDY, R. E. & JAMIESON, J. D. (1973) A heme-peptide labelled antibody fragment as a marker for intracellular antigens. *Fed. Proc.* 32, 962 (abstr. 4171)

KRAEHENBUHL, J. P., RACINE, L. & GALARDY, R. E. (1975) Localization of secretory IgA, secretory component, and α heavy chain in the mammary gland of lactating rabbits by immunoelectron microscopy. *Ann. N.Y. Acad. Sci.* 254, 190-202

MACH, J. P. (1970) *In vitro* combination of human and bovine free secretory component with IgA of various species. *Nature (Lond.)* 228, 1278-1282

RODEWALD, R. (1975) Intestinal transport of peroxidase-conjugated IgG fragments in the neonatal rat, in *Materno-fetal Transmission of Immunoglobulins* (Hemmings, W. A., ed.), pp. 137-153, Cambridge University Press, London

SCOTT, B. B. (1976) M.D. Thesis, London University

Antibodies in human serum and milk induced by enterobacteria and food proteins

S. AHLSTEDT*, B. CARLSSON, S. P. FÄLLSTRÖM, L. Å. HANSON, J. HOLMGREN, G. LIDIN-JANSON, B. S. LINDBLAD, U. JODAL, B. KAIJSER, A. SOHL-ÅKERLUND and C. WADSWORTH

Department of Immunology, Institute of Medical Microbiology and Department of Pediatrics, University of Göteborg, and Department of Pediatrics of Karolinska Institutet at St. Göran's Children's Hospital, Stockholm

Abstract Ingestion of *Escherichia coli* O83 bacteria by adults resulted in a transient irregular colonization leading to a serum antibody response in only four out of 14 cases examined. In all of three pregnant women, however, IgA antibodies against *E. coli* O83 antigen were released from colostral cells after similar bacterial ingestion although no serum antibody response was noted. The findings indicate a link between the antigenic exposure of the gut and secretory antibodies of the IgA class, presumably locally formed in the mammary gland.

Antibodies of the secretory IgA class registered in colostrum may, at least partly, reflect the antigenic exposure of the gut. These antibodies are probably important in protecting against *E. coli* infections in the neonate, as suggested by the findings of antibodies in human milk against O and K antigens of non-enteropathogenic as well as enteropathogenic serotypes of *E. coli*. Furthermore, in milk of women from low socio-economic groups in Pakistan, neutralizing antibodies were present against enterotoxins of *E. coli* bacteria and occasionally against *Vibrio cholerae* enterotoxins.

In addition, secretory IgA antibodies against food proteins were detected in human milk. This suggests that intestinal exposure to such antigens could stimulate a local immune response in the gut resulting in triggered lymphoid cells homing to the mammary gland. These human milk secretory IgA antibodies against bovine milk proteins may help to prevent cow's milk allergy in infants on mixed feeding, since these infants tend to have a lower serum antibody response to cow's milk proteins than infants fed mostly artificially. Furthermore, children suffering from cow's milk protein intolerance and gluten enteropathy may have higher serum levels of antibody to cow's milk protein antigens than normal children, possibly reflecting increased permeability of the intestinal mucosa for various antigens.

Intestinal exposure to antigens has been found to stimulate the immunological system in man as well as in animals (see Crabbé *et al.* 1970; Lodinová *et al.*

---

* *Present address:* Astra Läkemedel AB, Research and Development Laboratories, Södertälje, Sweden

1973; Sagie et al. 1974). The resulting immune response, mostly registered as an increase in antibody titre, may be local as well as systemic.

Immunity resulting from intestinal exposure to microbial antigens appears to be important in the body's defence against enteric infections. A protective role of acquired local immunity has been demonstrated in cholera where antibacterial as well as anti-enterotoxin antibodies have been found to be effective (Fubara & Freter 1973; Holmgren et al. 1975). Protection mediated by local antibodies against other enteric organisms such as *Escherichia coli*, *Salmonella* and *Shigella* has also been indicated (reviewed by Gerrard 1974 and Hanson et al. 1976a). Local immunity in the form of secretory IgA antibodies not only provides protection against mucosal adhesion of bacteria or toxins, but may also protect the mucosa from contact with potential allergens such as food proteins (Walker et al. 1972, 1974b, 1975; Soothill 1974, 1976). Furthermore, the local antibodies can serve a regulatory role with regard to their continued synthesis by abrogating further antigenic contact with the lymphoid cells in the gut mucosa (Fubara & Freter 1973; Walker et al. 1972, 1974b). Recent observations suggest a close relation between antigenic stimulation in the gut and the appearance of secretory IgA antibodies in the mammary secretion (Allardyce et al. 1974; Goldblum et al. 1975; Montgomery et al. 1974). This paper surveys studies of the relationship between the systemic serum antibody response and the local responses in the gut and the mammary gland against enteric microbial antigens and food proteins.

SERUM ANTIBODY RESPONSE AFTER INTESTINAL EXPOSURE TO E. COLI

Colonization of the gut in infants with *Escherichia coli* O83 bacteria gives rise to a specific serum antibody response if the *E. coli* O83 establishes itself as a resident strain dominating the aerobic faecal flora (Lodinová et al. 1973). In contrast, we found that if healthy adults were exposed to these bacteria by the ingestion of two doses, resulting in *E. coli* O83 as one of many transient strains in the gut, serum antibody responses were detectable in only four out of 11 individuals (Jodal et al. 1976) (Fig. 1).

Serum antibody responses presumably stimulated from the gut in healthy children as well as in adults may vary with the bacterial antigens involved. Thus, the anti-*E. coli* O6 serum antibody levels are lower than those against *E. coli* O2, O4 and O75 (Table 1) (Ahlstedt & Jodal 1976; Jodal et al. 1976). Yet the virulence of these bacteria of various types may be similar, as suggested by their relative frequency in urinary tract infections and in faecal flora (Grüneberg et al. 1968; K. Lincoln & G. Lidin-Janson, personal communication). Thus a tolerogenic effect of the O6 antigen, as previously observed in

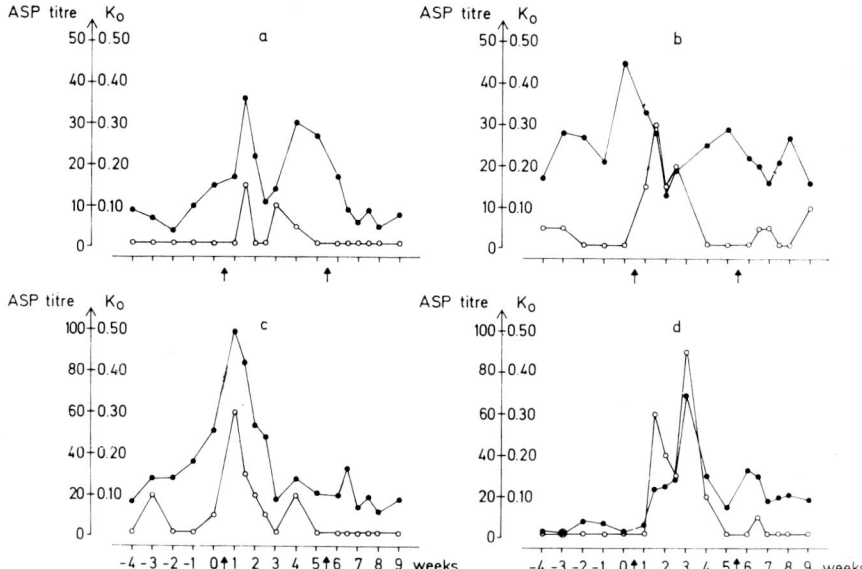

FIG. 1. The antibody titre (ASP) (— • —) and the antibody avidity (Ko) (— ○ —) to the *E. coli* O83 antigen in four healthy adults (*a–d*) after ingestion of the bacteria. Two ingestion times are indicated (↑).

TABLE 1

Mean serum antibody titre against *E. coli* O antigens, determined with the ASP technique

	Antibody titre against				
	O2	O4	O6	O75	O83
Children	54[a]	47[a]	35	46	not done
Adults	40[b]	40[b]	26	40²	22

[a] Differs significantly from O6 ($P < 0.05$).
[b] Differs significantly from O6 and O83 ($P < 0.01$).

parenterally immunized mice (Ahlstedt *et al.* 1973), might possibly explain the lower anti-O6 titres observed.

MILK ANTIBODY RESPONSE AFTER INTESTINAL EXPOSURE TO E. COLI

Microbial antigens induce a local response in the gut demonstrable as IgA coproantibodies (Crabbé *et al.* 1970; Holmgren *et al.* 1975; Lodinová *et al.* 1973). Such a response is difficult to study, because of the problems of obtaining representative material and the risk of enzymic degradation, even though laborious experimental systems have recently been successfully applied (e.g. Svennerholm & Holmgren 1976; Pierce & Sack 1976; Walker et al. 1974a). We have studied the link between the antigenic exposure of the gut and antibody release from the mammary gland. The results indicate a close relationship between the intestinal antigenic stimulation and the antibodies in the mammary secretion (Goldblum et al. 1975). This prompted us to study in greater detail lymphoid cells and antibodies in the human milk as a reflection of the maternal gut immunity.

Human milk contains considerable numbers of lymphoid cells, up to 8% of which secrete IgA antibodies to *E. coli* O antigens as detected with the plaque haemolysis-in-gel technique (Ahlstedt et al. 1975). This high frequency of cells producing antibodies against only one group of antigens present in the gut suggests that they may represent a rather selective lymphoid cell population. The triggering of this cell population may occur within the intestinal tract. Thus three pregnant women ingested bacteria of the harmless *E. coli* O83 strain used in about 200 neonates by Lodinová et al. (1973). One or two ingestions by the women of 10^9 bacteria resulted within a few days in strikingly high numbers of cells in their milk which formed antibodies against the O83 antigen (Fig. 2). Actually, between 0.1 and 1% of the milk cells formed anti-O83 antibodies, again indicating that the cells recorded belong to a selective cell population forming antibodies against enterobacterial antigens present in the gastrointestinal tract. Since we did not see any corresponding serum antibody response it is not likely that the local antibody response was due to the transport of antigen from the gut to the mammary gland. Therefore we favour the hypothesis that the observed IgA-producing cells were antigenically triggered in the Peyer's patches and then homed to the mammary gland. This is in accordance with the findings of Craig & Cebra (1971) that cells from the Peyer's patches can repopulate the intestinal mucosa of irradiated animals with IgA-producing lymphoid cells. It is also in agreement with the recent demonstration by Pierce & Sack (1976) that lymphoid cells containing antibodies against an antigen used for peroral immunization can be found in the thoracic duct lymph.

Human milk contains high levels of antibodies against many enterobacterial antigens. Thus Gindrat et al. (1972) found antibodies against numerous *E. coli* O antigens. Using the enzyme-linked immunosorbent assay (ELISA), we found such antibodies to be predominantly of the secretory IgA type, although IgG and IgM were also demonstrated (Ahlstedt et al. 1975).

Analysis of antibodies in milk from well-nourished healthy Swedish mothers and undernourished Pakistani mothers showed quite similar antibody levels to

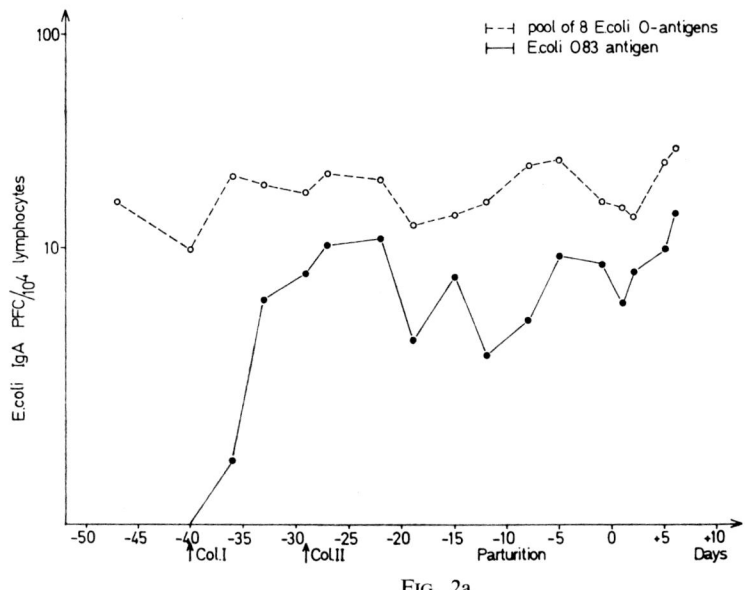

Fig. 2a

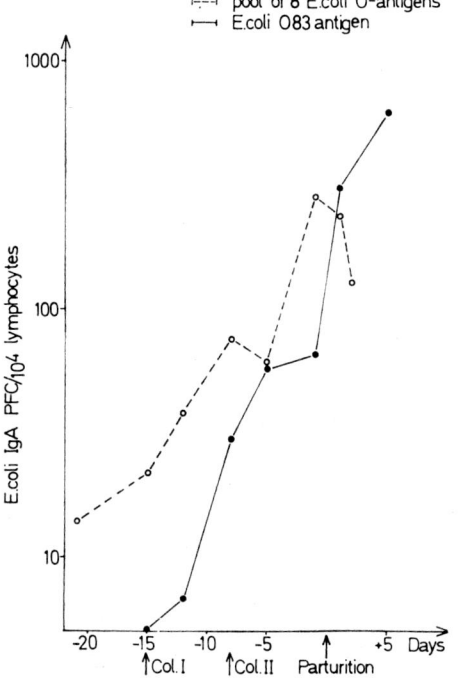

Fig. 2b

For legend, see p. 120

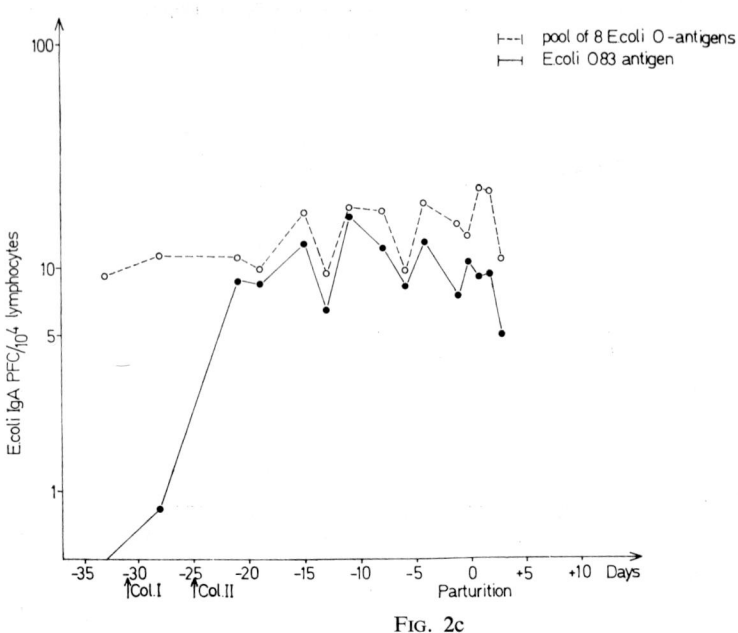

Fig. 2c

FIG. 2. Antibody-forming cells registered as plaques in colostrum samples from three women after ingestion of *E. coli* O83 bacteria. —●—, antibodies against the O83 antigen. --○--, antibodies against a pool of O antigens from the eight most frequent strains occurring in urinary tract infections. (*a*), (*b*) and (*c*) show the responses of the different women. (From Goldblum *et al.* (1975), by permission of the Editor of *Nature*.)

E. coli O antigens. This was noted regardless of whether a pool of the Swedish or Pakistani *E. coli* O antigens was used in the assays (Carlsson *et al.* 1976). Thus the finding that individuals suffering from protein calorie malnutrition are deficient in their secretory immune response (Sirisinha *et al.* 1974) could not be confirmed by studying the mammary gland secretion. There were indications, however, that the milk volumes were smaller from the undernourished Pakistani mothers than from the healthy Swedish mothers, resulting in a smaller output of the antibodies. In the Pakistani milk samples we also consistently found antibodies against the O antigens of enteropathogenic *E. coli* bacteria while such antibodies were less common in milk from Swedish mothers (Table 2).

Antibodies against the important virulence antigens of the capsule (K) of the *E. coli* bacteria are commonly present in the milk (Table 3 and Hanson *et al.* 1976*a*; Carlsson *et al.*, in manuscript). Of particular interest is the almost

TABLE 2

Milk antibody levels to enteropathogenic *E. coli* in Pakistani and Swedish mothers, measured with the enzyme-linked immunoabsorbent assay (ELISA)

Determined with antiserum against	Pakistani mothers (n = 13)		Swedish mothers (n = 20)		P
	$\bar{x}$	Range	$\bar{x}$	Range	
IgA	19.1	5.6–70.6	5.7	2.9–13.7	<0.01
SC[a]	27.1	0 –79.8	3.3	0 –22.3	<0.01
IgG	0.8	0 – 4.2	0.2	0 – 1.8	N.S.
IgM	2.9	0 –17.5	0	0	N.S.

[a] SC, secretory component.

TABLE 3

Antibodies to *E. coli* K antigens: ratio of antibody levels in milk/serum

	$\bar{x}$	Range	n
K1	3.36	0.48– 8.9	13
K3	4.70	0.98–15.3	13
K6	2.87	1.18– 6.7	12
K13	4.27	1.38–14.3	10
K52	2.68	0.97– 6.73	13

consistent presence of anti-K1 antibodies (Table 3) in spite of the previously shown poor immunogenicity of the K1 antigen (Kaijser et al. 1973). Since this K1 antigen has been found in 84% of the *E. coli* strains causing neonatal meningitis (Robbins et al. 1974), the presence of such antibodies may be of particular significance during the neonatal period.

Another antibody activity in human milk of potential biological importance is directed against the enterotoxins of *E. coli* and *Vibrio cholerae*. Striking differences were noticed between the milk specimens of Pakistani and Swedish women with regard to neutralizing activity against *E. coli* enterotoxin. This was tested with the adrenal cell morphology assay (Donta et al. 1974) using a few (2–5) minimal effective doses of enterotoxins and the milk samples diluted 1:50 to avoid non-specific cell reactions. Most of the Pakistani milk samples neutralized the enterotoxin of two different *E. coli* strains, whereas only a single Swedish milk sample had a partial neutralizing effect (Table 4). It seems likely that this difference reflects a more frequent intestinal exposure to enterotoxigenic *E. coli* of the Pakistani than of the Swedish women, resulting in the production of milk antibodies. Interestingly, neutralizing activity against *V.*

TABLE 4

Presence of neutralizing antibodies to *V. cholerae* and *E. coli* enterotoxins in human milk

Origin of milk	Neutralization of toxin from:		
	V. cholerae[a]	*E. coli I*[a]	*E. coli II*[a]
Pakistan	1/18	18/18	12/18
Sweden	0/16	1/16	1/16

Method: adrenal cell assay (Donta *et al.* 1974).
[a] 2-5 minimal effective doses of the enterotoxins were used.

cholerae enterotoxin was seen much less frequently (Table 4), indicating both that the anti-*E. coli* enterotoxin activity was specific rather than due to immunological cross-reactivity of cholera toxin antibodies, and that enterotoxigenic *E. coli* are much more common than *V. cholerae* as a 'normal' antigenic stimulus for the Pakistani population (Holmgren *et al.* 1976).

SERUM AND MILK ANTIBODY RESPONSE TO FOOD PROTEINS

The appearance of serum antibodies to food proteins such as cow's milk proteins has long been recognized. Thus Lippard *et al.* (1936) showed antibodies to bovine milk proteins in almost 100% of infants under one year of age who had been fed cow's milk. Investigating sera from healthy children with the ELISA (S. P. Fällström *et al.*, unpublished), we registered antibodies of the IgG and IgA classes to cow's milk proteins in most of the children. Antibodies of the IgE class were very rarely found (Fig. 3 and Table 5) while low levels of IgM antibodies were consistently present. Such findings are in accordance with previous observations (for review see Gerrard 1974). In children with acute gastroenteritis we noted the same levels of antibody to cow's milk proteins as in the healthy controls (Table 5).

Serum antibodies to cow's milk proteins have been shown by many techniques in patients with cow's milk protein intolerance (reviewed by Hanson & Johansson 1970). This has not been useful diagnostically, however, since discrimination from other patients and normals has been poor. Using the ELISA we also found rather variable patterns in infants with cow's milk protein intolerance and gastrointestinal symptoms (Table 5), even though they all had their diagnosis verified by provocation tests twice repeated. Increased levels of IgG, IgA and sometimes of IgE anti-cow's milk protein antibodies were noted in some individuals. However, no consistent antibody increase was found. Children with coeliac disease showed similar patterns to those of

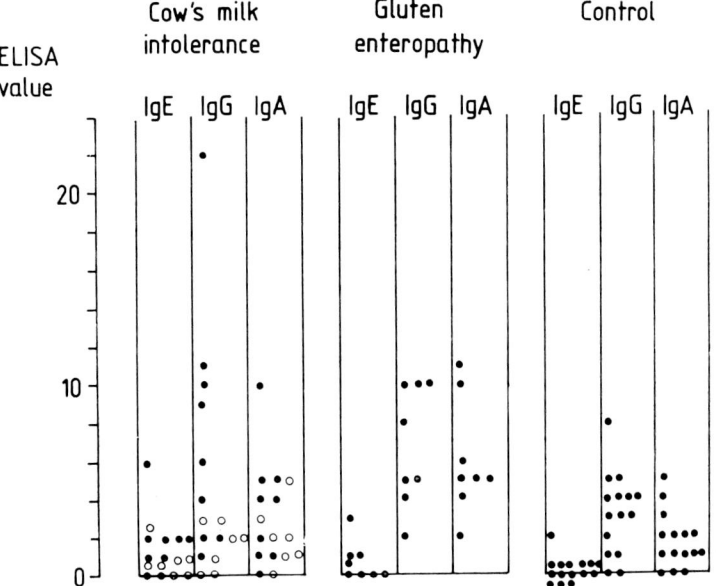

FIG. 3. Antibody levels in serum determined with the enzyme-linked immunoabsorbent assay (ELISA) to cow's milk protein antigens in children with cow's milk protein intolerance or gluten enteropathy and in healthy children. •, chronic disease; o, acute disease.

TABLE 5

Antibodies to cow's milk proteins determined with the enzyme-linked immunoabsorbent assay (ELISA) (median and range)

Protein	Ig	Cow's milk protein intolerance		Gluten enteropathy	Gastroenteritis	Control
		Chronic	Acute			
Cow's	E	1 (0–6)	0 (0–2)	0 (0–3)	0 (0)	0 (0–2)
milk	G	6 (0–22)	2 (0–5)	6.5 (2–10)	4 (1–5)	3 (0–8)
proteins	A	4 (0–10)	2 (0–5)	5 (2–11)	3 (0–7)	1 (0–6)
α-Casein	E	0 (0–2)	0 (0–1)	0.5 (0–2)	0 (0–1)	0 (0–1)
	G	4 (0–10)	3 (1–4)	4 (1–10)	4 (3–5)	3 (0–11)
	A	1 (0–7)	1 (0–2)	4 (1–8)	1 (1–5)	1 (0–4)
β-Casein	E	0 (0)	0 (0–1)	0 (0)	0 (0–1)	0 (0–1)
	G	1.5 (0–5)	3 (0–4)	0.5 (0–3)	1 (1–5)	1.5 (0–5)
	A	1 (0–3)	0 (0–1)	0 (0–2)	3 (1–5)	1 (0–2)
β-Lacto-	E	0 (0)	0 (0)	0 (0)	0 (0–1)	0 (0)
globulin	G	5 (0–6)	4 (1–5)	3.5 (1–5)	2 (1–3)	4 (0–5)
	A	0 (0–2)	0 (0–1)	2.5 (1–5)	1 (0–2)	2 (0–5)

children with cow's milk protein intolerance (S. P. Fällström *et al.*, unpublished), which presumably means that both groups of patients have a defective gut mucosa and perhaps an insufficient local immune response, permitting the penetration of various antigenic molecules. According to our hypothesis that antigenic exposure in the gut is important for antibody formation in the mammary gland, human milk should contain antibodies not only against microbial antigens but also against food material which may come into contact with the intestinal lymphoid tissue. Therefore we analysed human milk for the presence of antibodies to bovine milk proteins with the ELISA. In all 20 samples investigated we found considerable amounts of secretory IgA antibodies against bovine β-lactoglobulin and against α- and β-casein (Fig. 4) (S. P. Fällström *et al.*, unpublished). These studies illustrate the intimate relationship between food constituents and the gut mucosa, where resorption of native proteins may result in stimulation of immunocompetent cells within the Peyer's patches and in more central lymphoid tissues, thus inducing local as well as systemic immune responses (Lippard *et al.* 1936; Sagie *et al.* 1974; Soothill 1976; Walker 1976).

PROTECTIVE EFFECT OF MILK ANTIBODIES

A protective role of the secretory IgA antibodies from human milk detectable as coproantibodies with retained antibody activity in the breast-fed infant (Kenny *et al.* 1967; Gindrat *et al.* 1972) has been indicated against neonatal sepsis/meningitis (Winberg & Wessner 1971) and infantile intestinal infections caused by enteropathogenic species of *E. coli* and by *Shigella* (Mata & Urrutia 1971). Obviously it is a practical arrangement for the mother to provide the baby with secretory IgA antibodies against the enterobacteria she herself has been and is exposed to and which may colonize and eventually infect the neonate. Such protection would be of particular significance in developing areas of the world with undernutrition, because this condition seems linked with a defective first line of defence (Walker 1976).

Secretory IgA antibodies in the gastrointestinal tract probably protect primarily by preventing adhesion of the pathogens or their toxic products to the mucosa (Fubara & Freter 1973; Holmgren *et al.* 1976). Such a function of milk secretory IgA antibodies transferred from the mother to the infant could possibly be one of the determining factors behind the reported lower content of *E. coli* in the intestinal flora of the breast-fed than of the artificially fed infant (Bullen & Willis 1971). On the other hand, the anti-*E. coli* antibodies in milk directed against the O or the K antigens of *E. coli* do not appear to prevent bacterial colonization of the gut of the infant with the respective *E. coli* strains

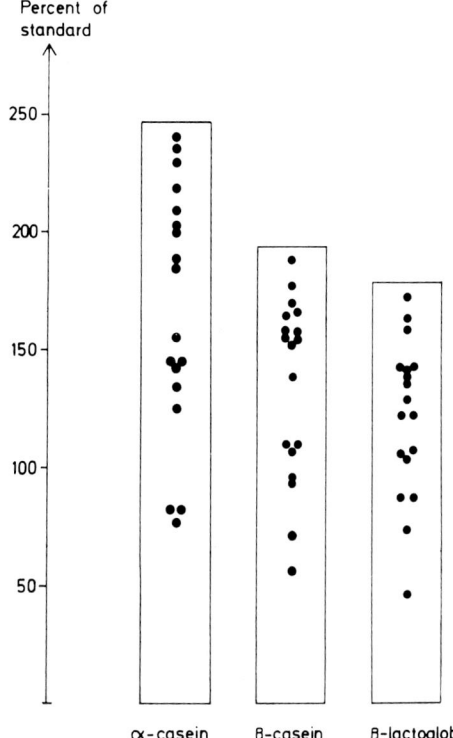

FIG. 4. Levels of antibody to cow's milk protein antigens in human milk from healthy mothers determined with the enzyme-linked immunoabsorbent assay (ELISA).

(Gothefors et al. 1976; B. Carlsson et al., unpublished). It is possible that the antibodies play a role by selecting mutants of relatively low virulence, as suggested by Gothefors et al. (1975) for babies fed with human milk.

That antibodies may induce continuous changes in an exposed bacterial flora has been indicated at the local level for V. cholerae in the mouse gut (Sack & Miller 1969), for V. fetus verseralis in the bovine vagina (Corbeil et al. 1975) and for E. coli in the human urinary tract (Olling et al. 1973; Hanson et al. 1976b,c). Such changes can be detected as variations in bacterial surface characteristics (Sack & Miller 1969; Hanson et al. 1976a,b; Olling et al. 1973; Lindberg et al. 1975b) and possibly by the extent of the symptoms induced by the infection (Lindberg 1975a; Verrier-Jones et al. 1975).

Since it is difficult to measure local secretory IgA antibody production in the gut directly it may be practical to use milk secretory IgA antibodies as a reflection of the antigenic exposure of the gut. Determination of milk secretory

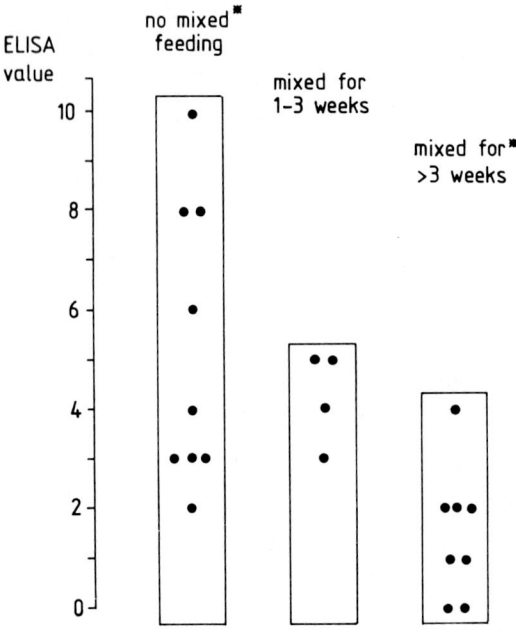

FIG. 5. Influence of breast-milk feeding on the serum IgG antibody response to cow's milk proteins in infants, as determined with the enzyme-linked immunoabsorbent assay (ELISA). *, difference significant at $P > 0.01$.

IgA antibodies may give a picture of the epidemiological situation by showing which microbial antigens have stimulated and are stimulating the antibody response in the gut.

The presence in human milk of antibodies against food antigens such as cow's milk proteins may also be important. These milk secretory IgA antibodies may prevent food allergies by hindering the absorption of the intact food proteins. In accordance with this hypothesis, a lower frequency of gastrointestinal allergies has been observed in children who are fed both breast milk and artificial nutrients as compared to those fed only artificial nutrients (Soothill 1974, 1976). The lower levels of antibodies to cow's milk proteins registered in sera from healthy children given mixed feeding, compared to sera from children given only artificial feeding, fits nicely with the proposed function of secretory IgA antibodies in human milk of preventing the absorption of intact immunogenic/allergenic food constituents (S. P. Fällström et al., in manuscript) (Fig. 5).

ACKNOWLEDGEMENTS

These studies were supported by grants from the Faculty of Medicine, University of Göteborg, the Swedish Medical Research Council (Project No. 215), the Wenner-Gren Foundation and the Ellen, Walter and Lennart Hesselman Foundation for Scientific Research.

References

AHLSTEDT, S. & JODAL, U. (1976) Antibodies against *Escherichia coli* O antigen. Antibody amount and avidities measured with ammonium sulphate precipitation technique. *Int. Arch. Allergy Appl. Immunol.* 50, 164-171

AHLSTEDT, S., HOLMGREN, J. & HANSON, L. Å. (1973) The primary and secondary antibody response to *Escherichia coli* O6 lipopolysaccharide analysed at the humoral and cellular level. Amount and avidity of the antibody in relation to protective capacity. *Immunology* 24, 191-202

AHLSTEDT, S., CARLSSON, B., HANSON, L. Å. & GOLDBLUM, R. G. (1975) Antibody production by human colostral cells. I. Immunoglobulin class, specificity and quantity. *Scand. J. Immunol.* 4, 535-539

ALLARDYCE, R. A., SHEARMAN, D. J. C., MCCLELLAND, D. B. L., MARWICK, K., SIMPSON, A. J. & LAIDLAW, R. B. (1974) Appearance of specific colostrum antibodies after clinical infection with *Salmonella typhimurium*. *Br. Med. J.* 3, 307-309

BULLEN, C. L. & WILLIS, A. T. (1971) Resistance of the breast-fed infant to gastroenteritis. *Br. Med. J.* 3, 338-343

CARLSSON, B., AHLSTEDT, S., HANSON, L. Å., LIDIN-JANSON, G., LINDBLAD, B. S. & SULTANA, R. (1976) *Escherichia coli* O antibody content in milk from healthy Swedish mothers and mothers from a very low socio-economic group of a developing country. *Acta Paediatr. Scand.* 65, 417-423

CORBEIL, L. B., SCHURIG, G. G. D., BIER, P. J. & WINTER, A. J. (1975) Bovine venereal vibriosis: antigenic variation of the bacterium during infection. *Infect. Immun.* 11, 240-244

CRABBÉ, P. A., NASH, D. R., BAZIN, H., EYSSEN, H. & HEREMANS, J. F. (1970) Immunohistochemical observations on lymphoid tissues from conventional and germ-free mice. *Lab. Invest.* 22, 448-457

CRAIG, S. W. & CEBRA, J. J. (1971) Peyer's patches: an enriched source of precursors for IgA-producing immunocytes in the rabbit. *J. Exp. Med.* 134, 188-200

DONTA, S. T., SACK, D. A., WALLACE, R. B., DUPONT, H. L. & SACK, R. B. (1974) Tissue-culture assay of antibodies to heat-labile *Esch. coli* enterotoxins. *N. Engl. J. Med.* 291, 117-121

FUBARA, E. S. & FRETER, R. C. (1973) Protection against enteric bacterial infection by secretory IgA antibodies. *J. Immunol.* 111, 395-403

GERRARD, J. W. (1974) Breast-feeding: second thoughts. *Pediatrics* 54, 757-764

GINDRAT, J.-J., GOTHEFORS, L., HANSON, L. Å. & WINBERG, J. (1972) Antibodies in human milk against *E. coli* of the serogroups most commonly found in neonatal infections. *Acta Paediatr. Scand.* 16, 587-590

GOLDBLUM, R. M., AHLSTEDT, S., CARLSSON, B., HANSON, L. Å., JODAL, U., LIDIN-JANSON, G. & SOHL-ÅKERLUND, A. (1975) Antibody-forming cells in human colostrum after oral immunization. *Nature (Lond.)* 257, 797-799

GOTHEFORS, L., CARLSSON, B , AHLSTEDT, S., HANSON, L. Å. & WINBERG, J. (1976) Influence of maternal gut flora and colostral and cord serum antibodies on presence of *Escherichia coli* in faeces of the newborn infant. *Acta Paediatr. Scand.* 65, 225-232

GOTHEFORS, L., OLLING, S. & WINBERG, J. (1975) Breast feeding and biological properties of faecal *E. coli* strains. *Acta Paediatr. Scand.* 64, 807-812

GRÜNEBERG, R. N., LEI, D. A. & BRUMFITT, W. (1968) *Escherichia coli* serotypes in urinary tract infection: studies in domiciliary antenatal and hospital practice, in *Urinary Tract Infection* (O'Grady, F. & Brumfitt, W., eds.), pp. 68-79, Oxford University Press, London

HANSON, L. Å. & JOHANSSON, B. G. (1970) Immunological studies of milk, in *Milk Proteins, Chemistry and Molecular Biology* (McKenzie, H. A., ed.), vol. I, pp. 45-123, Academic Press, New York

HANSON, L. Å., AHLSTEDT, S., CARLSSON, B., GOLDBLUM, R. M., KAIJSER, B. & LINDBLAD, B. S. (1976a) The antibodies of human milk, their origin and specificity, in *Swedish Nutrition Foundation Symposium XIII, Food and Immunology*, Almqvist & Wiksell International, Stockholm, in press

HANSON, L. Å., AHLSTEDT, S., FASTH, A., JODAL, U., KAIJSER, B., LARSSON, P., LINDBERG, U., OLLING, S., SOHL-ÅKERLUND, A. & SVANBORG-EDÉN, C. (1976b) *E. coli* antigens, human response and the pathogenesis of urinary tract infections, in *Proc. Symposium on Current Status and Prospects for Improved and New Bacterial Vaccines. J. Infect. Dis.* Suppl. in press

HANSON, L. Å., AHLSTEDT, S., GOLDBLUM, R. M., FASTH, A., HOLMGREN, J., JODAL, U., KAIJSER, B., LARSSON, P., LINDBERG, U. & SOHL-ÅKERLUND, A. (1976c) Immunology of the urinary tract infection, in *Third International Congress of Pyelonephritis, London. J Infect. Dis.* Suppl. in press

HOLMGREN, J., HANSON, L. A., CARLSSON, B., LINDBLAD, B. S. & RAHIMTOOLA, J. (1976) Neutralizing antibodies against *E. coli* and *V. cholerae* enterotoxins in human milk from a developing country. *Scand. J. Immunol. 5*, 867-872

HOLMGREN, J., SVENNERHOLM, A. M., OUCHTERLONY, Ö., ANDERSSON, Å., WALLERSTRÖM, G. & WESTERBERG-BERNDTSSON, U. (1975) Antitoxic immunity in experimental cholera protection, and serum and local antibody responses in rabbits after enteral and parenteral immunization. *Infect. Immun. 12*, 1331-1340

JODAL, U., AHLSTEDT, S., HANSON, L. Å., LIDIN-JANSON, G. & SOHL-ÅKERLUND, A. (1976) Intestinal stimulation of the serum antibody response against *Escherichia coli* O83 antigen in healthy adults. *Int. Arch. Allergy Appl. Immunol.*, in press

KAIJSER, B., JODAL, U. & HANSON, L. Å. (1973) Studies on antibody response and tolerance to *E. coli* K antigens in immunized rabbits and in children with urinary tract infection. *Int. Arch. Allergy Appl. Immunol. 44*, 260-273

KAIJSER, B. & OLLING, S. (1973) Experimental hematogenous pyelonephritis due to *Escherichia coli* in rabbits: the antibody response and its protective capacity. *J. Infect. Dis. 128*, 41-49

KENNY, J. F., BOESMAN, M. I. & MICHAELS, R. H. (1967) Bacterial and viral coproantibodies in breast-fed infants. *Pediatrics 39*, 202

LINDBERG, U., HANSON, L. Å., JODAL, U., LIDIN-JANSON, G., LINCOLN, K. & OLLING, S. (1975a) Asymptomatic bacteriuria in school girls. II. Differences in *Escherichia coli* causing asymptomatic bacteriuria. *Acta Paediatr. Scand. 64*, 432-436

LINDBERG, U., JODAL, U., HANSON, L. Å. & KAIJSER, B. (1975b) Asymptomatic bacteriuria in school girls. IV. Difficulties of level diagnosis and the possible relation to the character of infecting bacteria. *Acta Paediatr. Scand. 64*, 574-580

LIPPARD, V. W., SCHLOSS, O. M. & JOHNSON, P. A. (1936) Immune reactions induced in infants by intestinal absorption of incompletely digested cow's milk protein. *Am. Med. Assoc. J. Dis. Child. 51*, 562

LODINOVÁ, R., JONJA, V. & WAGNER, V. (1973) Serum immunoglobulins and coproglobulins and coproantibody formation in infants after artificial intestinal colonization with *Escherichia coli* O83 and oral lysozyme administration. *Pediatr. Res. 7*, 659-669

MATA, L. J. & URRUTIA, J. J. (1971) Intestinal colonization of breast-fed children in a rural area of low socio-economic level. *Ann. N.Y. Acad. Sci. 176*, 93

MONTGOMERY, P. C., ROSNER, B. R. & COHN, J. (1974) The secretory antibody response. Anti-DNP antibodies induced by dinitrophenylated type III pneumococcus. *Immun. Commun. 3*, 143-156

OLLING, S., HANSON, L. Å., HOLMGREN, J., JODAL, U., LINCOLN, K. & LINDBERG, U. (1973)

The bactericidal effect of normal human serum on *E. coli* strains from normals and from patients with urinary tract infections. *Infection 1*, 24-28

PIERCE, N. F. & SACK, R. B. (1976) Studies of the mucosal immune response to cholera toxoid. *J. Infect. Dis.* Suppl., in press

ROBBINS, J. B., MCCRACKEN, G. H., GOTSCHLICH, E. C., ØRSKOV, F., ØRSKOV, I. & HANSON, L. Å. (1974) *Escherichia coli* K-1 capsular polysaccharide associated with neonatal meningitis. *N. Engl. J. Med. 290*, 1216-1220

SACK, B. R. & MILLER, C. E. (1969) Progressive changes of vibrio serotypes in germ-free mice infected with *Vibrio cholerae*. *J. Bacteriol. 99*, 688-695

SAGIE, E., TARABULUS, J., MAEIR, D. M. & FREIER, S. (1974) Diet and development of intestinal IgA in the mouse. *Israel J. Med. Sci. 10*, 532-534

SIRISINHA, S., SUSKIND, R., EDELMAN, R., ASVAPAKA, C. & OLSON, R. E. (1974) Secretory and serum IgA in children with protein-calorie malnutrition, in *The Immunoglobulin A System* (Mestecky J. & Lawton, A. R., eds.) (*Adv. Exp. Med. Biol. 45*) pp. 389-398, Plenum Press, New York

SOOTHILL, J. F. (1974) Immunodeficiency and allergy. *Clin. Allergy 3* (Suppl.), 511-513.

SOOTHILL, J. F. (1976) Immunodeficiency, allergy and infant feeding, in *Swedish Nutrition Foundation Symposium XIII, Food and Immunology*, Almqvist & Wiksell International, Stockholm, in press

SVENNERHOLM, A. M. & HOLMGREN, J. (1976) Immunoglobulin and antibody synthesis *in vitro* by enteral and nonenteral lymphoid tissues after subcutaneous cholera immunization. *Infect. Immun.*, in press

VERRIER-JONES, E. R., MELLER, S. T., MCLACHLAN, M. S. F., SUSSMAN, M., ASSCHER, A. W., MAYON-WHITE, R. T., LEDINGHAM, J. G. G., SMITH, J. C., FLETCHER, E. W. L., SMITH, E. H., JOHNSTON, H. H. & SLEIGHT, G. (1975) Treatment of bacteruria in schoolgirls. *Kidney International 8*, S85-S89

WALKER, W. A. (1976) Host defense mechanisms in the gastrointestinal tract. *Pediatrics*, in press

WALKER, W. A., ISSELBACHER, K. J. & BLOCH, K. J. (1972) Intestinal uptake of macromolecules: effect of oral immunization. *Science (Wash. D.C.) 177*, 608-610

WALKER, W. A., ISSELBACHER, K. J. & BLOCH, K. J. (1974a) The role of immunization in controlling antigen uptake from the small intestine, in *The Immunoglobulin A System* (Mestecky, J. & Lawton, A. R., eds.) (*Adv. Exp. Med. Biol. 45*), pp. 295-303, Plenum Press, New York

WALKER, W. A., ISSELBACHER, K. J. & BLOCH, K. J. (1974b) Immunologic control of soluble protein absorption from the small intestine: a gut-surface problem. *Am. J. Clin. Nutr. 27*, 1434-1440

WALKER, W. A., WU, M., ISSELBACHER, K. J. & BLOCH, K. J. (1975) Intestinal uptake of macromolecules. III. Studies on the mechanism by which immunization interferes with antigen uptake. *J. Immunol. 115*, 854-861

WINBERG, J. & WESSNER, G. (1971) Does breast milk protect against septicaemia in the newborn? *Lancet I*, 1091-1094

Discussion

Porter: Your thesis was very nicely demonstrated by the work of Professor Bohl on pigs (Bohl *et al.* 1972). He has been interested in the transmissible gastroenteritis (TGE) virus. He found that sows that had suffered an enteric infection with TGE virus generated IgA antibodies in the colostrum and milk which subsequently gave solid protection of the neonate against deliberate infection with that virus, whereas sows that had been parenterally immunized with an attenuated virus developed IgG antibody which did not give solid protection in the neonate.

The IgA antibody demonstrated by Bohl was quite unassociated with serum antibody in the sow, so it was clear that there must have been a traffic of cells from the gut to the mammary gland to produce there locally the IgA which protected the neonate. In that respect, this work gives credence to your overall philosophy on this protective function.

Brandtzaeg: Haneberg (1974) has shown that it is probably only during the first month that colostral IgA antibodies survive passage through the gut of the infant. Do you have any ideas about this, Dr Ahlstedt?

Ahlstedt: Most studies dealing with antibodies in human colostrum and milk have been done on samples taken within a month after parturition. The protective capacity of the antibodies in this milk has been indicated but is not proved. Further, the protective effect of the antibodies in relation to that of other factors in the milk has to be established. If the antibodies are not of protective value for the infant after one month of age, why are they present in the milk? To protect the breast? But why then the close relation between antigenic exposure of the gut and antibodies in the milk?

Pierce: Survival of IgA through the gut may depend in part upon inhibition of gastric acid secretion. This inhibition occurs during the first few months of life in suckling children but not in children fed cow's milk (Maffei & Nobrega 1975), which suggests that either the suckling process or a component of the mother's milk is responsible. Inhibition of acid secretion would protect IgA from acid pepsin degradation.

Brandtzaeg: This shows up in the pH of the faeces of breast-fed children.

Pierce: The pH of the faeces reflects events that take place in the small intestine and colon, particularly lactose degradation. Faecal pH is not necessarily a direct reflection of what happened in the stomach.

Porter: On this point about the survival of IgA in the gut, in relation to whether gastric enzymes develop or not, the pig is a good model for the human infant!

We studied the passage of anti-*E. coli* IgA antibodies along the intestine in piglets fed sow's milk (Porter *et al.* 1970). The way the IgA separates from the milk clot in the stomach and passes into the small intestine and the speed at which this happens assists in the antibody activity in the gut. Within five minutes of feeding the milk the IgA appears in the duodenum, and it passes through the small intestine and appears in the ileum within one hour, so that the whole processes takes about ninety minutes. The piglet feeds about once every ninety minutes, so one has a fast passage of IgA and a continuous coating of maternal antibody. Going back to Bohl's observations, it is particularly interesting that where he took milk from sows immunized by the gut route with TGE virus and subsequently infected the neonate with the virus, he got total protection, with no pathological effects in the gut. When he fed milk from sows in which IgG antibody was present he found a massive degeneration in the mucosa of the neonate but the first yard of the intestine appeared to be protected, as though the IgG survived that far and thereafter protection was absent. It looks as if, in this species at least, IgA has physiological features that support the local maternal defence of the mucosa. I would suspect it is probably similar in the human.

André: We have some preliminary results that are relevant. We immunized pregnant guinea pigs by the oral route with sheep red cells on the day of parturition. IgA against sheep red cells was found in the milk ten days later. The newborn guinea pigs were fed with this milk. One or two months later they were injected with sheep red cells and compared to controls. Their response was markedly decreased (C. André, unpublished work 1975).

Lachmann: If you immunize into the mammary gland do you get a rise in IgA antibody in the gut?

André: We haven't tried this.

Pierce: Dr Ahlstedt, have you examined the morphology of the cells in milk which presumably contain or secrete IgA? Do they look like plasma cells or immunoblasts?

Ahlstedt: We have tried to study the morphology of the cells, but it is difficult to obtain good samples to examine. However, we do know that we have antibody specificity in the plaques, which indicates that the cells are of B cell type, probably plasma cells, and not epithelium cells.

Gowans: How do the cells reach the colostrum? What is the route they take from the capillaries to the acini?

Pepys: The mammary gland during lactation is not a nicely organized exocrine gland. It is an apocrine gland with shedding of cell fragments and whole cells, including lymphocytes, polymorphs and epithelial cells.

Evans: There are not many polymorphs in the interstitium of the lactating mammary gland, surely?

Soothill: We have certainly found both polymorphs and macrophages in human milk. How they get there, we don't know.

Cebra: I wonder if there is any contradiction between Dr Gowans' finding that secretory component does not bind to IgA immunoblasts and your being able to facilitate plaque formation by plasma cells in the milk with anti-SC. Is this just a matter of the stage in maturation of the IgA-secreting cells? Presumably the plasma cells have to obtain secretory component from outside sources, since they don't make it?

Ahlstedt: I don't know the stage in maturation since we haven't been able to do morphological studies, as I said. On the formation of *secretory* IgA plaques, we know that there is antigenic specificity in the plaque, indicating that the centrum cell is a plasma cell *making* IgA and not an epithelium cell *releasing* secretory IgA. However, we cannot exclude that the antibody coming out of the plasma cell takes up secretory component formed by an epithelium cell nearby and becomes a secretory IgA antibody, absorbing on to the red cell coated with antigen and picking up the developing anti-secretory component antiserum. I think we have epithelium cells present, since we have not found a good way of getting rid of them.

When culturing the milk cells we have found that the binding between the IgA molecule and the secretory component is very strong, confirming the findings of Dr Brandtzaeg. Further, the cultured cells produce dimeric secre-

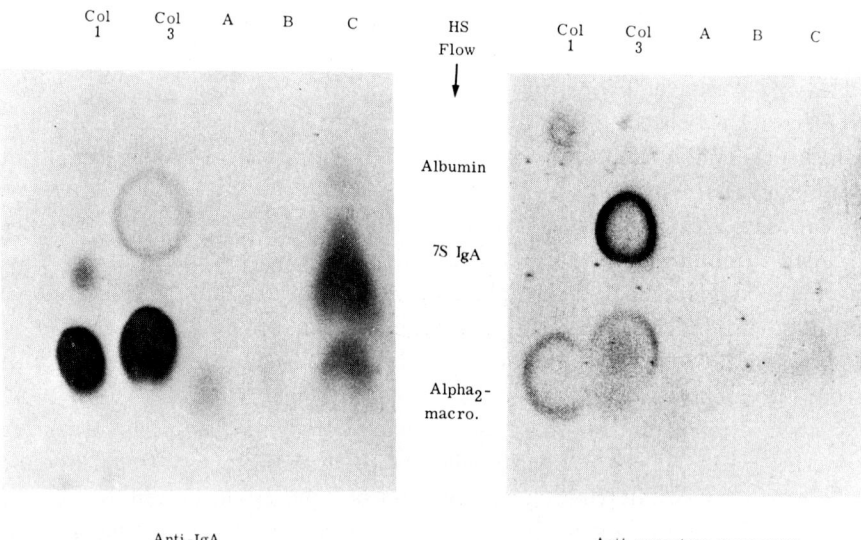

FIG. 1. (Ahlstedt). Thin layer immuno-gel filtration, using Sephadex G-200 superfine, of the supernatants A, B and C from 5-day cultures of IgA-producing cells from colostrum obtained two days *post partum*. Cols. 1 and 3 are colostrum obtained one and three days *post partum* from another woman. Comparison of these patterns shows that all five samples contain protein of the size of secretory IgA (heavily stained on the left and large rings on the right in Cols. 1 and 3). Although the colostrum samples contain fragments of IgA as well as secretory component filtering more slowly than secretory IgA, there are no indications that the secretory component was released from the IgA in the culture supernatants during the filtration. The filtration positions of some human serum proteins are indicated (centre). Cultures A and B contained 10^6 cells/ml and C, 3.9×10^6 cells/ml.

tory IgA, very little free secretory component and monomeric IgA. When a sample from a culture was run using the immuno-gel filtration method of Hanson *et al.* (1971) we found very little separation of the formed secretory IgA during filtration (Fig. 1). The secretory component of small molecular size demonstrable in Col. 1 in the figure is not seen in preparation C, although IgA in a similar filtration region was demonstrated in both Col. 1 and in preparation C.

Lachmann: You showed us that you do not get asymmetric overlapping plaques when you develop with antiserum to SC but that you get perfectly round plaques. Presumably this is because there is secretory piece everywhere. Might you not have expected that if you need cooperation between two cells making different components to obtain a plaque the plaques would be asymmetrical?

Ahlstedt: If we have two cells, one making IgA antibodies, which then attach to the antigen-coated red cells and pick up the secretory component formed by the other cell, perhaps the plaque would be somewhat askew, but probably not very much.

Lachmann: I would have expected that in some circumstances you would get haemolysis on one side only.

Ahlstedt: The diffusion rate of the secretory component is rather rapid and the distances are small between cells of varying types, giving a high probability for an even distribution of the secretory component.

Bienenstock: The problem of whether dimeric IgA has a selective transport advantage was briefly mentioned by Dr Brandtzaeg. The question of whether it really has, and whether the antibodies synthesized in the bowel, presumably circulating, can be selectively transported out into the secretions, is one on which I know of no direct evidence in man. The problem is that man has monomeric IgA, primarily in serum, and also dimeric IgA, primarily in secretions. Many animal species have dimeric IgA in the serum, and many people have shown transport advantages for IgA in the serum going out into the secretions. One of the continuing problems is why in man one has primarily monomeric IgA in the serum, and what that is due to, and whether dimeric IgA has a selective transport advantage from the serum into the gastrointestinal and other glandular secretions.

Brandtzaeg: According to Heremans' (1974) calculations, the level of dimeric IgA in human serum is about the same as the level in dog serum.

Vaerman: That study has been criticized by Rádl *et al.* (1975). It was previously said that there is about 10% polymeric IgA in normal human serum, but they now find that it is as low as perhaps 1%. They used three criteria to say that there were very few true polymers in serum, but rather some aggregates. These aggregates were not J-chain-containing, they did not bind secretory component, and thirdly they lacked a 'configurational polymeric' antigenic determinant. So we may have to revise our estimates.

References

BOHL, E. H., GUPTA, R. K. P., OLGUIN, M. U. F. & SAIF, L. J. (1972) Antibody responses in serum, colostrum and milk of swine after injection or vaccination with transmissible gastroenteritis virus. *Infect. Immun. 6*, 289-301

HANEBERG, B. (1974) Immunoglobulins in feces from infants fed human or bovine milk. *Scand. J. Immunol. 3*, 191-197

HANSON, L. Å., HOLMGREN, J. & WADSWORTH, C. (1971) A radial immuno-gel filtration method for characterization and quantitation of macromolecules. *Int. Arch. Allergy Appl. Immunol. 40*, 806-814

HEREMANS, J. F. (1974) Immunoglobulin A, in *The Antigens*, vol. 2 (Sela, M., ed.), p. 450, Academic Press, London

MAFFEI, H. V. L. & NOBREGA, F. J. (1975) Gastric pH and microflora of normal and diarrhoeic infants. *Gut 16*, 719-726

PORTER, P., NOAKES, D. E. & ALLEN, W. D. (1970) Secretory IgA and antibodies to *E. coli* in porcine colostrum and milk and their significance in the alimentary tract of the young pig. *Immunology 18*, 245-257

RÁDL, J., SWART, A. C. & MESTECKY, J. (1975) The nature of the polymeric serum IgA in man. *Proc. Soc. Exp. Biol. Med. 150*, 482-484

Immunological responses to bacterial plaque in the mouth

T. LEHNER

Department of Oral Immunology and Microbiology, Guy's Hospital Medical and Dental Schools, London

Abstract A heavy load of bacteria, referred to as dental plaque, accumulates at the junction between the teeth and gum. Bacterial plaque may be considered to have three functional components: (*a*) cariogenic organisms, (*b*) organisms inducing gingival inflammation and periodontal disease, and (*c*) adjuvant and tolerizing agents, such as lipopolysaccharides, dextrans and levans. Sequential investigation of plaque accumulation in man has shown a correlation between gingival inflammation and both lymphocyte transformation and macrophage migration inhibition. An adjuvant effect of *in vivo* plaque accumulation was manifested by the enhancement of T lymphocytes in the mixed leucocyte culture reaction and of B lymphocytes, as shown by the increased response to lipopolysaccharide. It may be significant that a substantial component of bacterial plaque consists of dextrans and levans, produced by certain streptococci and actinomyces, and lipopolysaccharides from Gram-negative bacteria. These bacterial products are B cell mitogens which may have an adjuvant or tolerizing effect on immune responses. The relationships between immunogenicity, mitogenicity, adjuvanticity and tolerogenicity of lipopolysaccharides, levan and dextran have not been clearly defined. However, important variables of the polyglycans are the molecular weight, type of branching, negative charge, epitope density, degradability, dosage and the sequence between mitogen and antigen. Dental plaque in man is a focus of B cell mitogens and T cell antigens which may modulate the immune responses in such a way as to induce a protective response in the development of caries and a damaging response in periodontal disease.

A heavy load of bacteria, referred to as dental plaque, may accumulate at the junction between the teeth and gum, containing 2.5×10^7 aerobic and 4.6×10^7 anaerobic organisms per mg of plaque (Gibbons *et al.* 1964). Bacterial plaque accumulates under the influence of a fine consistency, largely roughage-free diet, with a high content of refined sugars, prevalent in countries with Western dietary practices. The development of daily oral hygiene measures has attempted to limit the accumulation of dental bacterial plaque. If oral hygiene is deliberately not practiced, up to 50 mg of removable bacterial plaque will accumulate on the teeth and influence the immune responses to oral bacteria (Lehner *et al.* 1974*a*).

Dental plaque is deposited on the teeth, adjacent to the crevicular epithelium which is supplied by blood vessels possibly of the post-capillary venule type (Egelberg 1966) and through which passes a constant traffic of neutrophils, lymphocytes and monocytes (Attström & Egelberg 1970; Skapski & Lehner 1976). A conservative estimate of the total surface area of crevicular epithelium round 28 teeth is of the order of 760 mm^2 and this can increase up to about 7600 mm^2 in periodontal disease (Arne 1963). It is therefore evident that dental plaque, consisting of bacteria and their products, of which lipopolysaccharides (LPS; Mergenhagen *et al.* 1961), dextrans and levans (Wood 1967) are most important, is found adjacent to an extensive epithelial surface. This can be penetrated by bacterial products, as was shown by autoradiography after the application of tritiated LPS to the gingival sulci of dogs (Schwartz *et al.* 1972).

Bacterial plaque may be considered to have three functional components: (*a*) cariogenic organisms, of which *Streptococcus mutans*, *Lactobacilli* and *Actinomyces* are most important; (*b*) organisms inducing gingivitis and periodontitis, such as *Veillonella*, *Fusobacteria*, *Bacteroides* and *Actinomyces*; and (*c*) adjuvant and tolerizing agents, the most potent being lipopolysaccharides (Johnson *et al.* 1956), dextrans (Battisto & Pappas 1973; Howard *et al.* 1975) and levans (Miranda *et al.* 1972). The interaction of bacteria with the adjuvants and tolerizing agents in plaque may induce immune responses which could inhibit or enhance the development of caries and periodontal disease.

In this paper the results of studies on cell-mediated immune (CMI) responses to oral bacteria and their products will be discussed, with particular reference to the modulating effect of *in vivo* bacterial plaque on the *in vitro* CMI functions and their relationship to the disease indices of caries and gingival inflammation in man.

LYMPHOPROLIFERATIVE RESPONSES TO PLAQUE ORGANISMS

Peripheral blood lymphocytes in man are sensitized to dental plaque antigens and there is a significant correlation between the degree of lymphocyte stimulation and the periodontal index (Ivanyi & Lehner 1971; Horton *et al.* 1972*a*). A corresponding sensitization of lymphocytes to the following plaque bacteria has been shown: *Veillonella alcalescens*, *Actinomyces viscosus*, *Bacteroides melaninogenicus* and *Fusobacterium fusiforme* (Ivanyi & Lehner 1970). It appears that plaque bacteria can be chemically altered into mitogens, for when alkali-treated organisms were used to stimulate lymphocytes there was no differentiation between the proliferative response of lymphocytes from controls and patients with periodontal disease and some of the altered bacterial antigens induced greater stimulation than phytohaemagglutinin (Kiger et al. 1974).

The cells responding to plaque antigens are both T and B lymphocytes (Mackler et al. 1974) and this may be accounted for by the finding that protein antigens of *Veillonella* stimulate T lymphocytes, whereas the lipopolysaccharide from *Veillonella* elicits a response only in B lymphocytes (Ivanyi & Lehner 1974).

LYMPHOPROLIFERATIVE RESPONSES INDUCED BY B CELL MITOGENS

Lipopolysaccharides, dextrans and levans are mitogens which activate a broad spectrum of B lymphocytes (Gery et al. 1972; Greaves & Janossy 1972; Andersson et al. 1972; Coutinho & Möller 1973). These polymers are found in large amounts in dental plaque; lipopolysaccharides from Gram-negative bacteria, dextran synthesized by *Strep. mutans* and *sanguis* and levan formed by *Strep. salivarius* and *Actinomyces viscosus*. They induce a low but significant lymphoproliferative response in B lymphocytes in man (Ivanyi & Lehner 1974) and do not seem to be inhibited by the serum inhibitory factor in severe periodontitis. Levan induced the highest stimulation of lymphocytes, with a mean of 4.2 (± 0.7), followed by LPS (2.6 $\pm$ 0.5) and dextran (2.3 $\pm$ 0.3). Lymphocyte stimulation induced by levan and LPS was significantly increased in gingival and periodontal disease, as compared with controls ($P < 0.05$–0.01). However, the optimal doses were highest for levan (500 μg per ml of culture), followed by dextran (50 μg) and LPS (10 μg).

MODULATING FACTORS IN SERUM

Lymphocyte activity can be modulated *in vitro* by serum factors, by stimulating or inhibitory antibodies, or their immune complexes. Activation of lymphocytes by *Veillonella* seems to depend not only on the presence of sensitized lymphocytes but also on stimulating factors present in sera from patients with gingivitis or mild and moderate periodontitis (Ivanyi et al. 1973). A depression of lymphocyte transformation, in the presence of autologous serum from patients with severe periodontitis, has been ascribed to a serum inhibitory factor (Ivanyi et al. 1973). The response of these lymphocytes, however, can be restored by substituting autologous for homologous serum from patients with gingivitis or moderate periodontitis. These results can be interpreted by assuming that blocking antibodies on the surface of lymphocytes might be counteracted by deblocking antibodies, as is found in tumours (Hellström & Hellström 1970).

SOLUBLE MEDIATORS

Sensitized lymphocytes release macrophage migration inhibition factor (MIF; Ivanyi et al. 1972) which might serve to localize macrophages at the site of antigenic activation of lymphocytes. Furthermore, an osteoclast-activating factor is produced and this can cause bone resorption, as measured by the release of ^{45}Ca from fetal rat bone (Horton et al. 1972b).

CYTOTOXIC MECHANISMS

A cytotoxic assay has been described in which specific activation of sensitized lymphocytes causes non-specific cytotoxicity of target cells *in vitro* (Ivanyi et al. 1972). This mechanism is antibody-independent and probably different from lymphotoxin, which is released by lymphocytes and damages fibroblasts (Horton et al. 1973). Activated lymphocytes can thus damage fibroblasts and other cells and can cause destruction of the supporting bone. Antibody-dependent cytotoxicity by K cells has not yet been described in periodontal disease.

THE ROLE OF MACROPHAGES

Macrophages can be localized to the site of microbial attack by chemotaxis and by the release of MIF and chemotactic factor from lymphocytes, and they may take part in several functions. The cells are essential for the induction of an immune response and for lymphocyte differentiation and proliferation *in vitro* (Sjöberg et al. 1972). Removal of macrophages may impair T lymphocyte stimulation by *Veillonella* antigens and B lymphocyte stimulation by lipopolysaccharides, levan and dextran (Ivanyi & Lehner 1974).

Macrophages may play an important part in adjuvanticity, because bacterial adjuvants induce the formation of macrophage granulomata (Suter & White 1954), macrophage chemotactic factors (Wilkinson et al. 1973), sequestration of lymphocytes in lymphoid tissues, which appears to be macrophage dependent (Frost & Lance 1973), and the increased antibody formation resulting from transferring macrophages, containing adjuvant and antigen, to syngeneic mice (Allison 1973). Tolerance to T-dependent antigens induced by B cell mitogens might be mediated by macrophages (Ivanyi 1976), for the suppressive effect of LPS or levan on T cell proliferation induced by *Veillonella* or PPD is mediated by the interactions of LPS and levan with macrophages.

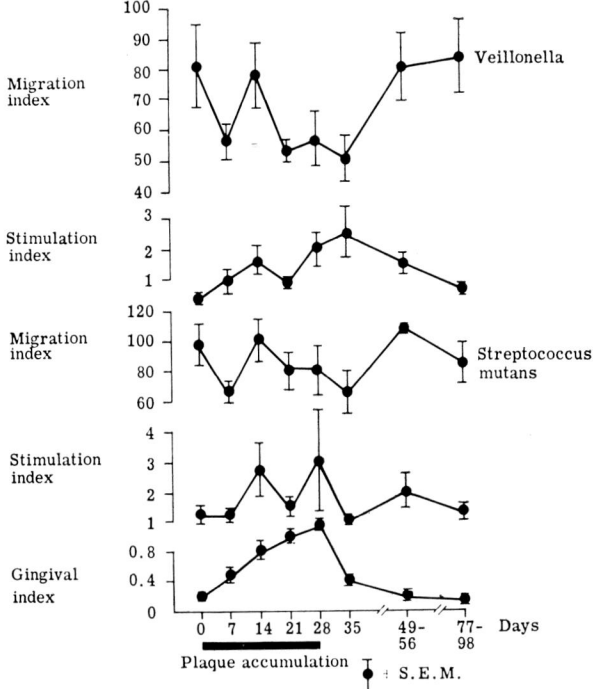

FIG. 1. Sequential cell-mediated immunity to *Streptococcus mutans* and *Veillonella alcalescens* induced by accumulation of bacterial plaque.

Dental plaque or endotoxin may stimulate macrophages directly to synthesize and release lysosomal hydrolases (Page *et al.* 1973). Activation of guinea-pig macrophages by endotoxin, however, requires B lymphocytes (Wilton *et al.* 1975). There is now evidence that endotoxin exerts a direct effect on macrophages, stimulating them to synthesize collagenase, though soluble mediators from B lymphocytes may enhance this response (Mergenhagen *et al.* 1976). The acid hydrolases and collagenase may be responsible for much of the tissue damage in periodontal disease.

SEQUENTIAL IMMUNE RESPONSES IN EXPERIMENTAL GINGIVITIS IN MAN

Sequential changes in CMI responses were examined in young healthy subjects who abstained from oral hygiene for 28 days, to find out whether the cellular responses were closely related to the clinical changes, or whether they were a consequence of long-standing bacterial stimulation (Lehner *et al.* 1974*a*). Accumulation of dental bacterial plaque and the associated gingival inflammation were correlated with an increase in lymphocyte transformation and release of MIF (Fig. 1). These were induced by sonicates of autologous bacterial plaque, a number of Gram-negative organisms, *A. viscosus*, and some unrelated antigens. Both cellular responses were of limited duration and had returned to base-line values 28 days after plaque was removed. The close temporal relationship between CMI and gingivitis suggests the following sequence: accumulation of a heavy antigenic load induces CMI responses which lead to the gingival inflammation and later periodontal destruction. This is substantiated by the evidence from the use of immunosuppressive and immunopotentiating drugs (see below, p. 146).

IMMUNOPOTENTIATION BY DENTAL PLAQUE IN VIVO

The possibility that dental plaque may exert an adjuvant effect *in vivo* has been raised on the basis that an increase in DNA synthesis and release of MIF by lymphocytes can be induced *in vitro* not only by related antigens but also by such unrelated stimulants as the mixed leucocyte culture reaction (MLC) and purified protein derivative of tuberculin (PPD) (Fig. 2; Lehner *et al.* 1974*a,b*). Although purified cell preparations were not examined, both T and B lymphocyte functions were enhanced in the subjects who had accumulated plaque for 28 days, as tested by the MLC reaction for T lymphocytes (Johnston & Wilson 1970) and lipopolysaccharide activation for B lymphocytes (Ivanyi & Lehner 1974). There was no detectable increase in antibody titres to the plaque bacteria but an increase in serum immunoglobulins was found. This is consistent with the view that LPS, dextran and levan act as polyclonal B cell activators (Coutinho & Möller 1973). It should, however, be noted that whereas immunogenicity and tolerogenicity to levan are dependent on macrophages and epitope density, this is not so with mitogenicity (Desaymard & Ivanyi 1976).

In view of these findings, it has been suggested that dental plaque may act as an endogenous adjuvant acting on both T and B lymphocytes. Among a multitude of antigens in dental plaque, lipopolysaccharides (Johnson *et al.* 1956) from Gram-negative bacteria, and dextran (Battisto & Pappas 1973) synthesized by *Strep. mutans* and *Strep. sanguis* have adjuvant properties. Dextran given to mice enhances the responses of lymphoid cells both to T-dependent (Concanavalin A) and T-independent mitogens (LPS; Alevy & Battisto 1976*a*). This is comparable to the enhanced responses of lymphocytes in man in the T-dependent (MLC) and T-independent (LPS) reactions induced by bacterial plaque accumulation *in vivo* (Lehner *et al.* 1974*b*). It is suggested that dextrans and other B cell mitogens found in dental plaque have a comparable function in man to that of dextran injected into mice. The proliferative response of human lymphocytes by *Veillonella* has been also potentiated *in vitro* by levan and LPS (Ivanyi 1976). The enhanced responses are mediated

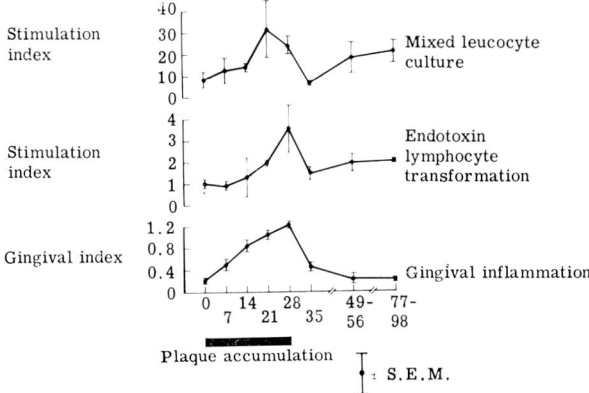

FIG. 2. Sequential responses of T and B lymphocytes in the mixed leucocyte culture reaction and to endotoxin induced by accumulation of bacterial plaque.

through soluble factors elaborated by T lymphocytes and some affect T cells and others, B cells; corresponding receptors are found on thymus cells and bone marrow cells, respectively (Alevy & Battisto 1976b). A similar but non-specific factor derived from T cells has been described in relation to LPS (Waldmann & Munro 1975).

Considerable quantities of LPS, dextran and levan are found in dental plaque and they may be responsible for the predominant B lymphocyte proliferation, resulting in plasma cells, in gingivitis. The relationship between mitogenicity and adjuvanticity has not been clarified, as LPS and dextran induce proliferation of B cells (Andersson et al. 1972; Coutinho & Möller 1973; Ivanyi & Lehner 1974) and yet the adjuvant effect may be T-cell dependent (Allison & Davies 1971; Battisto & Pappas 1974).

The mechanism of action of adjuvants is complex but four points need to be emphasized in relation to dental plaque. (a) The persistence of dental plaque along the gingival margin enables LPS, dextran and levan to be released continuously over an extensive epithelial surface. (b) Dental plaque or LPS are potent agents causing release of lysosomal hydrolases from macrophages and these may be involved in the action of adjuvants (Page et al. 1973; Spitznagel & Allison 1970). (c) In order for dextran to potentiate immune responses (Diamantstein & Blitstein-Willinger 1975) and to activate the alternative pathway of complement (Hadding et al. 1973), it must be negatively charged. Indeed, sulphated macromolecules are found in dental plaque, some of which are sulphated glycoproteins (Baumhammers & Stallard 1966; Rolla et al. 1975). Negatively charged polysaccharides can be formed by Strep. mutans and

Strep. sanguis which incorporate labelled phosphate into soluble and insoluble high molecular weight polysaccharides (Melvaer *et al.* 1974). In addition to the negative charge of dextrans which may be necessary for adjuvanticity, the α1–3, α1–6 and α1–4 linkages may influence their adjuvanticity, especially as the α1–3 linked dextran is resistant to degradation and is slowly metabolized. (*d*) Recruitment and proliferation of immunocompetent cells both in the gingival mononuclear cell infiltration and the draining lymph nodes may follow exposure to high local concentrations of antigens.

FUNCTIONAL RELATIONSHIP BETWEEN IMMUNOPOTENTIATION BY PLAQUE AND THE EFFECT ON CARIES AND GINGIVITIS

Increasing the load of oral microorganisms and their products by allowing plaque to accumulate has led to an enhanced lymphoproliferative response stimulated by *Veillonella*, which can be considered as a representative organism in the development of gingivitis, and by *Strep. mutans*, which is a principal cariogenic organism. Bacterial plaque was allowed to accumulate on the teeth of young healthy subjects for 28 days by abstention from any oral cleansing.

The proliferative response of lymphocytes to *Strep. mutans* and *Veillonella* was determined and the stimulation indices (SI) were plotted against each subject's 'decayed, missing and filled' caries index (DMF) and gingival index (GI) before and during plaque accumulation (Lehner *et al.* 1976a; Figs. 3 and 4). All but two of the SI before plaque accumulation were less than 2 and all the GI were less than 0.4, so that these could not be correlated. However, with plaque accumulation the SI of lymphocytes induced by the oral organisms increased and showed a negative correlation with the DMF and a positive correlation with the GI (Figs. 1 and 2). Significant negative correlations between the SI ($\log_{10}$) and the DMF index was found with *Strep. mutans* ($P < 0.01$) and *Veillonella* ($P < 0.05$). In the analysis of SI against GI the positive correlations with *Veillonella* also reached a significant level ($P < 0.02$).

It seems that the immunopotentiating effect of bacterial plaque may not only act as a polyclonal mitogen, but that the increase in the mitogenic response of lymphocytes may be governed by previous sensitization to the bacterial antigens. Thus, polyclonal activators might recall the immunological memory for a variety of antigens and these bear a functional relationship to the relevant diseases. A positive correlation of the SI of lymphocytes with the gingival index of inflammation is consistent with other features associating CMI with a damaging effect on the gingiva. The negative correlation between the response of lymphocytes to *Strep. mutans* and the DMF suggests a protective relationship between CMI and caries; it is similar to that between serum antibodies and

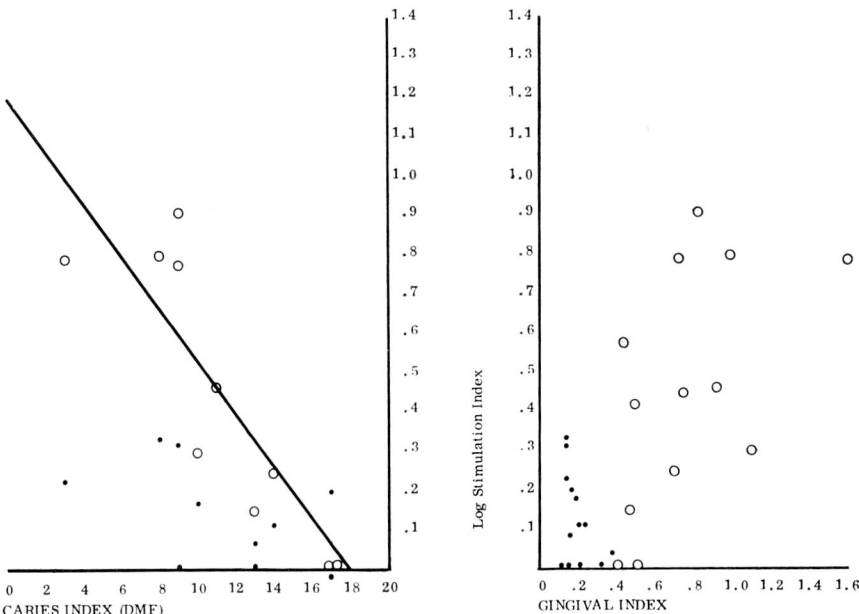

FIG. 3. Relationship between the stimulation indices of lymphocytes to *Streptococcus mutans* and the caries and gingival indices before (•) and during (o) plaque accumulation.

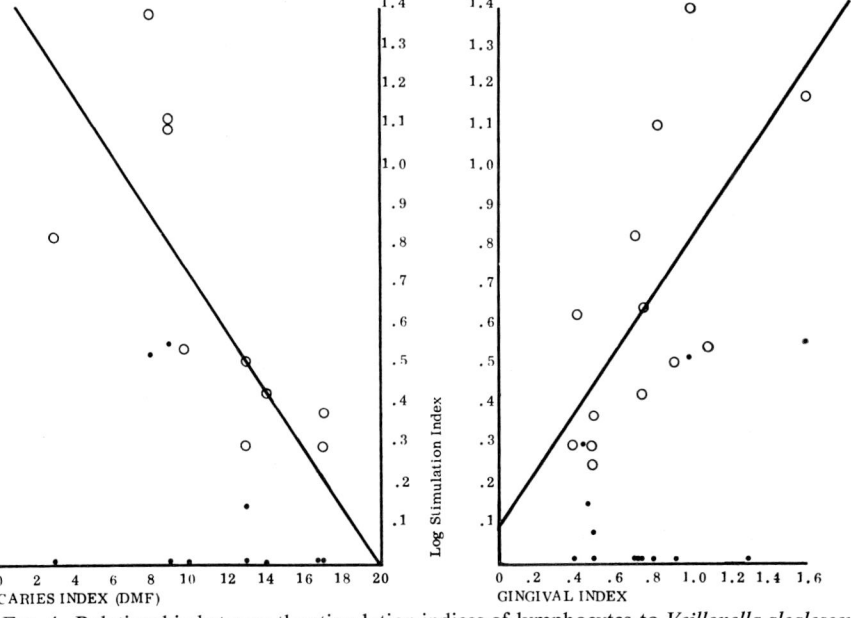

FIG. 4. Relationship between the stimulation indices of lymphocytes to *Veillonella alcalescens* and the caries and gingival indices before (•) and during (o) plaque accumulation.

DMF (Challacombe et al. 1973; Challacombe 1974; Challacombe & Lehner 1976), so that the lower the caries index, the higher are the serum antibody titres and responses of lymphocytes. Furthermore, a significant increase in lymphocyte proliferation and serum antibodies to *Strep. mutans* is found in monkeys immunized against dental caries (Lehner et al. 1976b). The CMI to cariogenic bacteria is recalled only under the immunopotentiating conditions of bacterial plaque and this might be a measure of the protective potential of the subject against dental caries. That the immunological recall may have some specificity is suggested by a lack of relationship between the proliferative response to PPD or PHA and the DMF and GI.

THE EFFECT OF BACTERIAL PLAQUE ON IMMUNOLOGICAL MEMORY

To test the hypothesis that dental bacterial plaque *in vivo* may both potentiate and recall previous sensitization to microorganisms, the plaque accumulation experiment was repeated in five subjects 210 days after plaque was removed and good oral hygiene reinstituted (Lehner et al. 1976a). Significant lymphocyte transformation was found earlier, it was greater in magnitude and it lasted longer in the second as compared with the first plaque accumulation experiment (Fig. 5). These immunological features are usually ascribed to secondary antibody responses, or to enhancement of an existing immune state. It suggests that bacterial plaque *in vivo* can induce a recall of immunological memory for plaque antigens on the cellular level. It is not clear at present whether this is a measure of T or B lymphocyte memory, but both might be involved, since pooled dental plaque and *Veillonella* specifically can stimulate T and B lymphocytes to undergo transformation into blast cells (Mackler et al. 1974; Ivanyi & Lehner 1974), though *Strep. mutans* seems to stimulate only T lymphocytes (unpublished obervations). It must be assumed that however good the oral hygiene might be, a small amount of dental plaque is always present from the time of eruption of the teeth—that is, from about four months of age. Indeed, there is now evidence that sensitization of fetal lymphocytes to plaque antigens might take place *in utero* in women with periodontal disease (Horton et al. 1976). Cord blood lymphocytes from these infants are stimulated by plaque antigens, and this has been interpreted to mean that plaque bacteria enter the vascular gingiva of the mother, cause a transient bacteraemia and then may cross the placenta to sensitize fetal lymphocytes.

IMMUNOSUPPRESSION INDUCED BY B CELL MITOGENS

Although LPS is best known for its adjuvant properties, it may also suppress

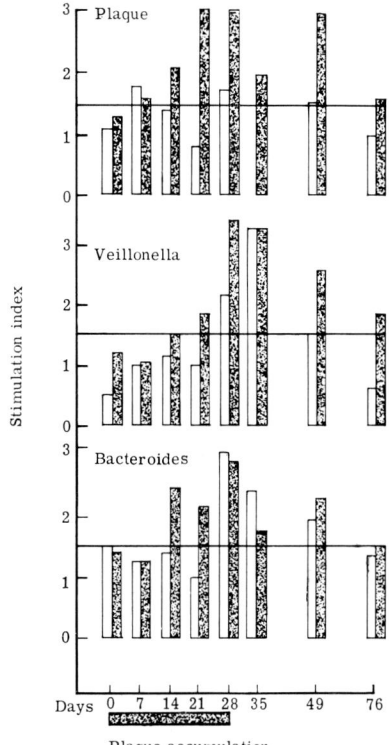

FIG. 5. Mean sequential lymphocyte transformation in five subjects with first (□) and second (■) episodes of experimental gingivitis.

immune responses if given before the antigen. LPS given to mice before sheep red cells causes a depression in food-pad swelling, but when given after the antigen it enhances the foot-pad reaction (Lagrange & Mackaness 1975). The *in vitro* findings with human lymphocytes are comparable with the *in vivo* effects of LPS on the T-cell mediated hypersensitivity in mice, for exposure of human lymphocytes to LPS or levan 24 hours before *Veillonella* results in suppression of *Veillonella*-induced T cell proliferation and, conversely, if the sequence of antigen and mitogen is reversed, T cell proliferation is enhanced (Ivanyi 1976).

High zone B cell tolerance can be induced in mice by polysaccharides; 1–10 mg of a branched native levan, with a molecular weight of 20×10^6, rapidly induces direct B cell tolerance, and if the levan is depolymerized to a molecular weight of 10 000 it still retains its tolerogenicity but not its immunogenicity

(Miranda et al. 1972). Low zone tolerance is induced by immunization with 10–100 µg of levan (Howard & Courtenay 1974). Dental plaque contains 1% dry weight of levan (McDougall 1964), it may account for about 5% of soluble hexose of the plaque matrix and *Strep. mutans* produces β-(2–1) linked soluble levan (Baird et al. 1973). High and low zone tolerance can also be induced with a predominantly α1–6 linked near-linear dextran and depolymerization reduces both immunogenicity and tolerogenicity, both of which are lost with a molecular weight of 20 000 (Howard et al. 1975). However, a more branched α1–3 linked dextran is a poor tolerogen and 10 mg of this dextran induces only minimal tolerance, although 1 mg is a potent immunogen (Howard & Courtenay 1975). Dental plaque contains about 8.5% of soluble dextran, having predominantly α1–6 linkages (Wood 1967) and about 1.4% of insoluble dextrans with predominantly α1–3 linkages (Hotz et al. 1972). *Strep. mutans* is capable of synthesizing a continuous series of dextrans with a variable proportion of α1–6 and α1–3 linkages (Guggenheim 1970; Lewicki et al. 1971; Baird et al. 1973) and these may have a complex effect on tolerance, though this has not been yet demonstrated against unrelated antigens. The net result between factors favouring enhancement and tolerance may then depend on the proportion of α1–3 and α1–6 linked dextrans, the negative charge these may carry, epitope density and on the sequence of adding mitogen and antigen.

THE EFFECT OF IMMUNOSUPPRESSIVE AND IMMUNOPOTENTIATING DRUGS ON GINGIVAL INFLAMMATION

The influence of CMI responses on gingival inflammation has been studied by using immunosuppressive and immunopotentiating drugs. Patients having long-term immunosuppressive treatment show decreased gingival inflammation (Schuller et al. 1973) and this is correlated with negative lymphoproliferative responses to oral microorganisms (L. Ivanyi & T. Lehner, unpublished). In contrast the immunopotentiating drug Levamisole, given to 50 subjects, induced a significant enhancement in the *in vitro* lymphoproliferative response stimulated by *Veillonella* ($P < 0.01$) and other antigens (Ivanyi & Lehner 1976); this was correlated with a significant increase in the gingival index of inflammation ($P < 0.001$). The inverse effects of immunosuppressive and immunopotentiating drugs on the *in vivo* gingival inflammation and the *in vitro* lymphoproliferative response strengthens the view that gingival inflammation is modulated by the cellular immune responses to plaque antigens and mitogens.

References

ALEVY, Y. G. & BATTISTO, J. R. (1976a) Dextran-triggered T cells heighten T- and B-cell reactions to mitogens. *Immunology 30*, 379-390

ALEVY, Y. G. & BATTISTO, J. R. (1976b) Characterization of dextran-activated T-cell factors. *Immunology 30*, 391-399

ALLISON, A. C. (1973) Effects of adjuvants on different cell types and their interactions in immune responses, in *Immunopotentiation (Ciba Found. Symp. 18)*, pp. 73-94, Elsevier/Excerpta Medica/North-Holland, Amsterdam

ALLISON, A. C. & DAVIES, A. J. S. (1971) Requirement of thymus-dependent lymphocytes for potentiation by adjuvants of antibody formation. *Nature (Lond.) 233*, 330-332

ANDERSSON, J., SJÖBERG, O. & MÖLLER, G. (1972) Induction of immunoglobulin and antibody synthesis *in vitro* by LPS. *Eur. J. Immunol. 2*, 99-101

ARNE, J. (1963) Root surface measurement and method for x-ray determination of root surface area. *Acta Odontol. Scand. 21*, 35-46

ATTSTRÖM, R. & EGELBERG, J. (1970) Emigration of blood neutrophils and monocytes into the gingival crevices. *J. Periodontal Res. 5*, 48-55

BAIRD, J. K., LONGYEAR, V. M. C. & ELLWOOD, D. C. (1973) Water insoluble and soluble glucans produced by extracellular glycosyltransferases from *Streptococcus mutans*. *Microbios 8*, 143-150

BATTISTO, J. R. & PAPPAS, F. (1973) Regulation of immunoglobulin synthesis by dextran. *J. Exp. Med. 138*, 176-193

BATTISTO, J. R. & PAPPAS, F. (1974) Dextran's regulatory effect on immunoglobulin synthesis is mediated through T cells. *Cell. Immunol. 10*, 489-495

BAUMHAMMERS, S. & STALLARD, R. E. (1966) Salivary mucoprotein contribution to dental plaque and calculus. *Periodontics 4*, 229-232

CHALLACOMBE, S. J. (1974) Serum complement fixing antibodies in human dental caries. *Caries Res. 8*, 84-95

CHALLACOMBE, S. J., GUGGENHEIM, B. & LEHNER, T. (1973) Antibodies to an extract of *Streptococcus mutans*, containing glucosyltransferase activity related to dental caries in man. *Arch. Oral Biol. 18*, 657-668

CHALLACOMBE, S. J. & LEHNER, T. (1976) Serum and salivary antibodies to cariogenic bacteria in man. *J. Dent. Res. 55*, 139-148

COUTINHO, A. & MÖLLER, G. (1973) B cell mitogenic properties of thymus independent antigens. *Nature (New Biol.) 245*, 12-14

DESAYMARD, C. & IVANYI, L. (1976) Comparison of *in vitro* immunogenicity, tolerogenicity and mitogenicity of dinitrophenyl levan conjugates with varying epitope density. *Immunology 30*, 647-653

DIAMANTSTEIN, T. & BLITSTEIN-WILLINGER, E. (1975) Relationship between biological activities of polymers. I. Immunogenicity, C3 activation, mitogenicity for B cells and adjuvant properties. *Immunology 29*, 1087-1092

EGELBERG, J. (1966) The blood vessels of the dento-gingival junction. *J. Periodontal Res. 1*, 163-179

FROST, P. & LANCE, E. M. (1973) The relation of lymphocyte trapping to the mode of action of adjuvants, in *Immunopotentiation (Ciba Found. Symp. 18)*, pp. 29-38, Elsevier/Excerpta Medica/North-Holland, Amsterdam

GERY, I., KRUGER, J. & SPIESEL, S. Z. (1972) Stimulation of B-lymphocytes by endotoxin. Reactions of thymus-deprived mice and karyotypic analysis of dividing cells in mice bearing T6 T6 thymus graft. *J. Immunol. 108*, 1088-1091

GIBBONS, R. J., SOCRANSKY, S. S., ARAUJO, W. C. DE & HOUTE, J. VAN (1964) Studies of the predominant cultivable microbiota of dental plaque. *Arch. Oral Biol. 9*, 365-370

GREAVES, M. F. & JANOSSY, G. (1972) Elicitation of selective T and B lymphocyte responses by cell surface binding ligands. *Transplant. Rev. 11*, 87-130

GUGGENHEIM, B. (1970) Enzymatic hydrolysis and structure of water-insoluble glucan produced by glucosyltransferases from a strain of *Streptococcus mutans. Helv. Odontol. Acta* 14, Suppl. 5, 89-108

HADDING, U., DIERICH, M., KONIG, W., LIMBERT, M., SCHLORLEMMER, H. U. & BITTER-SUERMANN, D. (1973) Ability of the T cell-replacing polyanion dextran sulfate to trigger the alternate pathway of complement activation. *Eur. J. Immunol.* 3, 527-529

HELLSTRÖM, K. E. & HELLSTRÖM, I. (1970) Immunological enhancement as studied by cell culture techniques. *Ann. Rev. Microbiol.* 24, 373-398

HORTON, J. E., LEIKIN, S. & OPPENHEIM, J. J. (1972a) Human lymphoproliferative reaction to saliva and dental plaque-deposits: an *in vitro* correlation with periodontal disease. *J. Periodontol.* 43, 522-527

HORTON, J. E., RAISZ, L. G., SIMMONS, H. A., OPPENHEIM, J. J. & MERGENHAGEN, S. E. (1972b) Bone resorbing activity in supernatant fluid from cultured human peripheral blood leukocytes. *Science (Wash. D.C.)* 177, 793-795

HORTON, J. E., OPPENHEIM, J. J. & MERGENHAGEN, S. E. (1973) Elaboration of lymphotoxin by cultured human peripheral blood leucocytes stimulated with dental plaque deposits. *Clin. Exp. Immunol.* 13, 383-393

HORTON, J. E., OPPENHEIM, J. J., CHAN, S. P. & BAKER, J. J. (1976) Relationship of transformation of newborn human lymphocytes by dental plaque antigen to the degree of maternal periodontal disease. *Cell. Immunol.* 21, 153-160

HOTZ, P., GUGGENHEIM, B. & SCHMID, R. (1972) Carbohydrates in pooled dental plaque. *Caries Res.* 6, 103-121

HOWARD, J. G. & COURTENAY, B. M. (1974) Induction of tolerance to polysaccharides in B lymphocytes by exhaustive immunization and during immunosuppression with cyclophosphamide. *Eur. J. Immunol.* 4, 603-608

HOWARD, J. G. & COURTENAY, B. M. (1975) Influence of molecular structure on the tolerogenicity of bacterial dextrans. II. The α 1–3 linked epitope of dextran B1355. *Immunology* 29, 599-610

HOWARD, J. G., COURTENAY, B. M. & VICARI, G. (1975) Influence of molecular structure on the tolerogenicity of bacterial dextrans. III. Dissociation between tolerance and immunity to the α 1-6 and α 1-3 linked epitopes of dextran B1355. *Immunology* 29, 611-619

IVANYI, L. (1976) Modulation of antigen-induced stimulation of human lymphocytes by LPS. *Clin. Exp. Immunol.* 23, 385-388

IVANYI, L. & LEHNER, T. (1970) Stimulation of lymphocyte transformation by bacterial antigens in patients with periodontal disease. *Arch. Oral Biol.* 15, 1089-1096

IVANYI, L. & LEHNER, T. (1971) Lymphocyte transformation by sonicates of dental plaque in human periodontal disease. *Arch. Oral Biol.* 16, 1117-1121

IVANYI, L. & LEHNER, T. (1974) Stimulation of human lymphocytes by B-cell mitogens. *Clin. Exp. Immunol.* 18, 347-356

IVANYI, L. & LEHNER, T. (1976) The effect of Levamisole on gingival inflammation in man. *Scand. J. Immunol.*, in press

IVANYI, L., WILTON, J. M. A. & LEHNER, T. (1972) Cell-mediated immunity in periodontal disease: cytotoxicity, migration inhibition and lymphocyte transformation studies. *Immunology* 22, 141-145

IVANYI, L., CHALLACOMBE, S. J. & LEHNER, T. (1973) The specificity of serum factors in lymphocyte transformation in periodontal disease. *Clin. Exp. Immunol.* 14, 491-500

JOHNSON, A. G., GAINES, S. & LANDY, M. (1956) Studies on the O antigen of *Salmonella typhosa*. V. Enhancement of antibody response to protein antigens by the purified lipopolysaccharide. *J. Exp. Med.* 103, 225-246

JOHNSTON, J. M. & WILSON, D. B. (1970) Origin of immuno-reactive lymphocytes in rats. *Cell. Immunol.* 1, 430-444

KIGER, R. D., WRIGHT, W. H. & CREAMER, H. R. (1974) The significance of lymphocyte transformation responses to various microbial stimulants. *J. Periodontol.* 45, 780-785

LAGRANGE, P. H. & MACKANESS, G. B. (1975) Effects of bacterial lipopolysaccharide on the induction and expression of cell-mediated immunity. II. Stimulation of the efferent arc. *J. Immunol. 114*, 447-451

LEHNER, T., WILTON, J. M. A., CHALLACOMBE, S. J. & IVANYI, L. (1974a) Sequential cell-mediated immune responses in experimental gingivitis in man. *Clin. Exp. Immunol. 16*, 481-492

LEHNER, T., CHALLACOMBE, S. J., IVANYI, L. & WILTON, J. M. A. (1974b) in *The Immunoglobulin A System* (Mestecky, J. & Lawton, A. R., eds.) (*Adv. Exp. Med. Biol. 45*), pp. 405-495, Plenum Press, New York & London

LEHNER, T., CHALLACOMBE, S. J., WILTON, J. M. A. & IVANYI, L. (1976a) Immunopotentiation by intrinsic microbial plaque and its relationship to oral disease in man. *Arch. Oral Biol. 21*, 749-753

LEHNER, T., WILTON, J. M. A., CHALLACOMBE, S. J. & CALDWELL, J. (1976b) Cellular and humoral immune responses in vaccination against dental caries in monkeys. *Nature (Lond.) 264*, 69-71

LEWICKI, W. J., LONG, L. W. & EDWARDS, J. R. (1971) Determination of the structure of a broth dextran produced by a cariogenic streptococcus. *Carbohydr. Res. 17*, 175-182

MCDOUGALL, W. A. (1974) Plaque studies. IV. Levans in plaque. *Aust. Dent. J. 9*, 1-15

MACKLER, B. F., ALTMAN, L. C., WAHL, S., ROSENSTREICH, D. L., OPPENHEIM, J. J. & MERGENHAGEN, S. E. (1974) Blastogenesis and lymphokine synthesis by T and B lymphocytes from patients with periodontal disease. *Infect. Immun. 10*, 844-850

MELVAER, K. L., HELGELAND, K. & ROLLA, G. (1974) A charged component in purified polysaccharide preparations from *Streptococcus mutans* and *Streptococcus sanguis*. *Arch. Oral Biol. 19*, 589-595

MERGENHAGEN, S. E., HAMPP, E. G. & SCHERP, H. W. (1961) Preparation and biological activities of endotoxins from oral bacteria. *J. Infect. Dis. 108*, 304-310

MERGENHAGEN, S. E., ROSENSTREICH, D. L., WILTON, J. M. A., WAHL, S. M. & WAHL, L. K. (1976) in *The Role of Immunological Factors in Infectious, Allergic and Autoimmune Processes (8th Miles Int. Symp.)*, Johns Hopkins University Press, Baltimore, Md.

MIRANDA, J. J., ZOLA, H. & HOWARD, J. G. (1972) Studies on immunological paralysis. X. Cellular characteristics of the induction and loss of tolerance to levan (polyfructose). *Immunology 23*, 843-855

PAGE, R. C., DAVIES, P. & ALLISON, A. C. (1973) Effects of dental plaque on the production and release of lysosomal hydrolases by macrophages in culture. *Arch. Oral Biol. 18*, 1481-1495

ROLLA, G., MELSEN, B. & SONJU, T. (1975) Sulphated macromolecules in dental plaque in the monkey *Macaca irus*. *Arch. Oral Biol. 20*, 341-343

SCHULLER, P. D., FREEDMAN, H. L. & LEWIS, D. W. (1973) Periodontal status of renal transplant patients receiving immunosuppressive therapy. *J. Periodontol. 44*, 167-170

SCHWARTZ, J., STINSON, F. L. & PARKER, R. B. (1972) The passage of tritiated bacterial endotoxin across intact gingival crevicular epithelium. *J. Periodontol. 43*, 270-276

SJÖBERG, O., ANDERSSON, J. & MÖLLER, T. (1972) Requirement for adherent cells in the primary and secondary immune response *in vitro*. *Eur. J. Immunol. 2*, 123-126

SKAPSKI, H. & LEHNER, T. (1976) A crevicular washing method for investigating immune components of crevicular fluid in man. *J. Periodontal Res. 11*, 19-24

SPITZNAGEL, J. K. & ALLISON, A. C. (1970) Mode of action of adjuvants: retinol and other lysosome-labilizing agents as adjuvants. *J. Immunol. 104*, 119-127

SUTER, E. & WHITE, R. G. (1954) The response of the reticulo-endothelial system to the injection of the 'purified wax' and the lipopolysaccharide of tubercle bacilli. *Am. Rev. Tuberculosis 70*, 793-805

WALDMANN, H. & MUNRO, A. (1975) The inter-relationship of antigenic structure, thymus-independence and adjuvanticity. IV. A general model for B-cell induction. *Immunology 28*, 509-522

WILKINSON, P. C., O'NEILL, G. J., MCINROY, R. J., CATER, J. C. & ROBERTS, J. A. (1973)

Chemotaxis of macrophages: the role of a macrophage-specific cytotaxin from anaerobic corynebacteria and its relation to immunopotentiation *in vivo*, in *Immunopotentiation (Ciba Found. Symp. 18)*, pp. 121-135, Elsevier/Excerpta Medica/North-Holland, Amsterdam

WILTON, J. M. A., ROSENSTREICH, D. L. & OPPENHEIM, J. J. (1975) Activation of guinea pig macrophages by bacterial lipopolysaccharide requires bone marrow-derived lymphocytes. *J. Immunol. 114*, 388-393

WOOD, J. M. (1967) The amount, distribution and metabolism of soluble polysaccharides in human dental plaque. *Arch. Oral Biol. 12*, 849-858

Discussion

Lachmann: Is the message that if we don't clean our teeth, we shall be protected against caries, but we shall get gum disease?

Lehner: No, one can't expect such protection, because eventually the large number of bacteria and the amount of acid produced would overcome the immunological defence mechanism.

Davies: Is the rate of accumulation of plaque dependent on diet? And is plaque accumulation only to be found in the human species?

Lehner: The answer to the second question is that it can be found in any animal, if you give it the appropriate diet. The Western, civilized diet—a soft, fibre-free diet—is conducive to the accumulation of plaque, and I suspect that in primitive times this was not the case. In fact, we know that in the developing countries the prevalence of caries is smaller than in the UK. In order for caries to be produced four factors may be involved: (*a*) a sugar-rich diet to be converted to acid; (*b*) acidogenic organisms; (*c*) the tooth itself; and (*d*) antibodies that may modulate caries formation.

Beeson: Did you always have the plaque removed mechanically in your subjects or did some of them merely begin brushing their teeth again?

Lehner: It was always removed mechanically by professional oral hygienists, so as to make quite certain that it was done thoroughly. It is an experiment which is highly reproducible in the sense that the inflammation appears with bacterial plaque accumulation, and disappears with removal of plaque.

Beeson: You don't think that the mechanical effect of brushing the gums might have something to do with it?

Lehner: I think you are probably right, in one sense. Back in the 1930's when focal sepsis was a popular subject, it was shown that trauma to the gum may cause a transient bacteraemia (Okell & Elliott 1935). If that was the case, as it almost certainly must have been, one should find immunization, instead of depression, during the bacteraemia caused by the removal of plaque.

Brandtzaeg: For the last experiments you mentioned that the caries index was recorded before plaque accumulation. Was the gingival index measured before or afterwards?

Lehner: The caries index, as you know, does not change within 28 days, so that would be constant. The gingival inflammation was measured before, during and after plaque accumulation, and maximum stimulation indices are given during the 28 days, mainly between 14 and 28 days. The gingival index was also the maximum index recorded.

Brandtzaeg: You implied that the influence on the immune system takes place in the mouth, by penetration of plaque components through the crevicular epithelium, but can you exclude that people with dirty mouths swallow a lot of mitogens and antigens, and that the immunological stimulation thus takes place in the gut?

Lehner: This is very much a possibility. You are right that the organisms, and therefore the polysacccharides, might well be swallowed and therefore the immune responses could take place through the gut. On the other hand, there is an extensive epithelial surface in the mouth, and all the relevant immunological cells are present at the site of plaque accumulation, in the gingival crevice epithelium, so that I wonder if we need to invoke another site for absorption.

Brandtzaeg: The surface will be small compared with the epithelial surface of the gut, however.

Lehner: Yes, except that because of the persistence of plaque and the inflammatory response it induces in the adjacent epithelium, the local permeability may be greatly increased.

White: Dr Brandtzaeg started to ask about the mechanism of polyclonal stimulation; how do you think the bacteria enter the blood? Okell & Elliott (1935) said that one had wobbly teeth and one wobbled them and the bacteria could be recovered by blood culture. Is that the mechanism?

Lehner: I think the situation is much more complex. First of all, even if you chew energetically on hard meat, you will probably produce a transient bacteraemia, and therefore you do not need to have loose teeth to force bacteria into the blood stream. Secondly, in an interesting study Horton *et al.* (1976) showed that cord blood lymphocytes are sensitized to maternal dental bacterial plaque antigens only from mothers with gingivitis associated with bacterial plaque. This suggested that fetal lymphocytes may get sensitized to dental bacterial plaque *in utero.* Furthermore, polyclonal stimulants, such as lipopolysaccharides, can penetrate the gingival epithelium in the rabbit and thereby presumably sensitize the animal (Schwartz *et al.* 1972).

White: I don't know what you would take as evidence of polyclonal stimulation in man, but to me this possibly arises in malaria, in trypanosomiasis, and in infectious mononucleosis. All these conditions, interestingly enough, are associated with the development of heterophile antibody to sheep red cells.

References

ALEVY, Y. G. & BATTISTO, J. R. (1976) Dextran-triggered T cells heighten T- and B-cell reactions to mitogens. *Immunology 30*, 379-390

ALLISON, A. C. & DAVIES, A. J. S. (1971) Requirement of thymus-dependent lymphocytes for potentiation by adjuvants of antibody formation. *Nature (Lond.) 233*, 330-332

CHALLACOMBE, S. J., GUGGENHEIM, B. & LEHNER, T. (1972) Serum and salivary antibodies to glucosyltransferase in dental caries in man. *Nature (Lond.) 238*, 219

COUTINHO, A. & MÖLLER, G. (1973) B cell mitogenic properties of thymus independent antigens. *Nature New Biol. 245*, 12-14

HORTON, J. E., OPPENHEIM, J. J., CHAN, S. P. & BAKER, J. J. (1976) Relationship of transformation of newborn human lymphocytes by dental plaque antigen to the degree of maternal periodontal disease. *Cell. Immunol. 21*, 153-160

IVANYI, L. & LEHNER, T. (1974) Stimulation of human lymphocytes by B-cell mitogens. *Clin. Exp. Immunol. 18*, 347-356

LEHNER, T., CHALLACOMBE, S. J., IVANYI, L. & WILTON, J. M. A. (1974) in *The Immunoglobulin A System* (Mestecky, J. & Lawton, A. R., eds.) (*Adv. Exp. Med. Biol. 45*), pp. 485-495, Plenum Press, New York

OKELL, C. C. & ELLIOTT, S. D. (1935) Bacteriaemia and oral sepsis with special reference to the aetiology of sub-acute endocarditis. *Lancet 2*, 869-872

OPPENHEIM, J. J. & PERRY, S. (1965) Effects of endotoxins on cultured leukocytes. *Proc. Soc. Exp. Biol. Med. 118*, 1014-1019

SCHWARTZ, J., STINSON, F. L. & PARKER, R. B. (1972) The passage of tritiated bacterial endotoxin across intact gingival crevicular epithelium. *J. Periodontol. 43*, 270-276

Sites of synthesis and localization of IgE in rats infested with *Nippostrongylus brasiliensis*

GRAHAM MAYRHOFER

MRC Cellular Immunology Unit, Sir William Dunn School of Pathology, University of Oxford

Abstract The tissue and cellular localization of IgE has been studied in normal rats and rats infested with the enteric parasite, *Nippostrongylus brasiliensis*. The results of the study do not support the suggestion that IgE is a secretory immunoglobulin with a physiology analogous to that of IgA. The lamina propria of the small intestine and the colonic and pulmonary mucosal surfaces contain numerous anti-IgE-binding cells, but these have been shown to be mast cells and not plasma cells. The major sites of IgE synthesis were the regional lymph nodes of the small intestine and the lungs, which contained large numbers of IgE-secreting plasma cells. Smaller numbers of IgE-secreting plasma cells were also found in peripheral lymph nodes, some of which were distant from tissues known to have direct contact with either larvae or adult worms. Peyer's patches, the intrapulmonary lymphoid tissue and the spleen contained few, if any, IgE-secreting plasma cells. The significance of the IgE which was readily demonstrated in germinal centres of Peyer's patches and several lymph nodes is not known. In contrast to infested animals, the lymphoid organs of normal rats rarely contained any IgE-containing cells. Thoracic duct lymph from infested animals contained only few IgE-containing large lymphocytes, similar in number to cells containing IgM or IgG but only 1/50 as many as those containing IgA. An unexpected observation was that mast cells in mucosal organs appear to contain intracellular IgE, differing in this respect from connective tissue mast cells. Mast cells lying between epithelial cells, the 'globule leucocytes', also appear to contain intracellular IgE and it is suggested that such cells may be responsible for the presence of IgE in exocrine secretions. This study highlights the need for careful identification of cells appearing to contain IgE and suggests reasons for the widely differing reports of the numbers of IgE-secreting plasma cells in human intestinal biopsies.

Antibodies of immunoglobulin class IgE have been shown to sensitize mast cells in man and a variety of other species for release of histamine and the subsequent manifestations of immediate-type hypersensitivity (type 1 hypersensitivity of Coombs & Gell 1963). Antibodies of this sort are variously referred to as homocytotropic, reaginic or anaphylactic antibodies. A protective role for such antibodies or for the hypersensitivity phenomenon to which they predispose has not been clearly demonstrated, while the pathological effects are the cause of considerable morbidity and mortality in medical practice.

In man, some 10% of the population are more or less severely afflicted by some symptom attributable to IgE/mast cell mediated hypersensitivity (Aaronson 1972). One is therefore provoked to ask why, in the face of a significant mortality produced by this mechanism, the trait persists at such a high level in the population. The answer must be that either now, or in man's relatively recent past, the capacity to mount strong IgE-mediated immune responses has held a selective advantage. The maintenance of this potentially harmful trait might be an example of a balanced polymorphism and it is therefore important to discover the circumstances where IgE antibodies are protective.

One possibility is that IgE and immediate-type hypersensitivity have importance in the host's immune response to parasites. During infestation with a variety of metazoan parasites, idiosyncratic factors affecting IgE responses appear to be largely over-ridden and most members of the population respond by producing large amounts of IgE. Populations of humans in areas where parasites are endemic have generally elevated levels of serum IgE (Bennich & Johansson 1971; Ogilvie & Jones 1973) and eradication of the parasites leads to a decline in circulating IgE (Grove *et al.* 1974). Similar observations in animals (Ogilvie 1967; Wilson & Bloch 1968; Jarrett & Bazin 1974) have also suggested that IgE antibodies may be important elements in the immune response to parasites but there has been no conclusive evidence that either proves or disproves this important possibility.

While systemic anaphylaxis may cause serious symptoms and death following injection of antigen into sensitized individuals, most manifestations of immediate-type hypersensitivity occur at mucosal surfaces of the body and are localized mainly at the site of contact with antigen. Sensitization to environmental and food antigens also occurs mainly at mucous membranes, although circulating homocytotropic antibody subsequently sensitizes mast cells throughout the body. It is therefore of interest to know where IgE antibodies are synthesized and whether they have a particular localization in mucous membranes and secretions. IgE has been detected in a variety of secretions (Ishizaka & Newcomb 1970; Hobday *et al.* 1971; Deuschl & Johansson 1974; Nakajima *et al.* 1975), with some suggestion that active secretion increases its concentration relative to that which would be found in a simple exudate of serum proteins. Ishizaka *et al.* (1969) and Tada & Ishizaka (1970) have investigated sites of IgE synthesis by immunofluorescence techniques and have concluded that IgE is mainly synthesized in the lamina propria and the regional lymph nodes of mucosal organs. An analogy has therefore been drawn between IgE and IgA, where the latter is undoubtedly a class of immunoglobulin specialized both chemically and by site of synthesis for incorporation into exocrine secretions. However, the case that IgE is a secretory immunoglobulin is by no means as strong as that for IgA. The recent availability of monoclonal rat IgE from myeloma serum (Bazin *et al.* 1974) stimulated an investigation of the sites of IgE synthesis in rats, using fluorescent antibody monospecific for rat IgE. The results of studies in normal rats and in rats infested with the nematode parasite *Nippostrongylus brasiliensis* do not support the contention that IgE is a secretory immunoglobulin with a physiology similar to that of IgA.

METHODS

Fourteen-week-old female Wistar *rats* were infested by subcutaneous injection on the dorsum of the neck with 2000 third-stage larvae of *N. brasiliensis*. The larvae were obtained from the Wellcome Laboratories, Beckenham, Kent and were produced by the method of Keeling (1960). Infestation of animals was confirmed by faecal egg counts, and faeces were virtually free of eggs by 12 days after injection of larvae. Some rats were given secondary and tertiary infestations by injection of 2500–3000 third-stage larvae 5 weeks and 30 weeks respectively after the primary infestation.

Purified monoclonal *rat IgE* was supplied by Dr H. Bazin (Brussels). *Rabbit anti-rat IgE* was raised against myeloma IR2 IgE and purified by Dr A. F. Williams (Oxford). The antibody was rendered monospecific by absorption with a Sepharose 4B column to which were coupled the proteins of normal rat serum and lymph together with purified IgG_2 and anti-idiotype antibody was removed by adsorption to and elution from a myeloma IR162 IgE-Sepharose 4B column. The purified antibody was conjugated with fluorescein isothiocyanate (FITC) and before use was absorbed with thymus and lymph node cells from specific pathogen-free rats. *Goat anti-rabbit Ig* (GAR) was obtained as a conjugate with FITC from Cappel Laboratories (Downingtown, Pa., USA). A 1:50 dilution of this serum was absorbed with mesenteric lymph node cells from a *Nippostrongylus*-infested rat before use. *Rabbit anti-rat IgA* was the same reagent as was used by Williams & Gowans (1975).

IgE was detected in tissue sections by incubation with *FITC-anti-IgE* followed by washing and further incubation with FITC-GAR to improve the fluorescence. Omission of the middle layer or replacement with normal rabbit IgG abolished fluorescence, as did absorption of the anti-IgE with a 2.5-fold excess of purified rat IgE. *IgA* was demonstrated by a direct method, essentially as described by Williams & Gowans (1975).

Where sections were for study of IgE-containing cells only, *tissue specimens* were fixed in cold ethanol and embedded in paraffin (modified from Brandtzaeg 1974). When identification of mast cells was also necessary, the tissues were fixed in cold Carnoy's fluid instead of ethanol. Non-specific eosinophil fluorescence was modified with Lendrum's stain (Johnston & Bienenstock 1974) and mast cells were demonstrated by their affinity for Alcian blue (Enerbäck 1966a, b). Tissue fixed in Carnoy's fluid could be stained with Alcian blue before incubation with fluorescent reagent without interfering with the fluorescence of FITC conjugates. Sections photographed for fluorescent cells could then be counterstained with Safranin and the same areas re-examined for mast cells by conventional microscopy.

Homocytotropic antibody responses against *N. brasiliensis* were measured by passive cutaneous anaphylaxis (PCA) in Wistar R rats by the method of Ovary (1964), using a saline extract of adult worms as the challenging antigen.

CELLS BINDING ANTI-IgE IN MUCOSAL ORGANS

The mucosal organ most extensively studied for secretory antibody production has been the small intestine. Food and bacterial antigens provide a stimulus for the population of the intestinal lamina propria with IgA-secreting plasma cells in newborn animals and in germ-free animals after exposure to a conventional environment (Crabbé *et al.* 1968, 1969, 1970). The small intestines of *normal rats* were therefore examined for plasma cells secreting either IgE or IgA. In sections stained with the indirect method for IgE, rare weakly fluorescent cells were seen in the lamina propria (Fig. 1). Although the nature of these cells has not been pursued, the intensity of fluorescence was much less than that of IgE-secreting plasma cells. In contrast, when sections from the same tissue blocks were stained by the direct method for IgA, large numbers of IgA-secreting plasma cells were present throughout the length of the small intestine (Fig. 2). Therefore, local synthesis of IgE does not occur to a significant extent in the normal small intestine. The lamina propria of the colon and of the bronchi in normal rats also lacked IgE-secreting plasma cells.

Two *hyperimmune rats* were killed 10 and 20 days after secondary infestation with *N. brasiliensis* (PCA titres 1:2048 and 1:128 respectively). The lamina propria of the small intestine in these animals contained large numbers of brightly fluorescent cells that appeared to contain IgE (Fig. 3). Although the worm burden is carried mainly in the proximal jejunum, the fluorescent cells were relatively uniformly distributed along the length of the small intestine. Many of the cells had the appearance of typical plasma cells, but several differences were noted from the IgA-secreting plasma cells in the lamina propria. IgA-secreting plasma cells mainly occupied the bases of villi, in an

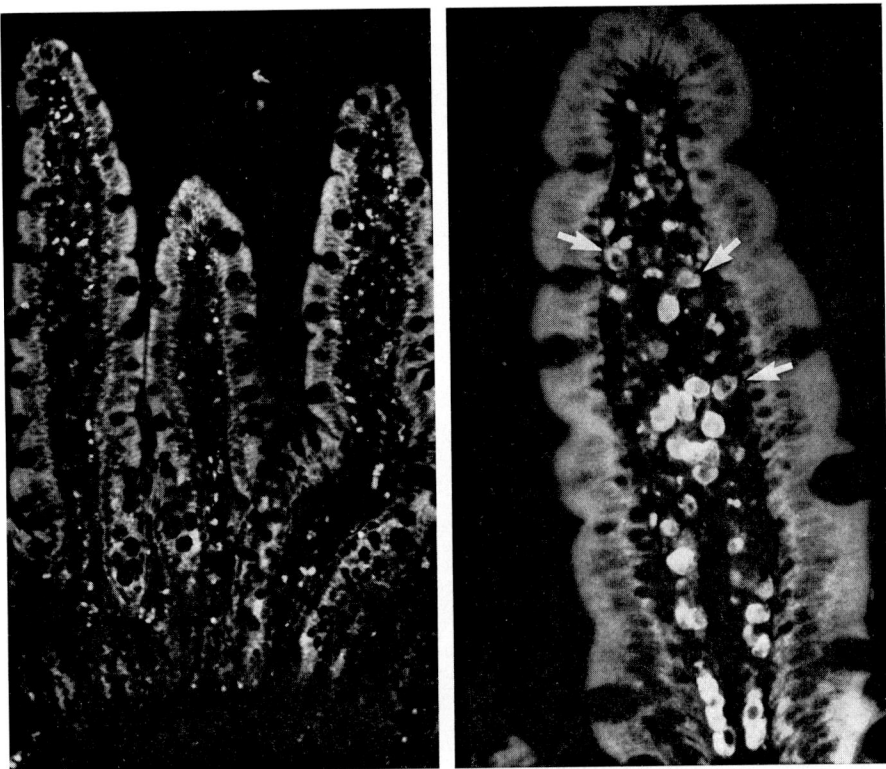

Fig. 1   Fig. 2

FIG. 1. Section of normal rat ileum, stained with FITC-anti-IgE and FITC-GAR. All fluorescence in the lamina propria comes from eosinophils. This, and the autofluorescence of the epithelium, are of quite different colour to the specific green fluorescence of FITC. No specifically fluorescent cells are present. Cf. Figs. 2 and 3. × 340.

FIG. 2. Section cut from the same block as Fig. 1 and stained with FITC-anti-IgA. Villus containing numerous IgA-secreting plasma cells. Note the axial position of the cells. Fluorescent objects in the tip of the villus and arrowed cells are eosinophils. × 830.

axial position, whereas the anti-IgE-binding cells were usually subepithelial and extended to the villus tips. Especially at the bases of villi and in the crypts, anti-IgE-binding cells were quite frequently found between cells of the epithelium. Although the cells appeared to contain IgE, their morphology and distribution was similar to that of mast cells in rats infested with *N. brasiliensis* (Miller & Jarrett 1971).

Mast cells could not be demonstrated in ethanol-fixed tissue by staining with either toluidine blue or Alcian blue, as was found by Enerbäck (1966a), and

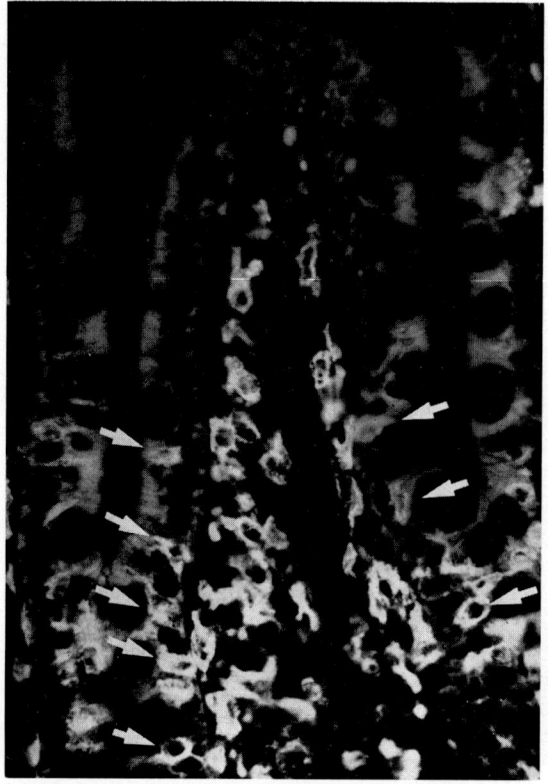

FIG. 3. Section of ileum from a rat 10 days after the second infestation with *N. brasiliensis*, stained with FITC-anti-IgE/FITC-GAR. Note the large number of specifically fluorescent cells in the lamina propria, occupying mainly subepithelial positions. Several cells *(arrowed)* lie between epithelial cells. × 840.

only weak staining was obtained with acridine orange (Jagatic & Weiskopf 1966). A rat was killed 10 days after a tertiary infestation (PCA titre 1:16 384) and its tissues were fixed with cold Carnoy's fluid. This fixative preserved the affinity of mucosal mast cells for Alcian blue (Enerbäck 1966a) and did not interfere with detection of immunoglobulins. As in the other hyperimmune animals, the lamina propria of the small intestine contained large numbers of anti-IgE-binding cells. Defined fields were photographed for fluorescence and then re-examined for the presence of Alcian blue-positive mast cells. Comparison of Figs. 4a and 4b shows that all fluorescent cells are also stained by Alcian blue. Few, if any, fluorescent cells in the lamina propria were not mast cells. Therefore, although there is greatly increased synthesis of IgE in rats

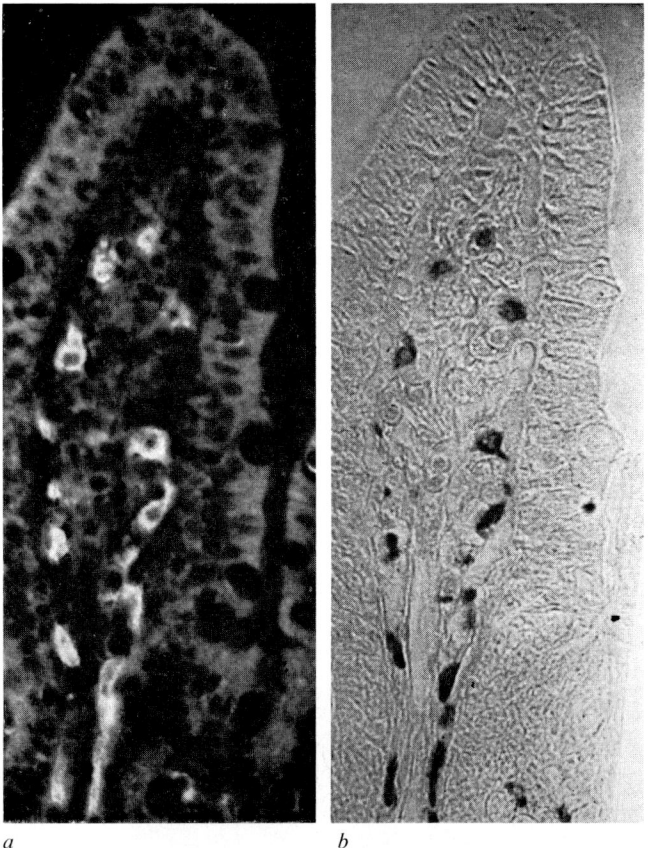

a   *b*

FIG. 4. Section of ileum from a rat 10 days after the third infestation with *N. brasiliensis*. The tissue was fixed with cold Carnoy's fluid and has been stained sequentially with Alcian blue and FITC-anti-IgE/FITC-GAR.

(*a*) Photographed for fluorescence. All cells are specifically stained.

(*b*) The same field as (*a*) after counterstaining with Safranin. All fluorescent cells are mast cells stained with Alcian blue. × 980.

infested with *N. brasiliensis*, synthesis of IgE antibodies does not occur locally in the lamina propria of the small intestine.

The colon is not infested by the parasite, although it may be exposed to antigen. The lamina propria in infested animals contained considerable numbers of fluorescent mast cells (Fig. 5), but no IgE-secreting plasma cells. Fluorescent mast cells (the so-called 'globule leucocytes') were also present between epithelial cells of the colonic glands.

The lungs of infested animals contained large numbers of fluorescent mast cells (Fig. 6). These had the same staining properties as intestinal mast cells

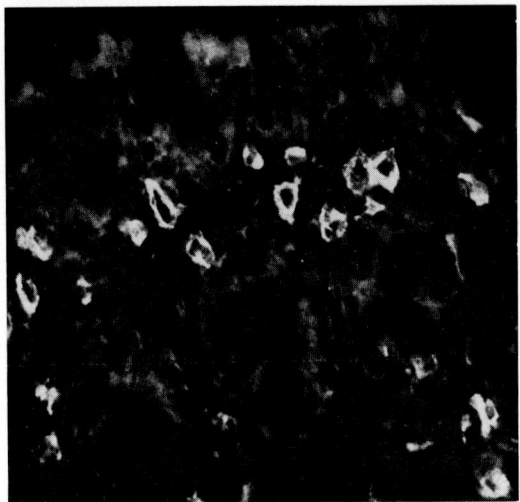

FIG. 5. Section of transverse colon from a rat 10 days after the second infestation, showing cells with specific fluorescence in the superficial layer of the lamina propria and between colonic glands. Fixed and stained as in Fig. 4. The fluorescent cells are mast cells. × 870.

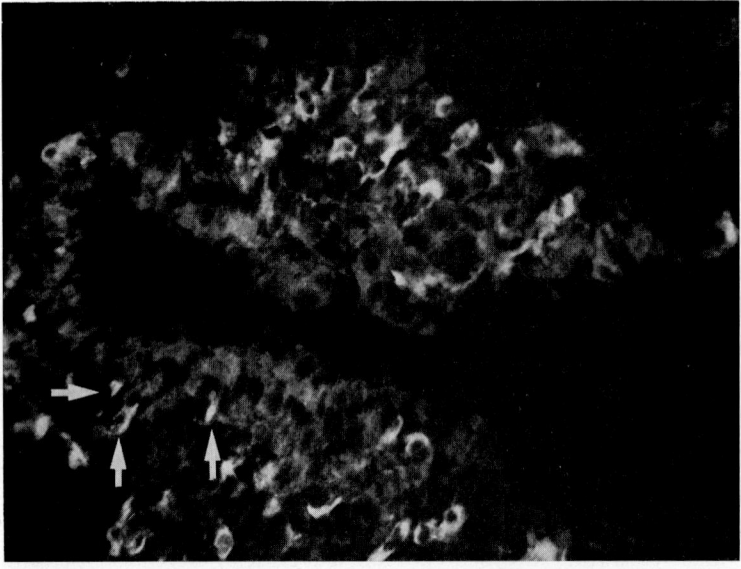

FIG. 6. Section of lung from a rat 10 days after the third infestation, showing a terminal bronchiole surrounded by specifically fluorescent cells. Three fluorescent cells lie between cells of the respiratory epithelium *(arrowed)*. Fixed and stained as in Fig. 4. The fluorescent cells are mast cells. × 830

and also appeared to contain IgE. In the bronchi, fluorescent mast cells were present in the lamina propria and between cells of the respiratory epithelium from the major bronchi down to the terminal bronchioles. No IgE-secreting plasma cells were seen either in the bronchial lamina propria or in the intrapulmonary lymphoid nodules. Granulomata produced in the lungs by the passage of larval worms (Taliaferro & Sarles 1939) contained large numbers of fluorescent mast cells. These foci of mast cells may explain the IgE-containing 'germinal centres' described by Ishizaka *et al.* (1969) in the parenchyma of the lungs of monkeys infested with a pulmonary parasite.

IgE AND MUCOSAL MAST CELLS

The fluorescence of the mucosal mast cells does not appear to be limited to the cell perimeter, but to emanate also from the cytoplasm of the cells (Fig. 7). This contrasts with the fluorescence of mature mast cells in connective tissues such as the capsules of lymph nodes, where the appearance is that of binding of the FITC conjugate to the cell membrane (Fig. 8). From these appearances of the fluorescent cells, it seems possible that mucosal mast cells may actually *contain* IgE, in addition to surface-bound IgE, while connective tissue mast cells may only have surface IgE. This suggestion is not wholly novel, as mast cells in dogs infested with *Ascaris* also have the appearance of cytoplasmic fluorescence when stained to demonstrate IgE (Halliwell 1973). Further studies are in progress to assess this possibility by more definitive criteria.

SITE OF IgE SYNTHESIS

Adult worms in the small intestine are thought to be the main source of immunizing antigen during infestation with *N. brasiliensis* (Ogilvie & Jones 1971). The most likely site of IgE synthesis is therefore the gut-associated lymphoid tissue. Normal *Peyer's patches* bound no anti-IgE. The Peyer's patches of hyperimmune rats did not contain mature IgE-secreting plasma cells but did bind anti-IgE. The mucosal poles of the germinal centres had bright fluorescence in a coarse dendritic pattern, while the serosal pole was unstained (Fig. 9). The mantle of small lymphocytes was stained in a fine reticular pattern, but the interfollicular T-dependent areas (Parrott & Ferguson 1974) and the sub-epithelial corona were unstained. The significance of the IgE in the germinal centres is not known, and although Peyer's patches may be important in the generation of the IgE response to the parasite, they do not appear to be sites of IgE secretion.

The *mesenteric lymph nodes* were major sites of IgE secretion in infested rats.

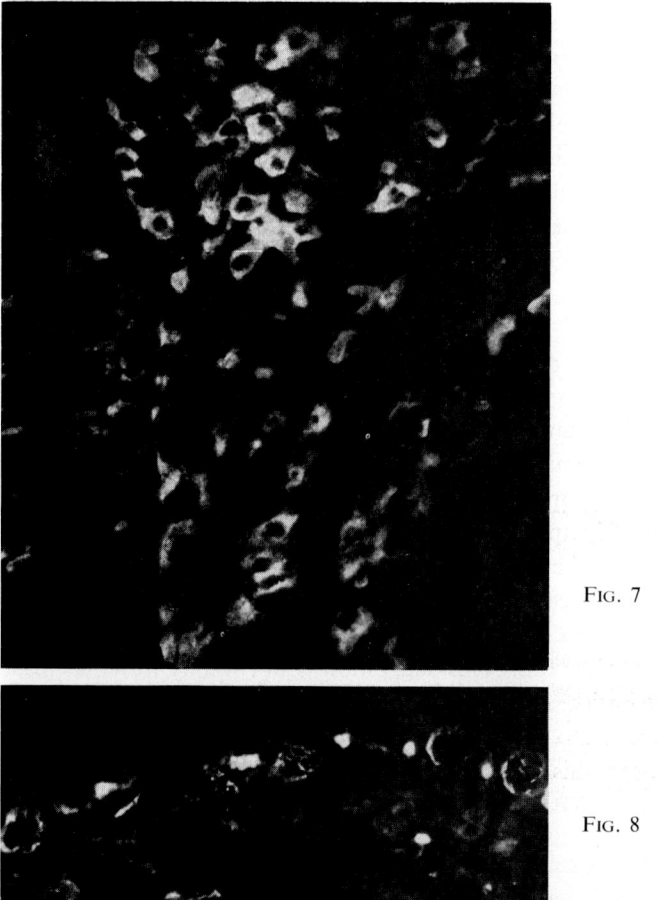

Fig. 7

Fig. 8

Fig. 7. Section from the same block as Fig. 4, stained in the same way. Many fluorescent cells are present in the lamina propria of the villus. The same cells were all also stained by Alcian blue. Note the similarity to plasma cells and the appearance suggesting that the cytoplasm of the cells is stained. × 840.

Fig. 8. Section of the capsule of an axillary lymph node from a rat 10 days after the second infestation stained with FITC-anti-IgE/FITC-GAR. Mature mast cells in the connective tissue stain in a pattern suggesting that only the cell membrane is stained. × 730.

Very few cells bound anti-IgE in normal lymph nodes, but in those from hyperimmune rats the medullary cords contained large numbers of brightly fluorescent cells. These had no affinity for Alcian blue and by exclusion are plasma cells (Fig. 10). Anti-IgE-binding cells were rare in the medullary sinuses and where present were found to be mast cells. This suggests that the

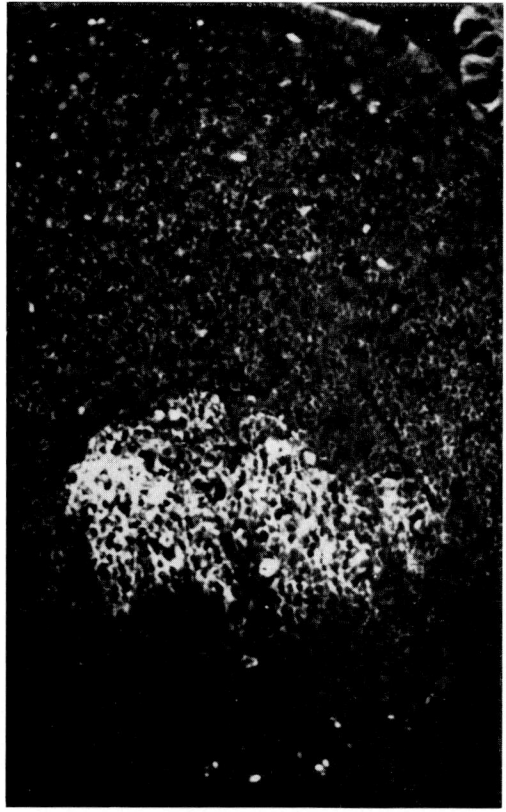

FIG. 9. A Peyer's patch from a rat 10 days after the second infestation, stained with FITC-anti-IgE/FITC-GAR. The mucosal pole of the germinal centre is brightly stained in a coarse dendritic pattern, while the serosal pole is unstained. The mantle of small lymphocytes is also stained, in a fine reticular pattern. $\times$ 330.

IgE-secreting cells in the medullary cords are a sedentary population that does not migrate into the efferent lymph. Many germinal centres of the lymph node had brightly fluorescent caps of a coarse dendritic pattern, but the medullary pole of the germinal centre was unstained. The small lymphocytes of the follicles had a fine reticular pattern of fluorescence while the interfollicular recirculatory areas and the paracortex were unstained.

The *lung* is an organ of passage and maturation of the larval parasite. However, the intrapulmonary lymphoid tissue associated with the large bronchi did not contain IgE-secreting plasma cells in either normal or hyperimmune rats. In further studies (on PVG/c rats), the mediastinal lymph nodes of hyperimmune rats were studied, as these hypertrophy during infestation.

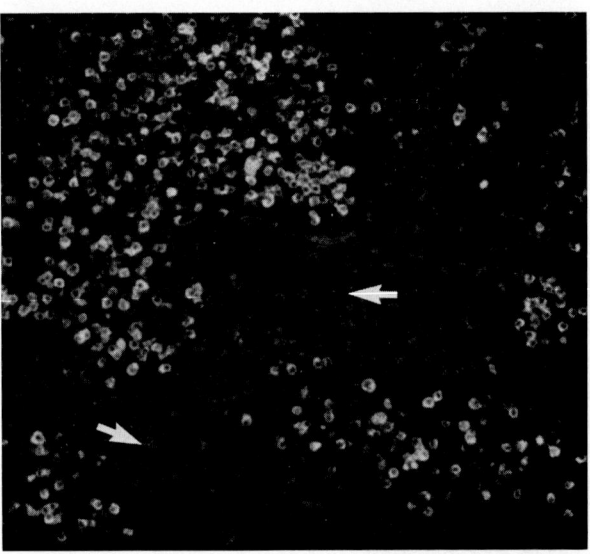

Fig. 10. Section of the medulla of the mesenteric lymph node of a rat 10 days after the third infestation, fixed and stained as in Fig. 4. The medullary cords contain large numbers of IgE-secreting plasma cells. Two large medullary sinuses *(arrowed)* do not contain any fluorescent cells. × 340.

Sections of these lymph nodes from a rat 10 days after a secondary infestation (PCA titre 1:2048) contained large numbers of IgE-secreting plasma cells in the medullary cords. The density of fluorescent cells and the appearance of the follicles was similar to the findings in the mesenteric lymph nodes of hyperimmune animals. It therefore appears that, as with the small intestine, IgE synthesis occurs in the draining lymph nodes of a mucosal organ and not locally in the lamina propria of the organ or in specialized lymphoid tissues closely associated with the mucosa.

The *spleen* was found to contain very few anti-IgE-binding cells in either normal or hyperimmune rats. *Peripheral lymph nodes* of normal rats contained no anti-IgE-binding cells. The axillary, para-aortic and popliteal lymph nodes of hyperimmune rats all contained fluorescent germinal centres and small numbers of IgE-secreting plasma cells in the medullary cords. The axillary lymph node drains the site of injection of larvae, but the other lymph nodes do not drain areas directly exposed to either larvae or adult worms. Synthesis and localization of IgE in these lymph nodes may result from a systemic antigenaemia during infestation, or from anomalous migration of larvae to extra-intestinal sites (Weinstein 1955).

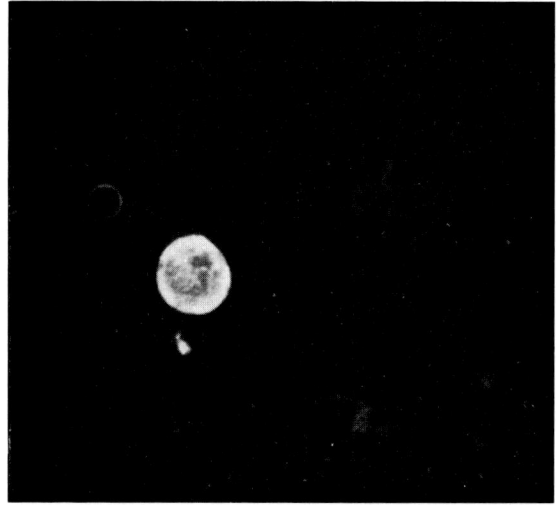

FIG. 11. A fluorescent large lymphocyte in a smear of thoracic duct lymph from a rat 7 days after the second infestation with *N. brasiliensis*. The smear was stained with FITC-anti-IgE and FITC-GAR. Most of the cells were unstained. × 1500.

IgE-CONTAINING CELLS IN THORACIC DUCT LYMPH

Plasma cells in the lamina propria of the gut are known to arise from precursors in thoracic duct lymph (TDL) that are large lymphocytes (Gowans & Knight 1964), and at least some of which contain internal IgA (Williams & Gowans 1975). At the point of cannulation in the abdomen, the thoracic duct drains the entire intestinal lymphatic bed and its associated lymphoid tissue. Approximately 40% of large lymphocytes in normal rat TDL contain internal IgA, and such cells constitute about 2–4% of all thoracic duct lymphocytes. Cells containing either IgM, IgG2a or IgG2b are very much rarer in normal animals, amounting to approximately 0.1% for IgM and 0.2% for these combined IgG subclasses. Plasma cells containing IgM, IgG2a or IgG2b are very rare in the intestinal lamina propria of normal rats (unpublished results). It was therefore of some interest to know whether TDL contained IgE-synthesizing large lymphocytes during infestation with *N. brasiliensis*. Smears of washed thoracic duct lymphocytes obtained from a PVG/c rat cannulated seven days after a secondary infestation were fixed in ethanol and stained to detect either IgE- or IgA-containing cells. 4.6% of all cells contained IgA at this time, while 0.1% of cells contained IgE. The IgE-containing cells had the morphology of large lymphocytes (Fig. 11). This observation, together with the absence of IgE-containing blast cells in the medullary sinuses of the mesenteric lymph node, shows that the traffic of IgE-containing cells in TDL is small compared to that of IgA-containing cells, even during a period of intense IgE synthesis. In this respect, IgE is similar to other classes of immunoglobulin that are not specialized for secretion, and the absence of IgE-secreting plasma cells from the lamina propria of the gut is also consistent with this generalization.

DISCUSSION

Two main conclusions can be drawn from this work. Firstly, IgE is not synthesized locally in the lamina propria of those mucosal organs of infested rats through which absorption of parasite antigens might be expected to occur. IgE antibodies made during infestation are synthesized by plasma cells in the regional lymph nodes of these organs. The second main conclusion is that although IgE-secreting plasma cells are absent from the lamina propria of the infested gut, large numbers of cells are present that appear to contain IgE. These cells have been shown by their histochemical properties to be mast cells.

Normal rats had few anti-IgE-binding cells in any of the mucosal organs examined. Even after challenging with *N. brasiliensis*, which stimulates synthesis of large amounts both of specific IgE (Ogilvie 1967; Wilson & Bloch 1968) and total IgE (Jarrett & Bazin 1974), IgE-secreting plasma cells were not found in the lamina propria of the small intestine although the main antigenic stimulus is thought to arise from adult worms in this organ (Ogilvie & Jones 1971). Similarly, although the lung has direct contact with the migratory larval stage of the infestation, no IgE-secreting plasma cells were detected in the lamina propria of the bronchi. Therefore, neither food and environmental antigens nor parasite antigens stimulate local IgE synthesis in the intestine or the lung. This finding contrasts with the local synthesis of IgA that occurs in the intestine following initial exposure to food and bacterial antigens (Crabbé *et al.* 1968, 1969, 1970; Tomasi & Grey 1972) or oral immunization with a specific antigen (Pierce and Gowans 1975).

The thoracic duct lymph of a rat undergoing a secondary response to infestation with *N. brasiliensis* contained only rare IgE-containing large lymphocytes. These were only 1/50th as numerous as cells containing IgA and were in about the same proportion to the total cells as are those containing IgM and IgG in normal TDL. Therefore, during a period of greatly accelerated IgE synthesis, IgE-containing cells were present in TDL only in numbers similar to those containing non-secretory classes of immunoglobulin in normal rats. At this time the mesenteric lymph node contained large numbers of IgE-secreting plasma cells and it is noteworthy that these were present in the medullary cords and absent from the medullary sinuses. These findings are in accordance with the absence of IgE-secreting plasma cells from the lamina propria of the intestine.

Synthesis of IgE occurred mainly in the mesenteric and mediastinal lymph nodes of the infested rats. This is in agreement with work of Ishizaka & Ishizaka (1975) and Ishizaka et al. (1976), where use of different methods led to the conclusion that these lymph nodes were major sites of IgE synthesis in *Nippostrongylus*-infested rats. These workers also found the spleen to contribute very little to the production of IgE in response to the parasite. However, it does appear that the spleen can be an important source of IgE when antigen and appropriate adjuvant are administered by a parenteral route (Ishizaka & Ishizaka 1975). In the present study, it was found that peripheral lymph nodes contained IgE-secreting plasma cells and IgE-containing germinal centres. Thus, although IgE may be synthesized predominantly in lymphoid tissue draining the gut and the lung when antigen is presented via these organs and in this way bears some resemblance to IgA, it is different from IgA in that its synthesis can be stimulated in the spleen and peripheral lymph nodes by appropriate immunization. Parenteral immunization usually elicits the appearance of very few IgA-containing specific antibody-forming cells (Crabbé et al. 1969) and weak serum IgA responses (Ogra et al. 1968; Newcomb et al. 1969).

In summary, IgE is not synthesized locally in the lamina propria of mucosal organs by plasma cells and no precursor large lymphocytes containing IgE are found in TDL. IgE does not share with IgA the property of binding secretory component (Newcomb & Ishizaka 1970) and therefore probably does not appear in secretions by a similar mechanism to that used by IgA. In addition, while IgE is synthesized mainly in the lymph nodes draining the gut and lungs during infestation with *N. brasiliensis*, it is also synthesized to a lesser extent in peripheral lymph nodes. Other workers have shown that parenteral immunization can cause the spleen to be a major source of IgE antibody. These considerations do not support the hypothesis that IgE is a secretory immunoglobulin with a physiology similar to that of IgA.

The observations already discussed raise several points for discussion in relation to other published work. One intriguing possibility raised by the present study is that intestinal mast cells, including 'globule leucocytes', may contain IgE in their cytoplasm in addition to any IgE that might be bound to the surface membrane. The mast cells of the lung appeared similar to those of the intestine. Some other work has also suggested that mast cells may contain immunoglobulin. Dobson (1966) found that 'globule leucocytes' in sheep could be stained with a conjugate of a polyvalent anti-sheep globulin serum, although he interpreted this finding to mean that these cells contained Russell bodies and were therefore plasma cells. Halliwell (1973) observed that mast cells in dogs infested with *Ascaris* appeared to contain cytoplasmic IgE and that this pattern of fluorescence could be imparted to mast cells of non-infested dogs by passive transfer of serum with a high titre of anti-*Ascaris* homocytotropic antibody.

The presence of fluorescent mast cells in sections of intestine and lung stained with anti-IgE may explain the differences in the numbers of presumptive IgE-secreting plasma cells that have been reported in human and monkey material. Ishizaka *et al.* (1969) and Tada & Ishizaka (1970) found considerable numbers of IgE-containing cells in the lamina propria of the intestine and lungs of both humans and monkeys. However, other studies by Hobbs *et al.* (1969), Savilahti (1972), Skinner & Whitehead (1974) and Brown *et al.* (1975) have found few or no IgE-containing cells in intestinal biopsies from humans. Although Tada & Ishizaka (1970) considered the possibility that the IgE-containing cells seen by them might be mast cells, the ethanol fixation method used by them would not be expected to preserve intestinal mast cells for staining with toluidine blue (Enerbäck 1966a). The present study suggests that anti-IgE-binding cells around peptic ulcers (Brown *et al.* 1975) may be mast cells, as these are common at sites of chronic inflammation. The IgE content of mast cells appears to be related to serum IgE levels (Halliwell 1973) and the reason for the absence of IgE-containing cells in some studies may be that the tissues were obtained from individuals with normal IgE levels. This possibility is supported by the results of recent studies on intestinal diseases with probable allergic aetiology, where serum IgE levels could be expected to be elevated. Large numbers of IgE-containing cells were present in the affected intestinal lamina propria (Shiner *et al.* 1975; Kilby *et al.* 1975; Heatley *et al.* 1975) and the possibility that these might be mast cells was not excluded although mast cells were common in biopsies from patients with cow's milk allergy (Shiner *et al.* 1975).

Although IgE does not appear to be locally synthesized, it is reported to be present in a number of exocrine secretions (Ishizaka & Newcomb 1970; Hobday *et al.* 1971; Bennich & Johansson 1971; Deuschl & Johansson 1974; Nakajima *et al.* 1975), and to be apparently locally synthesized in nasal polypi (Donovan *et al.* 1970). IgE appears to be present in secretions in higher concentrations relative to serum levels than either albumin or non-secretory immunoglobulin, suggesting a secretory mechanism, although this does not involve secretory component (Newcomb & Ishizaka 1970). It is noteworthy that IgE is found in the secretions of organs prone to immediate-type hypersensitivity phenomena, while it is absent from the secretions of the salivary glands (Nakajima *et al.* 1975), which are not usually the sites of allergic reactions. The finding of mast cells that appear to contain IgE in the lamina propria of mucosal organs may provide an explanation for the high concentration of IgE in nasal polyp fluid, as mast cells are common in these lesions. The presence of IgE-containing mast cells (globule leucocytes) apparently passing between epithelial cells of the gut and the lung may provide the mechanism by which IgE finds its way into secretions. Its release could be due to shedding of these cells or to their degranulation by contact with specific antigens.

The mucosal mast cells have several properties that set them apart from connective tissue mast cells and blood basophils. The mucosal mast cells of the intestine and the lungs had a different pattern of fluorescence from mature connective tissue mast cells when stained with anti-IgE. In the latter cells, the fluorescence appeared to be associated with the surface membrane rather than the cytoplasm. Mucosal mast cells also differ from connective tissue mast cells in their histochemical properties (Enerbäck 1966a, b) and in their response to compound 48/80 (Mota et al. 1956; Enerbäck 1966c). It is possible that these two sorts of mast cells also differ in their lineage and physiology and that predictions about the behaviour of mucosal mast cells cannot be made on the basis of studies on more accessible cells such as those of the peritoneal cavity.

Accumulation of large numbers of mast cells in the intestines of rats infested with *N. brasiliensis* and synthesis of specific homocytotropic antibody are coincident events which demand a consideration of the role of immediate-type hypersensitivity in immunity to this parasite. A number of arguments can be marshalled against the essential participation of this mechanism, at least in worm expulsion after primary infestation (Ogilvie & Jones 1973), but some immunological (Mulligan et al. 1965; Urquhart et al. 1965; Barth et al. 1966) and pharmacological (Murray et al. 1971a,b; Rothwell et al. 1971) studies suggest that IgE and mast cells participate in the events leading to worm damage and expulsion. There is general agreement that worms are damaged by antibodies in the normal course of infestation (Ogilvie & Hockley 1968), that this is necessary though not sufficient to cause expulsion (Jones & Ogilvie 1971), and that worm expulsion can be hastened by passive immunization with specific antisera (Mulligan et al. 1965; Barth et al. 1966; Jones et al. 1970). It appears that the antisera need not necessarily contain homocytotropic antibody (Jones et al. 1970).

Despite the apparent independence of IgE antibodies of the passive immune response, it is not yet clear whether mast cell degranulation and histamine release are necessary to allow access of non-secretory classes of immunoglobulin to the worms in the gut lumen—the 'leak–lesion' hypothesis of Urquhart et al. (1965). It is known that the number of mucosal mast cells in the intestine falls during the early stages of infestation (Miller & Jarrett 1971; Keller 1971) and there is some evidence that this is due to release of a mast cell degranulating factor by the worms (Miller & Jarrett 1971; Keller 1971). In the experiments in which passive antibody was administered, it is possible that the role of IgE was replaced by the worm degranulating factor. Specific antibody was present throughout the infestation whereas normally antibodies would not be synthesized until later, and would include specific homocytotropic antibody. The 'leak–lesion' may have operated despite the absence from the transferred serum of specific homocytotropic antibody.

Direct functional studies on the participation of mast cells in worm expulsion have not been made. Mast cell numbers in histological sections at various times during infestation do not give any indication of the rates of turnover of cells or of their pharmacological mediators. The evidence from such studies is not persuasive in either supporting or refuting the role of mast cells. In studies of the effects of passive antibody, the conditions in the intestine at the time of normal worm expulsion may not be reproduced because mast cells are present in normal intestine in relatively small numbers compared to the numbers during the late phases of infestation. This may explain the relatively weak effects of passive immunization. In experiments utilizing active immunization with immune lymphoid cells, the possibility has not been satisfactorily excluded that the transferred cells may contain B cells committed to IgE synthesis on the one hand or, on the other hand, cells capable of differentiating into mucosal mast cells or exerting inductive effects on mast cell differentiation.

One is therefore still able to entertain the possibility that IgE may have importance in immunity to parasites. The evidence discussed above relates entirely to immune mechanisms expelling worms from a primary infestation. Relatively little work has been done on the immunity to subsequent infestation and an important question in the present context is whether IgE and mast cells are involved in the destruction of migrating larvae (Taliaferro & Sarles 1939), possibly by intensifying the local inflammatory response. The present work raises the possibility that IgE itself may be important as an effector molecule, in addition to its function in sensitizing mast cells. If mucosal mast cells are indeed found to contain IgE, then specific degranulation of mast cells by worm antigens may release high local concentrations of IgE antibody, in addition to amines. The unexpected possibility that mast cells may concentrate IgE makes it important to re-examine the role of homocytotropic antibodies in immunity to parasites.

ACKNOWLEDGEMENTS

The author acknowledges the close and enjoyable collaboration with Professor J. L.

Gowans (Oxford) and Dr H. Bazin (Brussels) throughout the course of this work. He is indebted to Dr A. F. Williams (Oxford) for his generous gifts of purified antisera and to Mr J. E. D. Keeling of the Wellcome Laboratories, Beckenham, Kent for gifts of *N. brasiliensis* and advice on its maintenance.

References

AARONSON, D. W. (1972) Asthma: general concepts, in *Allergic Diseases* (Patterson, R., ed.), pp. 197-236, Lippincott, Philadelphia & Toronto

BARTH, E. E. E., JARRETT, W. F. H. & URQUHART, G. M. (1966) Studies on the mechanism of the self-cure reaction in rats infected with *Nippostrongylus brasiliensis*. *Immunology 10*, 459-464

BAZIN, H., QUERINJEAN, P., BECKERS, A., HEREMANS, J. F. & DESSY, F. (1974) Transplantable immunoglobulin-secreting tumours in rats. IV. Sixty-three IgE-secreting immunocytoma tumours. *Immunology 26*, 713-723

BENNICH, H. & JOHANSSON, S. G. O. (1971) Structure and function of human immunoglobulin E. *Adv. Immunol. 13*, 1-55

BRANDTZAEG, P. (1974) Mucosal and glandular distribution of immunoglobulin components. Immunohistochemistry with a cold ethanol-fixation technique. *Immunology 26*, 1101-1114

BROWN, W. R., BORTHISTLE, B. K. & CHEN, S.-T. (1975) Immunoglobulin E (IgE) and IgE-containing cells in human gastrointestinal fluids and tissues. *Clin. Exp. Immunol. 20*, 227-237

COOMBS, R. R. A. & GELL, P. G. H. (1963) The classification of allergic reactions underlying disease, in *Clinical Aspects of Immunology* (Gell, P. G. H. & Coombs, R. R. A., eds.), pp. 317-337, Blackwell Scientific Publications, Oxford

CRABBÉ, P. A., BAZIN, H., EYSSEN, H. & HEREMANS, J. F. (1968) The normal microbial flora as a major stimulus for proliferation of plasma cells synthesizing IgA in the gut. *Int. Arch. Allergy Appl. Immunol. 34*, 362-375

CRABBÉ, P. A., NASH, D. R., BAZIN, H., EYSSEN, H. & HEREMANS, J. F. (1969) Antibodies of the IgA type in intestinal plasma cells of germ-free mice after oral immunization or parenteral immunization with ferritin. *J. Exp. Med. 130*, 723-744

CRABBÉ, P. A., NASH, D. R., BAZIN, H., EYSSEN, H. & HEREMANS, J. F. (1970) Immunohistochemical observations on lymphoid tissues from conventional and germ-free mice. *Lab. Invest. 22*, 448-457

DEUSCHL, H. & JOHANSSON, S. G. O. (1974) Immunoglobulins in tracheo-bronchial secretion with special reference to IgE. *Clin. Exp. Immunol. 16*, 401-412

DOBSON, C. (1966) Immunofluorescent staining of globule leucocytes in the colon of the sheep. *Nature (Lond.) 211*, 875

DONOVAN, R., JOHANSSON, S. G. O., BENNICH, H. & SOOTHILL, J. F. (1970) Immunoglobulins in nasal polyp fluid. *Int. Arch. Allergy Appl. Immunol. 37*, 154-166

ENERBÄCK, L. (1966a) Mast cells in rat gastrointestinal mucosa. 1. Effects of fixation. *Acta Pathol. Microbiol. Scand. 66*, 289-302

ENERBÄCK, L. (1966b) Mast cells in rat gastrointestinal mucosa. 2. Dye-binding and metachromatic properties. *Acta Pathol. Microbiol. Scand. 66*, 303-312

ENERBÄCK, L. (1966c) Mast cells in rat gastrointestinal mucosa. 3. Reactivity towards compound 48/80. *Acta Pathol. Microbiol. Scand. 66*, 313-322

GOWANS, J. L. & KNIGHT, E. J. (1964) The route of re-circulation of lymphocytes in the rat. *Proc. R. Soc. Lond. B Biol. Sci. 159*, 257-282

GROVE, D. I., BURSTON, T. O. & FORBES, I. J. (1974) Fall in IgE levels after treatment for hookworm. *Clin. Exp. Immunol. 18*, 565-569

HALLIWELL, R. E. W. (1973) The localization of IgE in canine skin: an immunofluorescent study. *J. Immunol. 110*, 422-430

HEATLEY, R. V., RHODES, J., CALCRAFT, B. J., WHITEHEAD, R. H., FIFIELD, R. & NEWCOMBE, R. G. (1975) Immunoglobulin E in rectal mucosa of patients with proctitis. *Lancet 2*, 1010-1012

HOBBS, J. R., HEPNER, G. W., DOUGLAS, A. P., CRABBÉ, P. A. & JOHANSSON, S. G. O. (1969) Immunological mystery of coeliac disease. *Lancet 2*, 649-650

HOBDAY, J. D., CAKE, M. & TURNER, K. J. (1971) A comparison of the immunoglobulins IgA, IgG and IgE in nasal secretions from normal and asthmatic children. *Clin. Exp. Immunol. 9*, 577-583

ISHIZAKA, K. & NEWCOMB, R. W. (1970) Presence of γE in nasal washings and sputum from asthmatic patients. *J. Allergy 46*, 197-204

ISHIZAKA, T. & ISHIZAKA, K. (1975) Biology of immunoglobulin E. *Prog. Allergy 19*, 60-121

ISHIZAKA, K., ISHIZAKA, T. & TADA, T. (1969) Immunoglobulin E in the monkey. *J. Immunol. 103*, 445-453

ISHIZAKA, T., URBAN, J. F. & ISHIZAKA, K. (1976) IgE formation in the rat following infection with *Nippostrongylus brasiliensis*. 1. Proliferation and differentiation of IgE-bearing cells. *Cell. Immunol. 22*, 248-261

JAGATIC, J. & WEISKOPF, R. (1966) A fluorescent method for staining mast cells. *Arch. Pathol. (Chicago) 82*, 430-433

JARRETT, E. & BAZIN, H. (1974) Elevation of total IgE in rats following helminth parasite infection. *Nature (Lond.) 251*, 613-614

JOHNSTON, N. W. & BIENENSTOCK, J. (1974) Abolition of non-specific fluorescent staining of eosinophils. *J. Immunol. Methods 4*, 189-194

JONES, V. E. & OGILVIE, B. M. (1971) Protective immunity to *Nippostrongylus brasiliensis*: the sequence of events which expels worms from the rat intestine. *Immunology 20*, 549-561

JONES, V. E., EDWARDS, A. J. & OGILVIE, B. M. (1970) The circulating immunoglobulins involved in protective immunity to the intestinal stage of *Nippostrongylus brasiliensis* in the rat. *Immunology 18*, 621-633

KEELING, J. E. D. (1960) The effects of ultra-violet radiation on *Nippostrongylus muris*. 1. Irradiation of infective larvae: lethal and sublethal effects. *Ann. Trop. Med. Parasitol. 54*, 182-191

KELLER, R. (1971) *Nippostrongylus brasiliensis* in the rat: failure to relate intestinal histamine and mast cell levels with worm expulsion. *Parasitology 63*, 473-481

KILBY, A., WALKER-SMITH, J. A. & WOOD, C. B. S. (1975) Small intestinal mucosa in cow's milk allergy. *Lancet 1*, 531

MILLER, H. R. P. & JARRETT, W. F. H. (1971) Immune reactions in mucous membranes. 1. Intestinal mast cell response during helminth expulsion in the rat. *Immunology 20*, 277-288

MOTA, I., BERALDO, W. T., FERRI, A. G. & JUNQUEIRA, L. C. U. (1956) Action of 48/80 on the mast cell population and histamine content of the wall of the gastro-intestinal tract of the rat, in *Histamine (Ciba Found. Symp. 16)* (Wolstenholme, G. E. W. & O'Connor, C. M., eds.), pp. 47-50, Churchill, London.

MULLIGAN, W., URQUHART, G. M., JENNINGS, F. W. & NEILSON, J. T. M. (1965) Immunological studies on *Nippostrongylus brasiliensis* infection in the rat. The 'self-cure' phenomenon. *Exp. Parasitol. 16*, 341-347

MURRAY, M., MILLER, H. R. P., SANFORD, J. & JARRETT, W. F. H. (1971a) 5-Hydroxytryptamine in intestinal immunological reactions. Its relationship to mast cell activity and worm expulsion in rats infected with *Nippostrongylus brasiliensis*. *Int. Arch. Allergy Appl. Immunol. 40*, 236-247

MURRAY, M., SMITH, W. D., WADDELL, A. H. & JARRETT, W. F. H. (1971b) *Nippostrongylus brasiliensis*: histamine and 5-hydroxytryptamine inhibition and worm expulsion. *Exp. Parasitol. 30*, 58-63

NAKAJIMA, S., GILLESPIE, D. N. & GLEICH, G. J. (1975) Differences between IgA and IgE as secretory proteins. *Clin. Exp. Immunol. 21*, 306-317

NEWCOMB, R. W. & ISHIZAKA, K. (1970) Physicochemical and antigenic studies on human γE in respiratory fluid. *J. Immunol. 105*, 85-89

NEWCOMB, R. W., ISHIZAKA, K. & DEVALD, B. L. (1969) Human IgG and IgA diphtheria antitoxins in serum, nasal fluids and saliva. *J. Immunol. 103*, 215-224

OGILVIE, B. M. (1967) Reagin-like antibodies in rats infected with the nematode parasite *Nippostrongylus brasiliensis*. *Immunology 12*, 113-131

OGILVIE, B. M. & HOCKLEY, D. J. (1968) Effects of immunity on *Nippostrongylus brasiliensis* adult worms: reversible and irreversible changes in infectivity, reproduction, and morphology. *J. Parasitol. 54*, 1073-1084

OGILVIE, B. M. & JONES, V. E. (1971) *Nippostrongylus brasiliensis*: a review of immunity and the host/parasite relationship in the rat. *Exp. Parasitol. 29*, 138-177

OGILVIE, B. M. & JONES, V. E. (1973) Immunity in the parasitic relationship between helminths and hosts. *Prog. Allergy 17*, 93-144

OGRA, P. L., KARZON, D. T., RIGHTHAND, F. & MACGILLIVRAY, M. (1968) Immunoglobulin response in serum and secretions after immunization with live and inactivated poliovaccine and natural infection. *N. Engl. J. Med. 279*, 893-900

OVARY, Z. (1964) Passive cutaneous anaphylaxis, in *Immunological Methods (CIOMS Symposium)* (Ackroyd, J. F., ed.), pp. 259-283, Blackwell Scientific Publications, Oxford

PARROTT, D. M. V. & FERGUSON, A. (1974) Selective migration of lymphocytes within the mouse small intestine. *Immunology 26*, 571-588

PIERCE, N. F. & GOWANS, J. L. (1975) Cellular kinetics of the intestinal immune response to cholera toxoid in rats. *J. Exp. Med. 142*, 1550-1563

ROTHWELL, T. L. W., DINEEN, J. K. & LOVE, R. J. (1971) The role of pharmacologically-active amines in the resistance to *Trichostrongylus colubriformis* in the guinea-pig. *Immunology 21*, 925-938

SAVILAHTI, E. (1972) Immunoglobulin-containing cells in the intestinal mucosa and immunoglobulins in the intestinal juice in children. *Clin. Exp. Immunol. 11*, 415-425

SHINER, M., BALLARD, J. & SMITH, M. E. (1975) The small-intestinal mucosa in cow's milk allergy. *Lancet 1*, 136-140

SKINNER, J. M. & WHITEHEAD, R. (1974) The plasma cells in inflammatory disease of the colon: a quantitative study. *J. Clin. Pathol. 27*, 643-646

TADA, T. & ISHIZAKA, K. (1970) Distribution of γE-forming cells in lymphoid tissues of the human and monkey. *J. Immunol. 104*, 377-387

TALIAFERRO, W. H. & SARLES, M. P. (1939) The cellular reactions in the skin, lungs and intestine of normal and immune rats after infection with *Nippostrongylus muris*. *J. Infect. Dis. 64*, 155-192

TOMASI, T. B. & GREY, H. M. (1972) Structure and function of IgA. *Prog. Allergy 16*, 81-213

URQUHART, G. M., MULLIGAN, W., EADIE, R. M. & JENNINGS, F. W. (1965) Immunological studies on *Nippostrongylus brasiliensis* infection in the rat: the role of local anaphylaxis. *Exp. Parasitol. 17*, 210-217

WEINSTEIN, P. P. (1955) The effect of cortisone on the immune response of the white rat to *Nippostrongylus muris*. *Am. J. Trop. Med. Hygiene 4*, 61-74

WILLIAMS, A. F. & GOWANS, J. L. (1975) The presence of IgA on the surface of rat thoracic duct lymphocytes which contain internal IgA. *J. Exp. Med. 141*, 335-345

WILSON, R. J. M. & BLOCH, K. J. (1968) Homocytotropic antibody response in the rat infected with the nematode, *Nippostrongylus brasiliensis*. II. Characteristics of the immune response. *J. Immunol. 100*, 622-628

Discussion

Ogilvie: Rats vary enormously in their capacity to synthesize IgE in response to this parasite, and in some animals one can never detect any anti-parasite IgE antibodies in their circulation. It has always been argued that this may not mean anything because IgE may be produced locally in the gut wall. Can you shed any light on this point?

Mayrhofer: I don't think I can. I have also had rats that have responded normally to worm challenge, with expulsion of the parasites in the usual time, but in which the serum has been negative when tested for specific IgE antibodies against *Nippostrongylus* by passive cutaneous anaphylaxis (PCA) titration. I have not looked at the mesenteric lymph nodes of such animals to see whether IgE is being produced. In the context of the results I have presented, local production of IgE antibody in the gut mucosa is unlikely. However, an important factor could be the local concentration of IgE in association with mast cells in the lamina propria, and serum IgE antibody levels may be poor indicators of this.

Ogilvie: Do you know how IgE gets from the mesenteric node to the tissue mast cells?

Mayrhofer: No. There is certainly IgE in thoracic duct lymph of infested rats, as judged by PCA assay, but I am not sure how it compares with the serum concentration.

Soothill: We adopted a different approach in looking at local IgE production. We (Donovan *et al.* 1969) measured the concentration of IgE in nasal polyp fluid, which provides a readily available sample of tissue fluid. This fluid is not a secretion, of course. We found high concentrations of IgE in nasal polyp fluid, far higher than could be accounted for by the concentration in serum. The levels paralleled the degree of allergy in the patient. Do you think the mast cell in some way concentrates circulating IgE and then releases it into the fluid? Could our effect have been an effect of mast cell binding?

Mayrhofer: These tissues contain large numbers of mast cells, so it is possible. The suggestion from our fluorescence studies is that mast cells can concentrate IgE. It is interesting that not all exocrine secretions contain IgE, while IgA appears to be secreted into all that have been examined. Nakajima *et al.* (1975) found that nasal washings from atopic individuals contained IgE but that parotid gland secretions from the same individuals did not have detectable concentrations. The secretions reported to contain IgE by these and other workers (e.g. nasal, bronchial and intestinal secretions) come from organs where allergic manifestations are more or less common. On the other hand, the salivary glands are not usually affected by immediate-type hypersensitivity. It is therefore possible that the IgE in secretions arises from mast cells as a result of contact with allergen.

Davies: I wonder why you appear to exclude the possibility that at least some of the IgE is synthesized by mast cells?

Mayrhofer: I don't exclude that possibility, although it seems unlikely. The mast cell IgE could either be acquired passively from the circulation or synthesized by the cells. I have thought of trying to distinguish these possibilities by using the phenomenon of allelic exclusion. The rat has two light chain allotypes. If the IgE is made by the mast cells, then only a proportion of the total IgE-containing population in an F_1 hybrid possessing both allotypic markers should stain with a labelled antibody directed against one of the allotypic antigens. If passively acquired, the IgE in the mast cells would be a mixture of allotypes and all IgE-containing cells would also stain for allotype.

Davies: You could perhaps do it by passive immunization studies with an appropriately labelled antibody.

Mayrhofer: Yes. The inference from Halliwell's work is that mast cells take up IgE into the cytoplasm (Halliwell 1973). When serum was transfused from dogs with a high reaginic antibody titre against *Ascaris* into dogs with a low titre, the mast cells in the recipients became fluorescent when stained with fluorescein-conjugated anti-IgE.

Gowans: Is the implication of Dr Davies' comment that mast cells are derived from lymphocytes?

Davies: No; perhaps cells other than plasma cells can produce antibody.

Brandtzaeg: Feltkamp-Vroom *et al.* (1975) recently described IgE staining of human mast cells and showed that the intensity was not related to the serum content of IgE but to the atopic status of the patients.

Mayrhofer: That would correspond with Halliwell's observations in dogs. He found that the IgE content of mast cells correlated well with the skin reactivity of the dogs to *Ascaris* extract, but not so well with the serum IgE level.

Brandtzaeg: Why do you use the indirect technique for IgE and the direct method to show IgA?

Mayrhofer: The fluorescence obtained when FITC-anti-IgE was used alone was rather weak, especially when I was looking for IgE-containing cells in the lamina propria. The absence of brightly fluorescent plasma cells from the lamina propria of normal animals was worrying at first. I added the second fluorescent layer to increase the brightness of positive cells.

Brandtzaeg: You have some background, especially some non-specific staining of the epithelium.

Mayrhofer: I would contest that; with the conditions of illumination that I use, the yellowish autofluorescence of the epithelium is quite different in colour from the specific fluorescence of fluorescein. It is present even in unstained material.

Brandtzaeg: Is there a problem with eosinophilic granulocytes?

Mayrhofer: Yes, and for that reason I have routinely used Lendrum's stain (Johnston & Bienenstock 1974) to modify the fluorescence of the eosinophils so that it is readily distinguished from that of specifically stained cells.

Brandtzaeg: Have you checked on peroxidase in these fluorescent cells?

Mayrhofer: Yes. Neither the IgE-containing plasma cells in the mesenteric lymph node nor the fluorescent mast cells in the lamina propria contain endogenous peroxidase, when tested in paraffin-embedded tissues. Eosinophils, and macrophages in the lymph node medulla, were positive for peroxidase under the same conditions.

White: I would like to take up the question of the membrane of the mast cell and its affinity for Ig. One would expect, from all that we know about heterocytotropic hypersensitivity, that the mast cell membrane would have an affinity for a lot of immunoglobulins and that there would be a rapid dynamic equilibrium for IgG antibodies and a slower one for IgE. When we were trying to isolate the two immunoglobulins of the guinea pig, γ_1 and γ_2, we observed a difference relative to their attachment to mast cells. The γ_1 (but not the γ_2) would go onto rat or mouse mast cells in connective tissues exactly as you show, and give this curious pattern of scalloped fluorescence. So the non-specific fluorescence to which you referred is an interesting phenomenon. In other words, if you take a frozen section of tissue and expose it to immunoglobulin, it would go onto the surface of the mast cell because it has an affinity for it. This is something which in the case of the guinea-pig antibody (and one could narrow it down to a determinant group on the H2 domain of the Fc piece of guinea pig γ_1) is productive of a brilliant fluorescent reaction. Human IgG has this ability too. This appears to be class-specific for human immunoglobulins. So when you do a double-layer staining reaction in which you put rabbit antibody on (rabbit anti-rat IgE, as it were), I think you would be laying the ground for this kind of result.

Mayrhofer: I don't believe that the fluorescence of the mast cells is non-specific. One of the specificity controls that I used was to substitute purified normal rabbit IgG for the specific rabbit anti-rat IgE as the middle layer of the sandwich. When this was done, there was no fluorescence after the addition of the top layer of fluorescent goat anti-rabbit Ig.

Cebra: Ishizaka's group (J. S. Urban, T. Ishizaka & K. Ishizaka, unpublished work 1976) have recently shown that after *Nippostrongylus* infection in rats there is a sharp increase in the number of circulating IgE-containing cells. Have you looked at peripheral blood cells and, if so, have you stained these with Alcian blue? I wonder whether Ishizaka's group may not have been detecting basophils in the circulation.

Secondly, what is known about the specificity of the abundant IgE produced after the infection? Kishimoto & Ishizaka (1973) suggested that a distinctive set of 'helper' cells seems to be stimulated by worm cuticle carriers. Thereafter, no matter what determinant is placed on this cuticle, a certain amount of IgE is produced that is reactive with that hapten. I wonder whether such a worm infection might not simply stimulate any kind of responding B cells to express IgE?

Mayrhofer: I have not looked for IgE-containing cells in rat blood, but I do know that basophils are notably absent in this species. In a preliminary study, I have not seen a basophilia in rats during infestation with *Nippostrongylus*.

In answer to your second question, one of the outstanding problems is how much of the antibody formed during the parasite infestation is specific. A potentiation of homocytotropic antibody responses to unrelated antigens during helminth infestations has been clearly demonstrated (Orr & Blair 1969; Jarrett & Stewart 1972). However, because of the antigenic complexity of parasites, it is difficult to measure the fraction of the total IgE response to infestation that is antibody directed at parasite antigens and the fraction that is directed against an unknown number of normal environmental antigens. The question has an important clinical aspect. There are epidemiological studies that suggest that allergic diseases are almost absent in areas of the world where parasite infestation is universal (Bennich & Johansson 1971; Godfrey 1975). It has been suggested that the high levels of IgE in parasitized humans may be the result of potentiated reagin responses to environmental antigens. Dr Ogilvie (Ogilvie & Jones 1973) has suggested that the potentiated response may protect the individual from serious allergic reactions to parasite antigens by competing with parasite-specific IgE antibodies for binding sites on mast cells. On the other hand, one could explain the epidemiological evidence by assuming that most of the IgE in infested individuals is directed against parasite antigens and that this antibody protects against allergic responses to environmental antigens by the same mechanism. On the latter hypothesis, man's natural state is to be parasitized and allergy-free and it is hygiene that has caused a proportion of the population to become troubled by allergy. Resolution of this problem may provide clues for the prophylaxis of allergy.

Evans: You made some statements about the sensitivity of the mast cell in the rat to alcohol fixation which I didn't understand. If the mast cell were disrupted by fixation, presumably you wouldn't see the IgE?

Mayrhofer: I don't think that ethanol fixation disrupts the mast cells, but that the staining properties of the granules are altered. This may involve the interaction of the basic proteins and the acidic mucopolysaccharide, heparin, in the mast cell granules. Certain fixatives may preserve the acidic groups of heparin so that they are available for subsequent binding with dyes such as Alcian blue.

Evans: Can I ask you about the technique used for staining with toluidine blue? Some histochemists when they stain with toluidine blue avoid subsequent exposure of the specimen to alcohol.

Mayrhofer: It depends on the conditions of staining. I have found that connective tissue and peritoneal mast cells hold toluidine blue and their metachromasia even after reprocessing through alcohol if they are initially stained in an alcoholic solution of the dye (50% ethanol, pH 3.5).

Evans: What technique did you use for the Alcian blue staining?

Mayrhofer: I have followed the method used by Enerbäck (1966). Staining is done in 0.7N-HCl. At the pH of this solution, the only dye-binding groups remaining ionized are said to be the sulphates of sulphated mucopolysaccharides. In the gut, the only structures stained are the mast cells and the contents of goblet cells. After counterstaining with Safranin in 0.125N-HCl, Alcian blue is displaced from mucus and the mast cells alone are stained blue.

Evans: I believe that in the guinea pig Kurloff cells may be stained with Alcian blue in certain circumstances. Can one stain rat plasma cells with this dye?

Mayrhofer: I have stained mesenteric lymph node sections containing IgE-secreting plasma cells with the same method. Plasma cells in the medullary cords, and in particular those secreting IgE, do not stain with Alcian blue. It has been argued in the past that mucosal mast cells and 'globule leucocytes' are Russell body-containing plasma cells (Dobson 1966; Whur & Johnston 1967). To support this view one would have to argue that Russell body cells have histochemical properties different from plasma cells from which they are believed to arise.

Evans: The Kurloff cell inclusion looks rather like a Russell body (Marshall *et al.* 1971).

Mayrhofer: I think the most convincing distinction is that the mucosal mast cells have been shown to contain histamine and 5-hydroxytryptamine, and are therefore in this key respect related to mast cells elsewhere (Murray *et al.* 1968; Miller & Walshaw 1972).

Lehner: If IgE binds onto the membrane of mast cells, they must have Fc receptors for IgE. Have you looked for these?

Mayrhofer: No. To look with this sort of approach requires an *in vitro* system, and at present this means adopting either the blood basophil or the peritoneal mast cell as one's model. However, I am not convinced that they are the same as the mucosal mast cell, for reasons I mentioned in my paper.

Lachmann: You were suggesting that in the mucosal mast cells the IgE was intracytoplasmic. Wouldn't you have expected that staining to be granular, or at least outlined by the granules? Your micrographs show a diffuse staining.

Mayrhofer: Yes. I wouldn't like to say whether the IgE is in the granules or in the soluble cytoplasm. The granules are very small in these cells, and often closely packed.

Ferguson: You mentioned that mast cells are distributed throughout the length of the small intestine. My colleague Mr T. T. MacDonald (unpublished work 1975) has examined the changes in the numbers of intestinal mast cells during *Nippostrongylus brasiliensis* infection of rats. He has found expansion of the mast cell population not only along the entire small intestine but also in segments of small intestine which have been transplanted under the kidney capsules as fetal tissue (by the technique of Ferguson & Parrott 1972) and therefore completely isolated from antigenic stimulation via the lumen. It seems to me likely that the mast cells of the intestinal mucosa are derived from lymph and that their precursors follow the same migration pathways as immunoblasts.

Bienenstock: The Ishizakas found that if they put rat thymus into long-term tissue culture they obtained fairly pure colonies and the expansion of mast cells (Ishizaka *et al.* 1976). It has been suggested in the past that lymphocytes and mast cells are related. Miller (1971) said that the mastoblasts in animals infected with *Nippostrongylus* are indistinguishable from immunoblasts in these animals. We have shown T cell markers on rabbit basophils, which suggests that these two cell types may be related (Day *et al.* 1975). Burnet (1965) showed that the thymuses of NZB mice had huge infiltrations with what looked like colony expansion of mast cells. So the possibility is there.

Gowans: The origin of tissue mast cells, including those in the intestine of animals with intestinal parasites, is unknown and it should be emphasized that the evidence for an origin from lymphocytes is entirely circumstantial. This includes the Ishizaka studies which are a follow-up of the earlier work of Ginsburg & Sachs (1963).

References

BENNICH, H. & JOHANSSON, S. G. O. (1971) Structure and function of human immunoglobulin E. *Adv. Immunol. 13*, 1-55

BURNET, F. M. (1965) Mast cells in the thymus of NZB mice. *J. Pathol. Bacteriol. 89*, 271-284

DAY, R. P., SINGAL, D. P. & BIENENSTOCK, J. (1975) Presence of thymic antigen on rabbit basophils. *J. Immunol. 114*, 1333-1336

DOBSON, C. (1966) Immunofluorescent staining of globule leucocytes in the colon of the sheep. *Nature (Lond.) 211*, 875

DONOVAN, R., JOHANSSON, S. G. O., BENNICH, H. & SOOTHILL, J. F. (1969) Immunoglobulins in nasal polyp fluid. *Int. Arch. Allergy Appl. Immunol. 37*, 154

ENERBÄCK, L. (1966) Mast cells in rat gastrointestinal mucosa. 2. Dye-binding and metachromatic properties. *Acta Pathol. Microbiol. Scand. 66*, 303-312

FELTKAMP-VROOM, T. M., STALLMAN, P. J., AALBERSE, R. C. & REERINK-BRONGERS, E. E. (1975) Immunofluorescence studies on renal tissue, tonsils, adenoids, nasal polyps, and skin of atopic and nonatopic patients, with special reference to IgE. *Clin. Immunol. Immunopathol. 4*, 392-404

FERGUSON, A. & PARROTT, D. M. V. (1972) Growth and development of 'antigen-free' grafts of foetal mouse intestine. *J. Pathol. 106*, 95-101

GINSBURG, H. & SACHS, L. (1963) Formation of pure suspensions of mast cells in tissue culture by differentiation of lymphoid cells from the mouse thymus. *J. Natl. Cancer Inst. 31*, 1

GODFREY, R. C. (1975) Asthma and IgE levels in rural and urban communities of The Gambia. *Clin. Allergy 5*, 201-207

HALLIWELL, R. E. W. (1973) The localization of IgE in canine skin: an immunofluorescent study. *J. Immunol. 110*, 422-430

ISHIZAKA, T., ODUDAIRA, H., MAUSER, L. E. & ISHIZAKA, K. (1976) Development of rat mast cells *in vitro*. I. Differentiation of mast cells from thymus cells. *J. Immunol. 116*, 747-754

JARRETT, E. E. E. & STEWART, D. C. (1972) Potentiation of rat reaginic (IgE) antibody by helminth infection. Simultaneous potentiation of separate reagins. *Immunology 23*, 749-755

JOHNSTON, N. W. & BIENENSTOCK, J. (1974) Abolition of non-specific fluorescent staining of eosinophils. *J. Immunol. Methods 4*, 189-194

KISHIMOTO, T. & ISHIZAKA, K. (1973) Regulation of antibody response *in vitro*. VII. Enhancing soluble factors for IgG and IgE antibody response. *J. Immunol. 111*, 1194-1205

MARSHALL, A. H. E., SWETTENHAM, K. V., VERNON-ROBERTS, B. & REVELL, P. A. (1971) Studies on the function of the Kurloff cell. *Int. Arch. Allergy Appl. Immunol. 40*, 137-152

MILLER, H. R. P. (1971) Immune reactions in mucous membranes. The differentiation of intestinal mast cells during helminth expulsion in the rat. *Lab. Invest. 24*, 339-347

MILLER, H. R. P. & WALSHAW, R. (1972) Immune reactions in mucous membranes. IV. Histochemistry of intestinal mast cells during helminth expulsion in the rat. *Am. J. Pathol. 69*, 195-206

MURRAY, M., MILLER, H. R. P. & JARRETT, W. F. H. (1968) The globule leukocyte and its derivation from the subepithelial mast cell. *Lab. Invest. 19*, 222-234

NAKAJIMA, S., GILLESPIE, D. N. & GLEICH, G. J. (1975) Differences between IgA and IgE as secretory proteins. *Clin. Exp. Immunol. 21*, 306-317

OGILVIE, B. M. & JONES, V. E. (1973) Immunity in the parasitic relationship between helminths and hosts. *Prog. Allergy 17*, 93-144

ORR, T. S. C. & BLAIR, A. M. J. N. (1969) Potentiated reagin response to egg albumin and conalbumin in *Nippostrongylus brasiliensis* infected rats. *Life Sci. 8*, 1073-1077

WHUR, P. & JOHNSTON, H. S. (1967) Ultrastructure of globule leucocytes in immune rats infected with *Nippostrongylus brasiliensis* and their possible relationship to the Russell body cell. *J. Pathol. Bacteriol. 93*, 81-85

The immunological consequences of nematode infection

BRIDGET M. OGILVIE* and DELPHINE M. V. PARROTT**

*National Institute for Medical Research, Mill Hill, London and **Department of Bacteriology and Immunology, Western Infirmary, Glasgow

Abstract Nematode infections in the gut induce a strong immune response which is rapidly detected parenterally. The response is thymus-dependent and long-lasting and involves both antibodies and cell-mediated reactions. The immunological response to unrelated antigens, tumours and other infectious organisms is altered in animals infected with nematodes. Both antibodies and sensitized lymphocytes participate in the immune response which affects the nematodes themselves, and characteristically the lymphocyte-dependent step cannot act in lactating animals and is neither induced nor able to act in young animals. Present evidence suggests that, despite their well-known association with helminth infections, parasite rejection from the gut does not require the participation of IgE antibodies, mast cells or eosinophils.

Homing of lymphoblasts from the mesenteric lymph node or thoracic duct lymph to the small intestine is increased in rats and mice infected with *Nippostrongylus brasiliensis* or *Trichinella spiralis* and the increase is antigenically non-specific. In mice infected with *T. spiralis* this increase is represented mainly by thymus-derived lymphoblasts.

In the UK nematode infections of the gut are studied for two reasons, either because of their importance in reducing animal productivity or because they induce various pathological or immunological changes in the gut which are of interest for reasons unconnected with parasitism. Here we briefly discuss the pathological changes induced in the host before describing the immunological changes induced by nematodes. Their presence in the gut influences the host's response to other antigens and affects the homing of lymphoblasts from the mesenteric lymph node or thoracic duct lymph to the intestine. Worm expulsion is brought about by a complex interaction between various components of the immune response. This fails in young and lactating animals which in consequence do not expel their worms efficiently.

These aspects of nematode parasitism are illustrated mainly from studies with two nematodes of the small intestine, *Nippostrongylus brasiliensis* in rats and *Trichinella spiralis* in mice, rats or guinea pigs, but some reference is made to studies with other nematodes.

PATHOLOGICAL CHANGES INDUCED BY NEMATODES

It is well known that heavy infections of nematodes in the gut prevent weight gain by the host and frequently cause diarrhoea (Symons & Fairbairn 1962; Castro & Olson 1967). The changes induced by these parasites in the small intestine have been studied by Symons using the *N. brasiliensis*/rat model and Castro and colleagues with *T. spiralis* in guinea pigs. The pathological changes seen in the parasitized small intestine are not specific to nematode infections but appear to be similar to the changes found in bacterial infections (Sprinz 1962) or in malabsorption conditions such as coeliac disease (Symons & Fairbairn 1962; Castro *et al.* 1967). These changes include hyperplasia of the villi, which shorten and become irregularly shaped and oedematous (Symons 1957; Castro *et al.* 1967). Epithelial cells change in appearance (Castro *et al.* 1967; Symons *et al.* 1971) and their turnover rate increases (Symons 1965). Brush border enzymes such as maltase, leucine aminopeptidase and alkaline phosphatase are reduced (Symons & Fairbairn 1962, 1963). Digestion and absorption of sugars and protein is impaired at the sites where the parasites are found (Symons 1960; Symons *et al.* 1971; Castro *et al.* 1967) but there may be no overall fall in digestion and absorption if the infection is localized in the upper part of the gastrointestinal tract, as the rest of the gut may compensate by increased digestion and absorption (Symons 1960, 1961). This is not possible, however, when the infection occurs in the large bowel, for example in cattle infected with *Oesophagostomum radiatum*, which in consequence are severely affected (Bremner 1969).

These deleterious effects of nematode infections are enhanced by loss of appetite and plasma protein leakage into the gut (Mulligan 1972). The studies of Symons and his colleagues (largely with *Trichostrongylus colubriformis* in guinea pigs and sheep) have shown that, because loss of appetite is exacerbated by leakage of plasma protein into the gut at the parasitized site, protein catabolism exceeds protein synthesis. Protein synthesis in the liver is elevated by the increased synthesis of plasma proteins which occurs (Symons & Jones 1974) and is depressed elsewhere, especially in skeletal muscle and wool follicles (Symons & Jones 1971, 1972, 1975). Consequently, productivity measured, for example, by increases in muscle weight or wool growth, is severely affected, even by light infections of gut nematodes and especially in growing animals (Symons & Jones 1974, 1975).

Apparently all nematodes of the gut (with the exception of *Trichuris* species found in the large bowel, see p. 188) induce high levels of IgE in their hosts. The anaphylactic reactions induced by interaction of specific IgE with worm allergen at the infected site may well account at least in part for the efflux of plasma protein into the gut lumen (Barth *et al.* 1966). Light and electron microscopy have shown that junctional complexes between cells of the villi may break down in the parasitized gut, permitting abnormal leakage of proteins into the gut lumen (Murray *et al.* 1971). There are few studies of the pathology of these infections in immunologically incompetent hosts. Ferguson & Jarrett (1975) have suggested that the distortion of villi in the intestine of rats infected with *N. brasiliensis* is caused by a thymus-dependent immune reaction. Whether any of the other changes associated with these infections are immunologically induced is not known.

Infections with nematodes may also cause increased microbial growth in the gut (Cypess *et al.* 1974*c*; Rutter & Beer 1975). It is possible that the pathological changes found in the nematode-infected gut may be caused by this increase in bacteria at the site of infection rather than by the nematodes themselves. Rutter & Beer (1975) studied conventional and gnotobiotic pigs infected with *Trichuris suis*. The muco-haemorrhagic diarrhoea associated with this infection developed only in conventional pigs. Therefore the diarrhoea may be caused by the spirochaetes and vibrio-like organisms which were observed only in the conventional pigs, in which increased numbers of bacteria were found during the clinical phase of the disease (Rutter & Beer 1975).

EFFECT OF NEMATODES ON THE IMMUNE SYSTEM OF THE HOST

The presence of nematode parasites in the gut alters the ability of the host to respond immunologically to a variety of antigens (including other infections), mostly given parenterally. The changes reported to date are summarized in Table 1 and show that immunity may be enhanced or depressed. The remarkable effect of *N. brasiliensis* on IgE levels is thought to result from the production of special helper T cells which enhance IgE, or a lack of suppressor T cells (Jarrett & Ferguson 1974; Kojima & Ovary 1975). Otherwise, these results have been explained by suggesting that the nematodes have non-specific effects on the immune system, such as antigenic competition and enhanced macrophage activity (Cypess *et al.* 1974*a*; Lubiniecki & Cypess 1975). Recent studies of cell homing in infected animals (discussed later, p. 189) have shown changes which might explain some of these effects. The effects of *Syphacia* (Table 1) are noteworthy in that they were caused by naturally

TABLE 1

Influence of nematode infections on the ability of the host to respond to other antigens

Parasite and host	Effect on response	Reference
	(a) Increased	
Trichinella spiralis in mice and rats	Delayed hypersensitivity reaction to BCG Resistance to infection with Listeria Resistance to infection with trypanosomes	Cypess et al. 1974b Cypess et al. 1974a Meerovitch & Ackerman 1974
Nippostrongylus brasiliensis in rats and mice	IgE production Resistance to tumour growth	Orr & Blair 1969 Jarrett & Bazin 1974 Keller et al. 1971
	(b) Decreased	

T. spiralis in mice	Antibody response to
	  (1) sheep red blood cells
	  (2) Japanese B encephalitis virus
	Skin graft survival prolonged
		Faubert & Tanner 1971
		Lubiniecki & Cypess 1975
		
		Svet-Moldavsky et al. 1970

N. brasiliensis in rats	Enhanced tumour growth Enhanced Plasmodium berghei infection	Keller et al. 1971 Golenser et al. 1976
Syphacia oblevata in rats	Incidence of adjuvant arthritis reduced Antibody response to ovalbumin	Pearson & Taylor 1975 Pearson & Taylor 1975
Nematospiroides dubius in mice (Heligmosomoides polygyrus)	Antibody response to sheep red blood cells[a]	Shimp et al. 1975

[a] Sheep red blood cells given orally. In all other reports, antigen given parenterally.

occurring infections which might arise in rodents in all conventional laboratory animal houses.

Nematodes induce a mixed immunological response, evoking antibodies in several immunoglobulin classes, a strong cell-mediated response and an inflammatory reaction which includes may cell types—plasma cells, mononuclear cells, mast cells/basophils and eosinophils (Taliaferro & Sarles 1939). In rats infected with N. brasiliensis, IgE, IgG, and IgM antibodies against parasite antigens have been detected but no IgA antibodies have been reported (Ogilvie & Jones 1973). There is indirect evidence that antibodies begin to affect these worms on day 8 of the infection in rats and by day 10 the effects are severe (see review, Ogilvie & Jones 1973). However, antibodies have not been detected in the sera of rats before day 17, which is after the parasites have been expelled.

Antibodies directed against *T. spiralis* antigens are found in the IgG1, IgG2, IgA and IgM in sera from mice about 11–15 days after the infection (Crandall & Crandall 1972). IgE antibodies were never detected in some strains of mice and in others were found from the second week after the infection (Rivera-Ortiz & Nussenzweig 1976). Cells which will cause accelerated rejection of these parasites from syngeneic recipients are found in the thoracic duct lymph or mesenteric lymph nodes of infected rats by day 7–8 of a *N. brasiliensis* infection (Ogilvie *et al.* 1976) and by day 8 in the mesenteric lymph nodes of mice infected with *T. spiralis* (Wakelin & Lloyd 1976).

THE IMMUNOLOGICAL MECHANISM WHICH EXPELS THE WORMS

The mixed immunological response induced by nematodes may make them especially useful in the study of immune reactions in the gut, but it has complicated the analysis of the immune responses which control these helminths. Besides *N. brasiliensis* and *T. spiralis*, detailed studies of the immune mechanism which affects nematodes have been made with *Trichuris muris*, which is found in the large intestine of mice (Wakelin 1975; Wakelin & Selby 1976), and *Trichostrongylus colubriformis* in guinea pigs (Dineen & Wagland 1966; Rothwell *et al.* 1974). In all cases, a strong, long-lasting and thymus-dependent response is induced (Ogilvie & Jones 1973) and in the case of the first three parasites it is clear that their expulsion requires the sequential action first of antibodies and then of sensitized cells from the mesenteric lymph node (Ogilvie & Jones 1973; Ogilvie & Love 1974; Wakelin 1975; Love *et al.* 1976; Wakelin & Lloyd 1976; Wakelin & Selby 1976). There is a variety of evidence which supports the idea that a two-step mechanism is involved. Recipients given either antiserum or cells are partly protected against infection but a level of resistance approaching that induced by an active infection can be conferred on recipients only by giving them both antiserum and cells from infected donors. In the *N. brasiliensis*/rat model, antibodies (IgG1, Jones *et al.* 1970) affect the worms to make them susceptible to the expulsive action of cells but antibodies alone cause either no rejection or a slow rejection of the worms.

The evidence for this is as follows. Irradiated recipients of antiserum expel their worms slowly if at all, and lactating and young (7–9 weeks) rats do not expel their worms, yet their antibody response (both IgE and IgG1) is normal or increased. That is, serum from young or lactating animals will passively protect immunologically competent recipients from infection and their own worms are damaged by antibodies, so that when transferred into mature non-lactating rats they are susceptible to the cellular step (Ogilvie & Love 1974). The cellular step is brought about by cells which require the presence of the thymus for their induction and have no surface immunoglobulin (Keller & Keist 1972; Ogilvie *et al.* 1976). Therefore, it would seem reasonable to surmise that the effector cells are T cells. The cellular step is induced but cannot act in lactating animals and is not induced in young animals. Furthermore, sensitized cells obtained from mature infected donors do not cause worm expulsion when given to lactating or young recipients harbouring worms already affected by the antibody step (Ogilvie & Love 1974; Love & Ogilvie 1975). Exactly how these cells bring about worm expulsion is not known. They expel worms from rats given 750 rads within five days and these animals have few mast cells or eosinophils at the site of infection (Ogilvie *et al.* 1977). It has been postulated that the release of prostaglandin E is the final effector of immunity to *N. brasiliensis* (Dineen *et al.* 1974) but no explanation has been offered as to how T cells might induce release of prostaglandins. Progress in this area requires a much more detailed understanding of cell changes at the site of infection, information which may come from current studies of cell traffic in parasitized animals (see later, p. 189 *et seq.*).

THE EFFECT OF IgE ANTIBODIES ON NEMATODES

A prolonged, thymus-dependent IgE response is characteristic of nematode as of most helminth infections. Much of this is not directed against parasite antigens, but IgE levels in general are elevated, for reasons discussed earlier. It is, however, clearly established that IgE antibodies are not directly concerned in the expulsion of nematodes. They are often found in animals unable to expel their worms (for example, in lactating hosts) and sometimes are not detectable in hosts which are strongly immune. The best illustration of this is that IgE antibodies have never been found in mice infected with *Trichuris muris* (D. Wakelin, personal communication), nor in man infected with *Trichuris trichiura* (Rosenberg *et al.* 1971). The immune mechanism which expels *T. muris* (Wakelin 1975; Wakelin & Selby 1976) is probably identical with that which expels *N. brasiliensis* and, as outlined above, this requires IgG antibodies and sensitized T cells.

It is nevertheless possible that the anaphylactic reactions induced by IgE antibodies might have an enhancing effect on the immune mechanisms which actually affect the worms. Barth *et al.* (1966) showed that an ovalbumin-induced anaphylactic reaction may enhance the action of antibodies on *N. brasiliensis*. Also, the 'self-cure' reaction described in certain nematode infections appears to be an anaphylactic reaction, although whether an IgE–worm allergen interaction is the primary effector in this situation or dramatically enhances other mechanisms has not been formally demonstrated. 'Self-cure' occurs when animals already infected with a particular nematode ingest a large second infection. Within hours, all the parasites are expelled (reviewed in Ogilvie & Jones 1973). This reaction is not predictable, it occurs only in certain strains of hosts (Cypess & Zidian 1975), and hosts in which it occurs may not necessarily resist further infections.

In the *T. colubriformis*/guinea pig infection there is good evidence that 5-hydroxytryptamine (serotonin) acts directly on the worm to cause expulsion (Rothwell *et al.* 1974). The curious feature of this reaction is that it can be adoptively transferred to recipients only with lymphocytes and not with serum (Dineen & Wagland 1966). If IgE-allergen causes release of 5-hydroxytryptamine from basophils in this infection, the essential requirement for lymphocytes can be explained by suggesting that they are necessary for inducing basophil infiltration into the sites of infection.

INFLUENCE OF PARASITES ON THE TRAFFIC OF IMMUNOBLASTS TO THE SMALL INTESTINE

The main objective in following the traffic of immunoblasts to the small intestine in nematode infection is to study the expulsion mechanism but, as suggested earlier, it may be that a greater gain will be the resolution of those pathological changes which are a direct effect of the parasite itself and those which are a result of the host's response to the parasites. As already stated, the sources of cells which are most effective in transferring immunity to gut parasites are the mesenteric lymph node and thoracic duct lymph. These cell populations contain, particularly after infection, large numbers of activated blast cells which readily take up isotopically labelled DNA precursors or analogues of DNA precursors. As is well known, such cells have a propensity to extravasate into the mucosal layer of the small intestine (Gowans & Knight 1964; Hall *et al.* 1972; Parrott & Ferguson 1974). Immunoblasts could thus, in theory, make close if not direct contact with parasites in the gut, although contact between cells and the nematodes discussed here has never been reported.

In August rats infected with either *T. spiralis* or *N. brasiliensis* larger numbers of [^{125}I]iododeoxyuridine-labelled thoracic duct lymphoblasts accumulate in the small intestine than in uninfected controls (Love & Ogilvie 1977) and in NIH mice infected with *T. spiralis*, similar findings were obtained with mesenteric lymph node blasts (Rose *et al.* 1976*a*). The increase occurred early in mice, within 2–4 days of infection, and was due to increased retention of labelled cells within the whole animal and not redistribution from other sites (Rose *et al.* 1976*a*). It was not related to increase in gut size in infected animals and at the time of nematode expulsion, which occurs about nine days after infection, there was no difference in cell traffic between infected and uninfected mice. In rats the increase in blast cell traffic was somewhat later, not until 9–12 days, it was coincident with gross inflammation, but again was unrelated to increase in gut size. There was a clear indication of increased localization within segments of intestine with the highest worm counts in both rats and mice but none of the increases were antigenically specific. In rats and mice infected with these nematodes, blast cells activated by completely unrelated stimuli were as capable of homing in increased amounts as were cells from donors infected with the same parasite. In normal uninfected mice both T and B blasts home to the gut mucosa (Guy-Grand et al. 1974; Parrott et al. 1975; Sprent 1976). However, in mice infected with T. spiralis the early increased migration of blast cells is almost entirely composed of mesenteric lymph node T immunoblasts. The number of B blasts from mesenteric node suspensions migrating to the gut was the same in infected mice as in normal controls (Rose et al. 1976a).

Villous atrophy is one pathological change in the infected gut which preliminary observations justify linking with the increased arrival of mesenteric lymph blasts to the small intestine (M. L. Rose & D. M. V. Parrott, unpublished data). By day 4 in mice infected with T. spiralis there is a shortening of villi and an increase in intraepithelial lymphocytes in the first segment of the intestine where worm counts and labelled cell accumulation are highest, whilst changes in lower segments remain minimal. There was, however, no indication from autoradiographs of sections of gut that the injected labelled cells were in any way attracted to the worms, although some labelled cells were in the epithelial layer as well as in the lamina propria. At this time too, as preliminary studies show (D. M. V. Parrott, unpublished), there is little polymorph infiltration or other cellular change indicative of inflammation.

Many of the results of cell migration to the infected gut are reminiscent of other situations in which activated T blasts have been shown to cross blood vessels into local areas of inflammation. Newly formed thoracic duct T blasts which appear during an infection with *Listeria monocytogenes* will assemble very readily in an inflamed peritoneal cavity but in an entirely non-specific way (McGregor & Logie 1974). Similarly the induction of peritonitis may cause cells to be diverted from the intestine in nematode infection (Love & Ogilvie 1977). T blasts from lymph nodes draining the skin after the application of a contact sensitizer such as oxazolone will accumulate in sites inflamed by an irritant such as turpentine or an unrelated contact sensitizer as easily as into the site to which the priming chemical has been applied (Asherson et al. 1973; Parrott et al. 1975). Four days after T. spiralis infection large numbers of peripheral T blasts appear in the small intestine, providing the skin is not inflamed at the same time (Rose et al. 1976b). These cells do not accumulate in the normal gut (Parrott & Ferguson 1974; Parrott et al. 1975).

Even at this early stage these studies of cell traffic in parasitized animals have yielded results which enable us to suggest possible explanations for some of the phenomena described earlier in this paper. For example, the pathological changes usually ascribed to the presence of nematodes might be exacerbated as a result of activation of T blasts by unrelated co-existing infections such as *Listeria monocytogenes*. Non-specific trapping of circulating lymphocytes such as that occurring in the mesenteric lymph nodes of *T. spiralis*-infected mice (Rose et al. 1976b) could reduce the chances of lymphocyte–antigen interaction in peripheral sites, which might explain alterations in the responsiveness of nematode-infected animals to unrelated antigens. Decreased immune responsiveness might occur because effector T blasts are diverted to the gut in infected animals rather than to the site of antigen location. The absence of specificity in the increased flow of blast cell traffic could well explain the enhanced worm expulsion which occurs in appropriately timed dual infections (Bruce & Wakelin 1974).

Blast cell diversion might also explain the failure of lactating animals to expel nematodes. In rats there are the same number of blast cells in the intestine of lactating as of normal mothers although the gut of lactating animals is $2\frac{1}{2}$ times increased (Love & Ogilvie 1977). In lactating mice there is an increase in blast cell migration to the gut but there is as much if not more migration to the mammary glands (M. L. Rose & D. M. V. Parrott, unpublished data).

It is obvious that all these suggestions require the support of many more experimental data before they can be accepted as anything other than speculation. It is clear, however, that the study of nematode infections of the gut can yield ideas which may be valuable in understanding the role which immune reactions may have in pathological conditions of the gut and the effect of these conditions on the immunological competence of the animal concerned.

ACKNOWLEDGEMENTS

D.M.V.P. wishes to acknowledge a grant from the Medical Research Council and to thank colleagues for their permission to refer to unpublished data.

References

ASHERSON, G. L., ALLWOOD, G. G. & MAYHEW, B. (1973) Contact sensitivity in the mouse. IX. Movement of T blasts in the draining nodes to sites of inflammation. *Immunology* 25, 485-493

BARTH, E. E. E., JARRETT, W. F. H. & URQUHART, G. M. (1966) Studies on the mechanism of the self-cure reaction in rats infected with *Nippostrongylus brasiliensis*. *Immunology 10*, 459-464

BREMNER, K. C. (1969) Pathogenetic factors in experimental bovine oesophagostomosis. IV. Exudative enteropathy as a cause of hypoproteinemia. *Exp. Parasitol. 25*, 382-394

BRUCE, R. G. & WAKELIN, D. (1974) Immunity to *Trichuris muris* in mice infected with *Trichinella spiralis*. *Parasitology 69, xx*

CASTRO, G. A., OLSON, L. J. & BAKER, R. D. (1967) Glucose maladsorption and intestinal histopathology in *Trichinella spiralis*-infected guinea pigs. *J. Parasitol. 53*, 595-612

CASTRO, G. A. & OLSON, L. J. (1967) Relationship between body weight and food and water intake in *Trichinella spiralis*-infected guinea pigs. *J. Parasitol. 53*, 589-594

CRANDALL, R. B. & CRANDALL, C. A. (1972) *Trichinella spiralis:* immunologic response to infection in mice. *Exp. Parasitol. 31*, 378-398

CYPESS, R. H., LUBINIECKI, A. S. & SWIDWA, D. M. (1974a) Decreased susceptibility of *Listeria monocytogenes* in *Trichinella spiralis*-infected mice. *Infect. Immun. 9*, 477-479

CYPESS, R. H., MOLINARI, J., EBERSOLE, J. L. & LUBINIECKI, A. S. (1974b) Immunological sequelae of *Trichinella spiralis* infection in mice. II. Potentiation of cell-mediated response to BCG following infection with *Trichinella spiralis*. *Infect. Immun. 10*, 107-110

CYPESS, R. H., SWIDWA, D. W., KENNY, J. F. & YEE, R. B. (1974c) Influence of a metazoan infection in the mouse on enteric colonization and immune response to *Escherichia coli*. *J. Infect. Dis. 130*, 534-538

CYPESS, R. H. & ZIDIAN, J. L. (1975) *Heligmosomoides polygyrus (= Nematospiroides dubius):* the development of self cure and/or protection in several strains of mice. *J. Parasitol. 61*, 819-824

DINEEN, J. K. & WAGLAND, B. M. (1966) The cellular transfer of immunity to *Trichostrongylus colubriformis* in an isogenic strain of guinea pig. II. The relative susceptibility of the larval and adult stages of the parasite to immunological attack. *Immunology 11*, 45-57

DINEEN, J. K., KELLY, J. D., GOODRICH, B. S. & SMITH, I. D. (1974) Expulsion of *Nipostrongylus brasiliensis* from the small intestine of the rat by prostaglandin-like factors from ram semen. *Int. Arch. Allergy Appl. Immunol. 46*, 360-374

FAUBERT, G. & TANNER, C. E. (1971) *Trichinella spiralis:* inhibition of sheep hemagglutinins in mice. *Exp. Parasitol. 30*, 120-123

FERGUSON, A. & JARRETT, E. E. E. (1975) Hypersensitivity reactions in the small intestine: thymus independent reactions of experimental 'partial villous atrophy'. *Gut 16*, 114-117

GOLENSER, J., SPIRA, D. T. & SCHMUEL, Z. (1976) Mutual influence of infection with *Plasmodium berghei* and *Nippostrongylus brasiliensis*. *Parasitology 73, xiii*

GOWANS, J. L. & KNIGHT, E. J. (1964) The route of re-circulation of lymphocytes in the rat. *Proc. R. Soc. B Biol. Sci. 159*, 257-282

GUY-GRAND, D., GRISCELLI, C. & VASSALLI, P. (1974) The gut-associated lymphoid system: nature and properties of the large dividing cells. *Eur. J. Immunol. 4*, 435-443

HALL, J. G., PARRY, D. M. & SMITH, M. E. (1972) The distribution and differentiation of lymph-borne immunoblasts after intravenous injection into syngeneic recipients. *Cell Tissue Kinet. 5*, 269-281

JARRETT, E. E. E. & BAZIN, H. (1974) Elevation of total serum IgE in rats following helminth parasite infection. *Nature (Lond.) 252*, 612-613

JARRETT, E. E. E. & FERGUSON, A. (1974) Effect of T cell depletion on the potentiated reagin response. *Nature (Lond.) 250*, 421-422

JONES, V. E., EDWARDS, A. J. & OGILVIE, B. M. (1970) The circulating immunoglobulins involved in protective immunity to the intestinal stage of *Nippostrongylus brasiliensis* in the rat. *Immunology 18*, 621-633

KELLER, R. & KEIST, R. (1972) Protective immunity to *Nippostrongylus brasiliensis* in the rat: central role of the lymphocyte in worm expulsion. *Immunology 22*, 767-773

KELLER, R., OGILVIE, B. M. & SIMPSON, E. (1971) Tumour growth in nematode-infected animals. *Lancet 1*, 678-680

KOJIMA, S. & OVARY, Z. (1975) Effect of *Nippostrongylus brasiliensis* infection on anti-hapten IgE antibody response in the mouse. I. Induction of carrier specific helper cells. *Cell. Immunol. 17*, 383-391

LOVE, R. J. & OGILVIE, B. M. (1975) *Nippostrongylus brasiliensis* in young rats. Lymphocytes expel larval infections but not adult worms. *Clin. Exp. Immunol. 21*, 155-162

LOVE, R. J. & OGILVIE, B. M. (1977) *Nippostrongylus brasiliensis* and *Trichinella spiralis*: localization of lymphoblasts in the small intestine of parasitized rats. *Exp. Parasitol.*, in press

LOVE, R. J., OGILVIE, B. M. & McLAREN, D. J. (1976) The immune mechanism which expels the intestinal stage of *Trichinella spiralis* from rats. *Immunology 30*, 7-15

LUBINIECKI, A. S. & CYPESS, R. H. (1975) Immunological sequelae of *Trichinella spiralis* infection in mice: effect on the antibody responses to sheep erythrocytes and Japanese B encephalitis virus. *Infect. Immun. 11*, 1306-1311

MCGREGOR, D. D. & LOGIE, P. S. (1974) Localisation of sensitized lymphocytes in inflammatory exudates. *J. Exp. Med. 139*, 1415-1430

MEEROVITCH, E. & ACKERMAN, S. J. (1974) Trypanosomiasis in rats with trichinosis. *Trans. R. Soc. Trop. Med. Hyg. 68*, 417

MULLIGAN, W. (1972) The effect of helminthic infection on the protein metabolism of the host. *Proc. Nutr. Soc. 31*, 47-51

MURRAY, M., JARRETT, W. F. H., JENNINGS, F. W. & MILLER, H. R. P. (1971) Structural changes associated with increased permeability of parasitized mucous membranes to macromolecules, in *Pathology of Parasitic Diseases* (S. M. Gaafar, ed.), p. 197, Purdue University Studies, Lafayette, Indiana

OGILVIE, B. M. & JONES, V. E. (1973) Immunity in the parasitic relationship between helminths and hosts. *Prog. Allergy 17*, 93-144

OGILVIE, B. M. & LOVE, R. J. (1974) Cooperation between antibodies and cells in immunity to a nematode parasite. *Transplant. Rev. 19*, 147-168

OGILVIE, B. M., LOVE, R. J., JARRA, W. & BROWN, K. N. (1976) *Nippostrongylus brasiliensis* in rats: the cellular requirement for worm expulsion. *Immunology*, in press

ORR, T. S. C. & BLAIR, A. M. J. N. (1969) Potentiated reagin response to egg albumin and conalbumin in *Nippostrongylus brasiliensis* infected rats. *Life Sci. 8*, 1073-1077

PARROTT, D. M. V. & FERGUSON, A. (1974) Selective migration of lymphocytes within the mouse small intestine. *Immunology 26*, 571-588

PARROTT, D. M. V., ROSE, M. L., SLESS, F., DE FREITAS, A. & BRUCE, R. G. (1975) Factors which determine the accumulation of immunoblasts in gut and skin, in *Future Trends in Inflammation II* (Girond, J. P., Willoughby, D. A. & Velo, D. P., eds.), pp. 32-39, Birkhauser Verlag, Basel

PEARSON, D. J. & TAYLOR, G. (1975) The influence of the nematode *Syphacia oblevata* on adjuvant arthritis in the rat. *Immunology 29*, 391-396

RIVERA-ORTIZ, C. & NUSSENZWEIG, R. (1976) *Trichinella spiralis*: anaphylactic antibody formation and susceptibility in strains of inbred mice *Exp Parasitol. 39*, 7-17

ROSE, M L., PARROTT, D. M. V. & BRUCE, R. G. (1976a) Migration of lymphoblasts to the small intestine I. Effect of *Trichinella spiralis* infection on the migration of mesenteric lymphoblasts and mesenteric T lymphoblasts in syngeneic mice. *Immunology. 31*, 723-730

ROSE, M. L., PARROTT, D. M. V. & BRUCE, R. G. (1976b) Migration of lymphoblasts to the small intestine. II. Divergent migration of mesenteric and peripheral immunoblasts to sites of inflammation in the mouse. *Cell. Immunol.*, in press

ROSENBERG, E. B., POLMAR, S. H. & WHALEN, G. E. (1971) Increasing circulating IgE in trichinosis. *Ann. Intern. Med. 75*, 575-578

ROTHWELL, T. L. W., PRITCHARD, R. K. & LOVE, R. J. (1974) Studies on the role of histamine and 5-hydroxytryptamine in immunity against the nematode *Trichostrongylus colubriformis*. I. *In vivo* and *in vitro* effects of the amines. *Int. Arch. Allergy Appl. Immunol. 46*, 1-13

RUTTER, J. M. & BEER, R. J. S. (1975) Synergism between *Trichuris suis* and the microbial flora of the large intestine causing dysentery in pigs. *Infect. Immun. 11*, 395-404

SHIMP, R. G., CRANDALL, R. B. & CRANDALL, C. A. (1975) *Heligmosomoides polygyrus* (= *Nematospiroides dubius*): suppression of antibody response to orally administered sheep erythrocytes in infected mice. *Exp. Parasitol. 38*, 257-269

SPRENT, J. (1976) Fate of H2-activated T lymphocytes in syngeneic hosts. I. Fate in lymphoid tissues and intestines traced with ^{3}H-thymidine, ^{125}I-deoxyuridine and ^{51}-chromium. *Cell. Immunol. 21*, 278-302

SPRINZ, H. (1962) Morphological response of intestinal mucosa to enteric bacteria and its implication for sprue and Asiatic cholera. *Fed. Proc. 21*, 57-64

SVET-MOLDAVSKY, G. J., SHAGHIJIAN, G. S., CHEENYAKHOVSKAYA, I. Y., OZERETSKOVSKAYA, N. N. & KADAGHIDZE, Z. G. (1970) Inhibition of skin allograft rejection in *Trichinella* infected mice. *Transplantation 9*, 69-70

SYMONS, L. E. A. (1957) Pathology of infestation of the rat with *Nippostrongylus muris* (Yokagawa). I. Changes in the water content, dry weight and tissues of the small intestine. *Aust. J. Biol. Sci. 10*, 374-383

SYMONS, L. E. A. (1960) Pathology of infestation of the rat with *Nippostrongylus muris* (Yokagawa). V. Protein digestion. *Aust. J. Biol. Sci. 13*, 578-583

SYMONS, L. E. A. (1961) Pathology of infestation of the rat with *Nippostrongylus muris* (Yokagawa). VI. Absorption *in vivo* from the distal ileum. *Aust. J. Biol. Sci. 14*, 165-171

SYMONS, L. E. A. (1965) Kinetics of the epithelial cells and morphology of villi and crypts in the jejunum of the rat infected by the nematode *Nippostrongylus brasiliensis*. *Gastroenterology 49*, 158-168

SYMONS, L. E. A. & FAIRBAIRN, D. (1962) Pathology, absorption, transport and activity of digestive enzymes in rat jejunum parasitized by the nematode, *Nippostrongylus brasiliensis*. *Fed. Proc. 21*, 913-918

SYMONS, L. E. A. & FAIRBAIRN, D. (1963) Biochemical pathology of the rat jejunum parasitized by the nematode *Nippostrongylus brasiliensis*. *Exp. Parasitol. 13*, 284-304

SYMONS, L. E. A. & JONES, W. O. (1971) Protein metabolism. I. Incorporation of ^{14}C-L-leucine into skeletal muscle and liver proteins of mice and guinea pigs infected with *Nematospiroides dubius* and *Trichostrongylus colubriformis*. *Exp. Parasitol. 29*, 230-241

SYMONS, L. E. A. & JONES, W. O. (1972) Protein metabolism. 2. Protein turnover, synthesis and muscle growth in suckling, young and adult mammals infected with *Nematospiroides dubius* or *Trichostrongylus colubriformis*. *Exp. Parasitol. 32*, 335-342

SYMONS, L. E. A. & JONES, W. O. (1974) Protein metabolism. 3. Relationship between albumin metabolism and elevated liver protein synthesis in the guinea pig infected with *Trichostrongylus colubriformis*. *Exp. Parasitol. 35*, 492-502

SYMONS, L. E. A. & JONES, W. O. (1975) Skeletal muscle, liver and wool protein synthesis by sheep infected by the nematode *Trichostrongylus colubriformis*. *Aust. J. Agric. Res. 26*, 1063-1072

SYMONS, L. E. A., GIBBINS, J. R. & JONES, W. O. (1971) Jejunal maladsorption in the rat infected by the nematode *Nippostrongylus brasiliensis*. *Int. J. Parasitol. 1*, 179-187

TALIAFERRO, W. H. & SARLES, M. P. (1939) The cellular reactions in the skin, lungs and intestine of normal and immune rats after infection with *Nippostrongylus muris*. *J. Infect. Dis. 64*, 157-192

WAKELIN, D. (1975) Immune expulsion of *Trichuris muris* from mice during a primary infection: analysis of the components involved. *Parasitology 70*, 397-406

WAKELIN, D. & LLOYD, M. (1976) Accelerated expulsion of adult *Trichinella spiralis* in mice given lymphoid cells and serum from infected donors. *Parasitology 72*, 307-316

WAKELIN, D. & SELBY, G. R. (1976) Immune expulsion of *Trichuris muris* from resistant mice: suppression by irradiation and restoration by transfer of lymphoid cells. *Parasitology 72*, 41-50

Discussion

Bienenstock: Guy-Grand's work (Guy-Grand et al. 1974) and that of Sprent (1976) suggests that T blasts have preferential localization in and homing to the gut epithelium, as opposed to the B blasts which do not reach the epithelium, in this infection.

Parrott: I have found some labelled T cells in the epithelial layer, but they don't occur so very often. Most of them are still in the lamina propria, when one uses [^{125}I]iododeoxyuridine labelling. If I had used [^{3}H]thymidine and looked at longer times after infection, I might have found more T cells in the epithelial layer. This procedure has proved successful in other experiments (Parrott et al. 1975).

Bienenstock: The obvious question is whether these T cells have anything to do with what is going on in the lumen.

Parrott: In nematode infections the T blasts don't appear to be interested in the worms in the gut. There is no inflammatory response near the nematodes, and we don't see any localization or clustering of T cells around the worm.

Gowans: When you refer to the homing of T cells, which kind of T cell are you talking about? Are you referring to T-blasts which can be labelled *in vitro* with [^{125}I]iododeoxyuridine or [^{3}H]thymidine, or to small, non-dividing T cells which can be labelled *in vitro* with radioactive precursors of RNA?

Parrott: In the studies referred to here (Rose et al. 1976) we labelled the blasts; one can of course also label ordinary T cells and trace them by autoradiography but I haven't seen any small T lymphocyte labelled by [^{3}H]-adenosine or [^{3}H]uridine in the lamina propria, with the exception of the area immediately around the Peyer's patches (Parrott & Ferguson 1974).

Lehner: Dr Ogilvie, you suggested that in the first 10 days of infection antibodies are produced which act on the nematodes, and then lymphocytes take over. Is this an *in vivo* sequence of the immune response, or are you implying that *in vitro* the lymphocytes could affect the worms?

Ogilvie: Unfortunately it is difficult to study the effect of antibodies or lymphocytes on this parasite *in vitro*. Fully sensitized and competent lymphocytes are found in rats as early as seven days after infection. If you transfer lymphocytes from a 7-day infected rat to another rat infected simultaneously with antibody-damaged worms they will expel the worms from the recipient within two or three days. But in the rat from which the cells came, lymphocytes apparently cannot act on the worms until the antibody step affects the worms, which does not happen until day 10. I dont' know why it is necessary for worms to be damaged by antibodies before cells can have their effect.

Lehner: Is the antibody acting on its own, or is it opsonizing the worms for phagocytosis?

Ogilvie: I think the antibody interferes with the parasites' feeding and they become rather unhappy worms! One can mimic all the effects of antibody by simply taking worms out of an infected rat before antibodies affect them and putting them into culture without antibodies. Twenty-four to 48 hours later we find all the changes which we normally associate with antibody action in the cultured worms, including sensitivity to lymphocyte action when cultured worms are put into rats again (Love *et al.* 1975). It seems that when worms are made less fit, either by the action of antibodies or by being kept *in vitro*, they become susceptible to lymphocyte attack.

Lehner: When the lymphocytes come along, are the worms killed?

Ogilvie: The worms are never killed. If you collect them as they come out of the intestine and put them back they behave like antibody-damaged worms (Love *et al.* 1975).

Lehner: Is the lymphocyte response antibody-independent or antibody-dependent?

Ogilvie: I think it is antibody-independent. To test the effect of the second step we take antibody-damaged worms from donors (or damage them in culture, as just described) and put them into an irradiated rat. Into that animal we put thoracic duct cells that have been run down a column of plastic beads coated with anti-rat globulin. The cells which are not retained on the column cause rejection of these worms within five days. I do not think antibodies are involved in the rejection of worms by lymphocytes in this experimental situation (Ogilvie *et al.* 1977).

Evans: Do you get the same result with lymphocytes that have been cultured?

Ogilvie: This experiment has not been done.

Mayrhofer: I find it difficult to imagine what causes the expulsion of the worms. We know that antibody damages them and that perhaps lymphocytes do also, but what makes them move down the gastrointestinal tract? Is it gut motility? I ask this because it is well known that the motility and tone of smooth muscle is reduced under the hormonal influences of pregnancy. Could the effect of lactation be similar, acting at a non-immunological level in a sequence of events with an earlier immunologically activated trigger?

Ogilvie: The work of Dineen *et al.* (1974) suggests that the final effect is due to prostaglandin E. When prostaglandins were introduced directly into the gut of these animals the parasites were expelled very quickly and, conversely, infected rats given inhibitors of prostaglandins were unable to expel their worms. So the final effect may be due to prostaglandin, released presumably from macrophages or T cells, or eosinophils.

Schmidt: Is there any evidence that macrophages play a role in your system?

Ogilvie: There is no evidence for their involvement, but if Dineen *et al.* (1964) are correct and the final effect is due to prostaglandins, the macrophage may be a source of prostaglandins.

Mayrhofer: It is difficult to argue from such experiments unless one knows the final step in worm expulsion. Failure to expel worms may be attributed to an early event, such as failure of mast cell accumulation or degranulation, whereas the defect may lie at the end of the chain of events.

On a different point, the temporal correlation between mast cell accumulation in the lamina propria and the onset of worm expulsion (or the failure to find such a correlation) has been held to support (or refute) the role of mast cells in immunity to *Nippostrongylus*. However, mast cell numbers as such may not be important. For instance, in the lactating rat, the presence of large numbers of mast cells despite failure to expel worms does not necessarily indicate normal mast cell function. Accumulation may be normal but degranulation or cell turnover may be defective. On the other hand, it is not necessarily correct to argue that mast cells are not involved in worm expulsion from those experiments where mast cells were not found to accumulate until after the expulsive phase. The low numbers during expulsion may in fact reflect intense mast cell activity and rapid cell turnover.

Ogilvie: I agree that the reported difference in time of appearance of mast cells in the gut is by itself probably not important; I also accept your comments that the mast cells in lactating rats may not be able to function exactly as they do in non-lactating rats. However, in our more recent experiments we get rapid expulsion of parasites from irradiated rats that have no mast cells in the lamina propria of their intestines (Ogilvie *et al.* 1977).

White: What could be the stimulus for the mast cells? Is it a worm-specific stimulus?

Ogilvie: I don't think anybody knows the answer to this interesting question.

White: How do you account for the finding that a heterologous anaphylactic reaction expels worms?

Ogilvie: I suspect that the experiments to which you refer (Barth *et al.* 1966) may have no relevance to the normal sequence of events in this infection. An important reason for my scepticism about the significance of this work is that lactating rats which produce anti-parasite antibodies and in which a violent, parasite-specific anaphylactic reaction can be induced in the intestine (Connan 1973) nevertheless do not expel their worms. This makes me think that the results of Barth *et al.* (1966) (which showed that an anaphylactic reaction induced by a non-parasite antigen enhanced expulsion of worms from rats passively immunized with antiserum) may be no guide to the mechanism which normally operates.

Booth: You mentioned the enlargement of the gut in the lactating rat. This enlargement is almost all accounted for by villous hyperplasia. I don't know any evidence that when there is hyperplasia of the intestine there is hyperplasia of the lamina propria tissue. But is there likely to be any hyperplasia, for example, of plasma cell or lymphocyte populations?

Ogilvie: We have not assessed these cell populations in lactating animals. It would be interesting to do this.

Booth: The other question is nutrition. When there is loss of protein from the gut, it is our impression from human and animal studies that it never produces a depletion of anything other than *serum* proteins. This situation is completely comparable to nephrotic syndrome with protein in the urine. The rest of the body protein is normal. This would fit in with your concept that whatever disease occurs in these rats results in lack of appetite and lack of intake, and therefore in a kwashiorkor-like picture in the animal. If that is the case, what is the effect on the immune response?

Ogilvie: In acute infections, there wouldn't be time for any interference in nutrition to influence the outcome, but in malnourished animals immunity is profoundly affected and this is almost certainly one reason why nematode infections are so important in endemically infected human populations or animals at pasture.

Ferguson: In the case of parasites which do not attach to the surface epithelium, I wonder if villi of a certain length are necessary to allow the parasites to remain in one area of the intestine. In *Nippostrongylus* infection, a couple of days before the parasite is expelled the villi are damaged by an immune reaction giving a flat or convoluted surface (Symons 1965; Ferguson & Jarrett 1975). I have always thought that this would be simply an unavoidable side-effect of the immune response, although it is clinically important in reducing the surface area available for absorption—in fact in some animals the appearances are similar to those found in the flat mucosa of coeliac disease. However, it could be that by destroying the villi a cell-mediated immune reaction can stop the worms from having something to twist around. In lactating animals the villi are longer than normal (Craft 1970) and perhaps in such animals the villi do not totally disappear during parasite infection.

Some other species of worm actually penetrate the gut. Is it known how these are expelled? Do they simply fall off the mucosa to be removed by peristalsis also?

Ogilvie: Trichuris spp. nematodes penetrate the gut mucosa and immunity to *T. muris* in the mouse has been studied in detail by Wakelin (1975). This work suggests that the immune mechanism operating in this model is similar to that postulated for *N. brasiliensis*, in that both antibodies and lymphocytes but not IgE antibodies are required.

Parrott: In the histological sections I have looked at, the villi although shortened aren't absolutely flat as in coeliac disease. Perhaps the parasites haven't such a good handhold, but they still have something to wind round.

Ferguson: I have never seen a patient with untreated coeliac disease and a flat mucosa who also has a parasite infection. However, these infections are uncommon in Britain. Paediatricians in other parts of the world might have epidemiological information on this.

Booth: I can't remember having seen parasitic infection in coeliac disease. In tropical sprue we find it, but the morphological change is quite different from that in coeliac disease. If you consider *Strongyloides* infection in man, there are a host of unanswered problems. Firstly, you get an acute reaction with eosinophilia, a type I response and malabsorption, just as you have described. The second type is the endemic one in populations which appear to be immune but where biopsies reveal worms inside the mucosa, nicely wrapped up, and no immune response at all. In between fall patients who may have chronic infections with *Strongyloides* for 10 years and suddenly develop a hyperinfection and die from it.

Ogilvie: I would suggest that this is because their cell-mediated immunity is being depressed at that time.

Pierce: What is the distribution and class of antibody found on these worms? This might help to elucidate its mechanism of action.

Ogilvie: Nematodes have a surface of modified collagen with no cellular structure. This passively absorbs immunoglobulins of a variety of classes. The beginning and end of the gut is also lined with this collagen and has adsorbed immunoglobulin. Nobody knows what antibodies are there.

Pierce: These worms have no demonstrated mechanism of attachment, but does that rule out some more or less specific adherence mechanism which might be analogous with the mucosal adherence factors on certain bacteria? And might not mucosal antibody interfere with such an adherence mechanism? I find it difficult to imagine that anything can hang onto the mucosa unless it has some specific adherence mechanism.

Ogilvie: *Nippostrongylus* does not have any obvious adherence mechanism and the worms are found twined between the villi. Even worms such as hookworms which do attach to the mucosa change their position in the gut.

Lehner: I think Dr Ferguson might inadvertently have described yet another lymphokine (p. 198)! If this were so, could you reproduce your results using not the whole cell, the Fc-negative lymphocyte you described, but a soluble mediator prepared from it?

Ogilvie: I have tried that kind of experiment, with no success so far.

Porter: One of the natural defence mechanisms of the gut is the peristaltic flow. Is there any evidence of stasis preceding infection?

Ogilvie: There has been much discussion about this, but the only good experimental study has only just been completed. Castro *et al.* (1976) have shown that the passage of ingesta through the intestine of rats is increased in rats infected with *Trichinella spiralis*.

Porter: In pigs with *E. coli* infections, when the animals were weaned onto cow's milk there was substantial stasis of the intestine which would contribute to colonization.

Schmidt: Why doesn't the lymphocyte defence mechanism function in lactating rats?

Ogilvie: Presumably lymphocyte function is impeded by the direct or indirect action of hormones, possibly resulting in increased cortisol levels which affect the cells. Suppression of cell-mediated reactions at or near parturition has long been known to occur. For example, it has been known for many years by the farming community that if you want to get your cow past the tuberculin test you take her when she is in the early stages of lactation. The farmers knew long before the immunologists that cell-mediated immune reactions are severely depressed early in lactation!

References

BARTH, E. E. E., JARRETT, W. F. A. & URQUHART, G. M. (1966) Studies on the mechanism of the self-cure reaction in rats infected with *Nippostrongylus brasiliensis*. *Immunology 10*, 459-464

CASTRO, G. A., BADIAL-ACEVES, F., SMITH, J. W., DUDRICK, S. J. & WEISBRODT, N. W. (1976) Altered small bowel propulsion associated with parasitism. *Gastroenterology 71*, 620-625

CONNAN, R. M. (1973) The immune response of the lactating rat to *Nippostrongylus brasiliensis*. *Immunology 25*, 261-267

CRAFT, I. L. (1970) The influence of pregnancy and lactation on the morphology and absorptive capacity of the rat small intestine. *Clin. Sci. 38*, 287-295

DINEEN, J. K., KELLY, J. D., GOODRICH, B. S. & SMITH, I. D. (1974) Expulsion of *Nippostrongylus brasiliensis* from the small intestine of the rat by prostaglandin-like factors from ram semen. *Int. Arch. Allergy Appl. Immunol. 46*, 360-374

FERGUSON, A. & JARRETT, E. E. E. (1975) Hypersensitivity reactions in the small intestine. 1. Thymus-dependence of experimental partial villous atrophy. *Gut 16*, 114-117

GUY-GRAND, D., GRISCELLI, C. & VASSALLI, P. (1974) The gut-associated lymphoid system: nature and properties of the large dividing cells. *Eur. J. Immunol. 4*, 435-443

LOVE, R. J., OGILVIE, B. M. & McLAREN, D. J. (1975) *Nippostrongylus brasiliensis:* further properties of antibody damaged worms and induction of comparable damage by maintaining worms *in vitro*. *Parasitology 71*, 275-283

OGILVIE, B. M., LOVE, R. J., JARRA, W. & BROWN, K. N. (1977) *Nippostrongylus brasiliensis* infection in rats: the cellular requirement for worm expulsion. *Immunology 32*, in press

PARROTT, D. M. V. & FERGUSON, A. (1974) Selective migration of lymphocytes within the mouse small intestine. *Immunology 26*, 571

PARROTT, D. M. V., TILNEY, N. L. & SLESS, F. (1975) The different migratory characteristics of lymphocyte populations from a whole spleen transplant. *Clin. Exp. Immunol. 19*, 459

ROSE, M. L., PARROTT, D. M. V. & BRUCE, R. G. (1976) Migration of lymphoblasts in the small intestine. I. Effect of *Trichinella spiralis* infection on the migration of mesenteric lymphoblasts and mesenteric T lymphoblasts in syngeneic mice. *Immunology 31*, 723-730

SPRENT, J. (1976) Fate of H2-activated T lymphocytes in syngeneic hosts. I. Fate in lymphoid tissues and intestine traced with ^{3}H-thymidine, ^{125}I-deoxyuridine and ^{51}chromium. *Cell. Immunol. 21*, 278-302

SYMONS, L. E. A. (1965) Kinetics of the epithelial cells and morphology of villi and crypts in the jejunum of the rat infected by the nematode *Nippostrongylus brasiliensis*. *Gastroenterology 49*, 158-168

WAKELIN, D. (1975) Immune expulsion of *Trichuris muris* from mice during a primary infection: analysis of the components involved. *Parasitology 70*, 397-406

Role of the eosinophil

PAUL B. BEESON

Veterans Administration Hospital, Seattle, Washington

Abstract The gut wall is one of the conspicuous sites of eosinophil accumulation, presumably because of local chemotactic stimuli. It is reasonable to assume that one chemotactic factor is released by the mast cell, which is often found in proximity to the eosinophil. The association of eosinophils and eosinophilia with allergic disorders has long been recognized, and recent work has shown that increased eosinophil production is mediated by the lymphocyte. That process shares characteristics with other immunological actions. An increased rate of eosinophil tissue accumulation and destruction may be the factor which initiates the mechanism for increased production. None of many hypotheses about the 'function' of the eosinophil is substantiated; nevertheless it seems likely that this member of the immunological apparatus, which tends to be distributed in the front line (mucosal and cutaneous tissues), fulfils some normal protective or homeostatic function. Aside from that assumed normal function, there is growing clinical evidence that eosinophils can at times cause host injury, for example in such states as eosinophilic gastroenteritis and endomyocarditis.

Inasmuch as the eosinophil appears to be a component of the immune system, and one of its conspicuous sites of localization is the wall of the stomach and intestine, it seems appropriate that consideration be given to this cell in a symposium on Immunology of the Gut. While eosinophil function cannot yet be described with confidence, much progress has been made within the past decade, and some patterns of its behaviour are beginning to emerge.

The eosinophil is formed in the marrow and circulates briefly in the blood before being deposited in tissues throughout the body. The relative numbers in marrow, circulation and tissues, as estimated from studies in rodents, are of the order of 300-1-300 (Rytömaa 1960; Hudson 1968). It can thus be seen that the number in the circulation at any one time furnishes an inadequate guide to the interplay of processes that accelerate or depress the rate of production in the marrow, or of the local forces that tend to extract the cells from the circulation. The inaccuracy of blood levels is further compromised by diurnal fluctuations, together with the error involved in the customary clinical method of quantifying these cells by differential count of 100 leucocytes in stained smears of peripheral blood.

In many clinical reports emphasis is laid on changes in the number of circulating cells within a few hours of a given event; this could only be a result of redistribution of preformed cells, and should not be interpreted as a sign of accelerated or diminished bone marrow production. Extensive experience with laboratory rodents indicates that about two days must elapse before an acceleration in the rate of marrow production can perceptibly raise the number of eosinophils in circulation (Spry 1971).

We can say with confidence that this cell differs markedly from the polymorphonuclear neutrophil in its behaviour, despite some resemblances in morphology, phagocytic capacity and enzyme content. Two examples are evident in their responses to adrenal glucocorticoid administration and to acute infection. In both circumstances, blood neutrophils usually increase, whereas eosinophils tend to diminish. Bass showed that these eosinopenic responses are independent, since the eosinopenia of acute infection is not prevented by adrenalectomy (1975a,b).

CLINICAL ASSOCIATIONS

Clinicians have long recognized eosinophilia as characteristic of certain allergic states such as drug reactions, asthma and eczema, and have equated the finding of an eosinophil marker—the Charcot-Leyden crystal—with intense local accumulations of eosinophils in the tissues affected. The appearance of eosinophils in response to the application of suspected allergens, in the Rebuck skin window test, has been useful in the diagnosis of allergy to drugs or pollens (Fowler & Lowell 1966).

As to the behaviour of the eosinophil in disorders other than allergies, the literature now amounts to tens of thousands of articles. I have studied a great many of these over the past decade, trying to discern some unifying theme. As is well known, eosinophilia accompanies most infestations by metazoan parasites, some skin diseases, some neoplastic diseases, and a number of poorly understood pulmonary infiltrations. There is no obvious common factor in this peculiar group of associations, beyond such vague suggestions as 'reaction to foreign protein or altered host tissue'. We should note too some rather surprising exceptions. Bacterial and viral infections, certain diffuse skin diseases such as psoriasis, lymphomas other than Hodgkin's disease, serum sickness, necrotizing vasculitis, many granulomatous diseases, infectious mononucleosis, chronic urticaria, rheumatic fever and graft rejection are all disorders which might be expected to be accompanied by eosinophilia, yet are not.

The eosinophil in diseases of the gut

Food allergy may be associated with blood and tissue eosinophilia. The best studies of this subject have been carried out in infants with milk allergy, where the occurrence of increased numbers of eosinophils in blood, as well as local infiltration of gut mucosa in response to milk feeding, has been well substantiated (Waldmann *et al.* 1967; Shiner *et al.* 1975).

Carcinoma of the oesophagus, stomach, pancreas, liver and colon has been associated with blood eosinophilia, as is of course true of cancer arising in other tissues (Isaacson & Rapoport 1946; Banerjee & Narang 1967). Eosinophilia may accompany chronic relapsing pancreatitis (Mullin *et al.* 1968), and has been noted during the course of chronic ulcerative colitis (Wright & Truelove 1966).

The entity of *eosinophilic gastroenteritis* deserves special attention here. This designation applies to a group of syndromes characterized by eosinophilic infiltration of one or more layers of the wall of the stomach or small intestine, together with substantial increases in the number of circulating eosinophils (Klein *et al.* 1970; Greenberger & Gryboski 1973). The syndromes seem to divide into three types, depending on the part of the gut wall affected. If the principal accumulation of eosinophils is in the serosa, the clinical manifestation may be eosinophilic ascites. Infiltration of the muscular coat may cause visible thickening or even local tumour formation, leading to partial obstruction, most often in the region of the gastroduodenal junction. Infiltration predominant in the mucosa may cause protein-losing enteropathy, anaemia, and malabsorption. Leinbach & Rubin (1970) made an intensive study of a young man with this disease. Over a period of months they examined scores of samples of gastric and small intestinal mucosa, which revealed a peculiar patchiness of the eosinophilic infiltrations. Where the accumulations were greatest and nearest the surface, there was loss of overlying mucosal villi. Eosinophils and Charcot-Leyden crystals were found in this patient's faeces throughout the period of observation. In most cases of eosinophilic gastroenteritis where suitable tests have been made, the blood level of IgE has been found to be elevated. Affected patients often have histories of food allergy, asthma and eczema.

EOSINOPHIL CHEMOTAXIS

Much study has been devoted to eosinophil chemotaxis, using the Boyden chamber technique, or modifications of it. It is obvious that many materials, some derived from lymphocytes and complement fractions, some from basophils and mast cells, and some from normal or diseased organs, can, under a variety of circumstances, exert strong chemotactic attraction for eosinophils. During the 1960's much interest was shown in the demonstration that certain kinds of immune complex attracted eosinophils, and were ingested by them (Litt 1964). This evidence has been reviewed by Parish (1974) and Kay (1974). One of the first defined substances to be assigned the property of eosinophil chemotaxis was histamine; nevertheless this matter is not yet settled, because studies employing different techniques and different hosts have given inconsistent results or have required concentrations of histamine or eosinophils that may not characterize the living host (Felarca & Lowell 1968; Clark et al. 1975). A possible source of confusion is that the mast cell, which is the principal source of histamine, probably also liberates one of the most active chemotactic substances.

THE RATE OF EOSINOPHIL PRODUCTION IN BONE MARROW

So far, I have focused on the behaviour of eosinophils in tissues. We know from clinical experience that tissue eosinophilia is often accompanied by blood eosinophilia, which in turn must be a reflection of accelerated production of the cells in the marrow. Until recently, nothing was known of the connection between these phenomena—that is, of the nature of the mechanism which increases the rate of production of eosinophils. This subject was investigated by several of us at Oxford between 1967 and 1973. Our experimental model was the blood and marrow eosinophil response to challenge of rats or mice by the nematode *Trichinella spiralis*. Inasmuch as that work has never been summarized, the main findings will now be listed.

In trichinosis the parasite, though encysted in striated muscle, causes prolonged eosinopoiesis in the bone marrow. The stimulus must be transmitted in the blood. Our first step was to look for evidence of a humoral eosinopoietic factor which would stimulate eosinophil production when injected into normal recipients. All tests gave negative results.

Clear evidence was then obtained that circulating lymphocytes played a part in the eosinophilic reaction: (*a*) eosinophilia was obliterated or greatly diminished by injection of antilymphocyte serum, prolonged thoracic duct drainage, or neonatal thymectomy; (*b*) thoracic duct lymphocytes from an animal in the intestinal phase of trichinosis caused eosinophilia when injected into syngeneic recipients; (*c*) the eosinophilic response involved cooperation of lymphocytes and bone marrow cells. Rats given whole-body irradiation and then reconstituted with lymphocytes alone, or with bone marrow cells alone, failed to develop eosinophilia when challenged; whereas animals reconstituted with both lymphocytes and bone marrow cells did develop eosinophilia when challenged (Basten & Beeson 1970).

In collaboration with A. J. S. Davies and his group, it was shown that thymus-deficient mice, which give normal neutrophil responses to acute infection, showed markedly defective eosinophil responses to trichinosis. Controls reconstituted by grafts of thymus tissue gave normal eosinophil responses to trichinosis (Walls *et al.* 1971).

Much of our work employed a test system in which muscle-stage *Trichinella* larvae, too large to pass through a capillary bed, were injected intravenously. This led to the formation of granulomatous inflammatory lesions containing numerous eosinophils wherever parasites were trapped in the lungs (Boyer *et al.* 1971). In this situation the parasite does not survive, and can be seen to be disintegrating within a day or two. An increase in blood eosinophils is detectable on the second or third day, reaches its peak about the seventh day, and disappears by the tenth to the fourteenth day. This method of producing a sharp burst of eosinophil production by a single injection of foreign material has advantages over previously used systems, nearly all of which involved repeated injections of antigen. It enabled us to examine the bone marrow eosinophil response with tests analogous to those used to study antibody formation. We found, for example, that an enhanced response resulted from a second injection of larvae, resembling a secondary antibody response. Immunological specificity was indicated by the absence of cross-reactivity between the eosinophilic response to dextran beads and that to the parasite larvae (Walls & Beeson 1972a).

Another kind of study permitted by the model of intravenous injection of muscle-stage larvae was to test the effect of immunosuppressive agents on the eosinophil response. The results fell in a pattern consistent with that known to characterize the antibody response to a single injection of antigen (Berenbaum 1967). Certain immunosuppressants, such as cortisone and antilymphocyte serum, were effective when given a few hours before the intravenous injection, but had no effect if given 24 hours later. Other agents, such as methotrexate and cyclophosphamide, ineffective before antigen administration, suppressed the eosinophil response if given 24 hours later (Boyer *et al.* 1970). Here was evidence of interference with sequential steps leading to accelerated marrow production.

There was no eosinophil response to intravenous injection of the larval material if the parasites were first ground in a tissue grinder, reducing them to fragments small enough to pass through the pulmonary vessels, presumably to be arrested by fixed macrophages elsewhere in the body. This refutes an oft-made suggestion that the eosinophilia of parasitic infestations is attributable to some unique constituent of parasites. Our findings, on the contrary, provided evidence that a key factor in the genesis of eosinophilia is the processing of foreign material by cells attracted to its site of lodgement in tissues—that is, in areas other than the reticuloendothelial system (Walls & Beeson 1972b).

Kinetic studies of the bone marrow response were made by Spry (1971), who counted labelled mitoses and the relative numbers of labelled cells making up the recognizable stages in marrow development. This revealed quickening of all phases of production, beginning with the earliest detectable precursors. After parasite challenge the mean cell cycle time in the marrow was shortened from 30 to 9 hours. Spry calculated that over a period of six days this could result in an output of mature eosinophils 64 times greater than would be produced in normal unstimulated animals.

Evidence linking the lymphocyte to eosinophil production or function has since come from other laboratories (McGarry *et al.* 1971; Ponzio & Speirs 1974; Schriber & Zucker-Franklin 1975). Colley (1973) has described a lymphokine which stimulates migration of eosinophils in a semi-solid medium. He used an immune system produced by schistosomal infection of mice. Similar results were reported by Kazura *et al.* (1975), also employing schistosomal infection.

HYPOTHESIS

As things stand at the moment, I feel that the most attractive scheme to link local concentrations of eosinophils with increased blood levels would be one which postulates a feedback system:

Chemotactic factors produced in tissues, from pre-existing cell components or formed during immunologically mediated inflammatory reactions, cause local deposition of circulating eosinophils in the affected tissues. The presence or destruction of excessive numbers of eosinophils affects lymphocytes so that they release a lymphokine which acts in the bone marrow to accelerate eosinophil production. This in turn causes the number of circulating eosinophils to rise.

THE EOSINOPHIL AND THE MAST CELL

The interrelation between the eosinophil and the tissue mast cell appears to to be of central importance. They are often found in association; the mast cell elaborates a potent eosinophil chemotactic agent; the eosinophil ingests mast cell granules, and neutralizes histamine, a mast cell product. Very probably another mediator, slow-reacting substance of anaphylaxis (SRS-A), which has been shown to be a product of a close relative of the mast cell, the basophil (Lewis et al. 1975), is also part of this functional interrelationship. The mast cell is a source of heparin, and it has been claimed that eosinophils contain plasminogen (Barnhart & Riddle 1963), so they may also collaborate in tissue processes involving coagulation.

Particularly impressive is the evidence that the tissue mast cell can liberate a powerful eosinotactic agent. The chemical structure of this eosinophil chemotactic factor of anaphylaxis (ECF-A) has now been identified by Goetzl & Austen as a tetrapeptide (1975). These workers have also demonstrated ECF-A in the blood basophil. Mann has published photographs of eosinophils clustering about degranulating mast cells and ingesting mast cell granules (1969). The human disease called urticaria pigmentosa is characterized by excessive numbers of mast cells in the subcutaneous tissue. Sufferers are liable to develop urticarial wheals after slight injury to the skin. Serial biopsies in such patients have shown massive influx of eosinophils occurring within fifteen minutes of light stroking of the skin (Prakken & Woerdeman 1952).

The special relationship between eosinophil and mast cell is also emphasized by the occurrence of blood eosinophilia following measures which cause mast cell degranulation. Hungerford (1964) and Fernex (1968) showed that repeated injections of Compound 48/80, a mast cell degranulator, will evoke marked elevation of the blood eosinophil level after four days. The timing and extent of the elevation are consistent with an increase in rate of marrow production. A comparable phenomenon is observed when rats are acutely deprived of dietary magnesium, a procedure which also causes mast cell degranulation. The animals develop a distinctive syndrome within one or two days, characterized by reddening of the skin, obvious itching, and high blood and urine levels of histamine (Bois et al. 1963). Within four days they exhibit blood eosinophilia (Hungerford & Karson 1960). Again we appear to be observing this chain of events: mast cell degranulation → eosinophil chemotaxis → accelerated eosinophil production.

THE EOSINOPHIL AS A MODULATOR OF IMMUNE RESPONSES

Regardless of whether histamine exerts a chemotactic influence, there is good evidence that eosinophils can exert some protection against its toxic effects (Kovacs 1950; Vercauteren & Peeters 1952; Lee 1969). Hubscher (1975) has evidence that the eosinophil accomplishes this by elaborating prostaglandins

E_1 and E_2. Much study has also been made of another factor, released during IgE-dependent immune reactions: SRS-A. This agent, which contracts smooth muscle and alters vascular permeability, is inactivated by arylsulphatase, a component of the eosinophil (Wasserman *et al.* 1975). So, a case is developing that the eosinophil can be attracted to a locality where an IgE-mediated immune reaction has occurred, and that it may be capable of modulating the actions of some products of the allergic inflammation. One of its 'functions', then, may be to act as a homeostatic agent, preventing excessive and continuing spread of an inflammatory reaction.

THE EOSINOPHIL AND TISSUE INJURY

It is not surprising, considering its content of proteolytic enzymes, that the eosinophil seems to be capable of damaging the host under certain circumstances. An interesting example of this was found in the so-called 'Gordon test' introduced in the 1930's, and regarded for a brief period as a specific test for Hodgkin's disease (Gordon 1933). When homogenized lymph node material from patients with that disease was injected intracerebrally in rabbits or guinea pigs, the animals developed a distinctive encephalitis, mainly due to destruction of Purkinje cells of the cerebellum. Subsequent investigation revealed that the test was not specific for Hodgkin's disease, but was simply an indicator of the presence of eosinophils in the lymph nodes, since the same phenomenon could be demonstrated by injecting buffy coat material from patients with blood eosinophilia (Seiler *et al.* 1969).

In clinical medicine, tissue destruction may be observed in sites where eosinophils seem to be the principal invaders. Examples are eosinophilic gastroenteritis, eosinophilic granuloma of bone and Löffler's endomyocarditis. In the last disease there is endocardial thickening due to fibrosis and eosinophilic infiltration, most prominent on the left side of the heart. The destructive process extends into the adjacent myocardium. Reports of endomyocardial fibrosis associated with prolonged high blood levels of eosinophils due to different causes have now appeared (Ive *et al.* 1967; Roberts *et al.* 1969; Borer *et al.* 1973; Brockington & Olsen 1973; Blatt *et al.* 1974; Frenkel *et al.* 1975). The cardiac lesion has been likened to that of carcinoid heart disease where an agent produced by the carcinoid tumour causes endocardial fibrosis (Zucker-Franklin 1971).

SUMMARY

We seem to be emerging from the period when the role of the eosinophil was called an enigma. There is a good basis for looking on this cell as a component of the immune system, recruited by lymphocytes in response to increased tissue utilization. One of its function seems to be to act as a modulator of inflammatory responses, notably those involving IgE and mast cell degranulation. In some instances of marked eosinophilia associated with neoplasia or certain other clinical states, the cell may be responding to a 'false signal', due to chance development of chemotactic factors, or of lymphokines which act directly on the bone marrow. A high and prolonged concentration of eosinophils can probably cause local tissue injury.

References

BANERJEE, R. N. & NARANG, R. M. (1967) Haematological changes in malignancy. *Br. J. Haematol. 13*, 829-843

BARNHART, M. I. & RIDDLE, J. M. (1963) Cellular localization of profibrinolysin (plasminogen). *Blood 21*, 306-321

BASS, D. A. (1975a) Behavior of eosinophil leukocytes in acute inflammation. I. Lack of dependence on adrenal function. *J. Clin. Invest. 55*, 1229-1236

BASS, D. A. (1975b) Behavior of eosinophil leukocytes in acute inflammation. II. Eosinophil dynamics during acute inflammation. *J. Clin. Invest. 56*, 870-879

BASTEN, A. & BEESON, P. B. (1970) Mechanism of eosinophilia. II. Role of the lymphocyte. *J. Exp. Med. 131*, 1288-1305

BERENBAUM, M. C. (1967) Immunosuppressive agents and the cellular kinetics of the immune response, in *Immunity, Cancer and Chemotherapy: Basic Relationships on the Cellular Level* (Mihich, E., ed.), p. 217, Academic Press, New York & London

BLATT, P. M., ROTHSTEIN, G., MILLER, H. L. & CATHEY, W. J. (1974) Löffler's endomyocardial fibrosis with eosinophilia in association with acute lymphoblastic leukemia. *Blood 44*, 489-493

BOIS, P., GASCON, A. & BEAULNES, A. (1963) Histamine-liberating effect of magnesium deficiency in the rat. *Nature (Lond.) 197*, 501-502

BORER, J. S., HENRY, W. L. & DALE, D. C. (1973) Echocardiographic findings in patients with idiopathic hypereosinophilic syndrome. *Clin. Res. 21*, 406

BOYER, M. H., BASTEN, A. & BEESON, P. B. (1970) Mechanism of eosinophilia. III. Suppression of eosinophilia by agents known to modify immune responses. *Blood 36*, 458-469

BOYER, M. H., SPRY, C. J. F., BEESON, P. B. & SHELDON, W. H. (1971) Mechanism of eosinophilia. IV. The pulmonary lesion resulting from intravenous injection of *Trichinella spiralis*. *Yale J. Biol. Med. 43*, 351-357

BROCKINGTON, I. F. & OLSEN, E. G. J. (1973) Löffler's endocarditis and Davies' endomyocardial fibrosis. *Am. Heart J. 85*, 308-322

CLARK, R. A. F., GALLIN, J. I. & KAPLAN, A. P. (1975) The selective eosinophil chemotactic activity of histamine. *J. Exp. Med. 142*, 1462-1476

COLLEY, D. G. (1973) Eosinophils and immune mechanisms. I. Eosinophil stimulation promoter (ESP): a lymphokine induced by specific antigen or phytohemagglutinin. *J. Immunol. 110*, 1419-1423

FELARCA, A. B. & LOWELL, F. C. (1968) Failure to elicit histamine eosinophilotaxis in the skin of atopic man. Description of an improved technique. *J. Allergy 41*, 82-87

FERNEX, M. (1968) *The Mast-Cell System*, pp. 138-139, Williams & Wilkins, Baltimore

FOWLER, J. W. III & LOWELL, F. C. (1966) The accumulation of eosinophils as an allergic response to allergen applied to the denuded skin surface. *J. Allergy 37*, 19-28

FRENKEL, R., GRIECO, M. H. & GARRET, R. (1975) Löffler's endomyocarditis associated with bronchial asthma and eosinophilia. *Ann. Allergy* 34, 213-218

GOETZL, E. J. & AUSTEN, K. F. (1975) Purification and synthesis of eosinophilotactic tetrapeptides of human lung tissue: identification as eosinophil chemotactic factor of anaphylaxis. *Proc. Natl. Acad. Sci. U.S.A.* 72, 4123-4127

GORDON, M. H. (1933) Hodgkin's disease. A pathogenic agent in the glands, and its application in diagnosis. *Br. Med. J.* 1, 641-644

GREENBERGER, N. & GRYBOSKI, J. D. (1973) Allergic disorders of the intestine and eosinophilic gastroenteritis, in *Gastrointestinal Disease* (Sleisenger, M. H. & Fordtran, J. S., eds.), pp. 1066-1082, Saunders, Philadelphia

HUBSCHER, T. (1975) Role of the eosinophil in the allergic reactions. II. Release of prostaglandins from human eosinophilic leukocytes. *J. Immunol.* 114, 1389-1393

HUDSON, G. (1968) Quantitative study of the eosinophil granulocyte. *Seminars Haematol.* 5, 166-186

HUNGERFORD, G. F. (1964) Role of histamine in producing the eosinophilia of magnesium deficiency. *Proc. Soc. Exp. Biol. Med.* 115, 182-185

HUNGERFORD, G. F. & KARSON, E. F. (1960) The eosinophilia of magnesium deficiency. *Blood* 16, 1642-1650

ISAACSON, N. H. & RAPOPORT, P. (1946) Eosinophilia in malignant tumors: its significance. *Ann. Intern. Med.* 25, 893-902

IVE, F. A., WILLIS, A. J. P., IKEMA, A. C. & BROCKINGTON, I. F. (1967) Endomyocardial fibrosis and filariasis. *Q. J. Med.* 36, 495-515

KAY, A. B. (1974) Chemotaxis of eosinophil leucocytes in relation to immediate-type hypersensitivity and the complement system. *Antibiot. Chemother.* 19, 271-283

KAZURA, J. W., MAHMOUD, A. A. F., KARB, K. S. & WARREN, K. S. (1975) The lymphokine eosinophil stimulation promoter and human schistosomiasis mansoni. *J. Infect. Dis.* 132, 702-706

KLEIN, N. C., HARGROVE, R. L., SLEISENGER, M. H. & JEFFRIES, G. H. (1970) Eosinophilic gastroenteritis. *Medicine* 49, 299-319

KOVACS, A. (1950) Antihistaminic effect of eosinophil leukocytes. *Experientia* 6, 349-350

LEE, D. (1969) Antihistamine activity of the eosinophil. *J. Pathol.* 99, 96-98

LEINBACH, G. E. & RUBIN, C. E. (1970) Eosinophilic gastroenteritis: a simple reaction to food allergens? *Gastroenterology* 59, 874-889

LEWIS, R. A., GOETZL, E. J., WASSERMAN, S. I., VALONE, F. H., RUBIN, R. H. & AUSTEN, K. F. (1975) The release of four mediators of immediate hypersensitivity from human leukemic basophils. *J. Immunol.* 114, 87-92

LITT, M. (1964) Studies in experimental eosinophilia. VI. Uptake of immune complexes by eosinophils. *J. Cell Biol.* 23, 355-361

MANN, P. R. (1969) An electron-microscope study of the relations between mast cells and eosinophil leucocytes. *J. Pathol.* 98, 183-186

MCGARRY, M. P., SPEIRS, R. S., JENKINS, V. K. & TRENTIN, J. J. (1971) Lymphoid cell dependence of eosinophil response to antigen. *J. Exp. Med.* 134, 801-814

MULLIN, G. T., CAPERTON, E. M., Jr, CRESPIN, S. R. & WILLIAMS, R. C., Jr (1968) Arthritis and skin lesions resembling erythema nodosum in pancreatic disease. *Ann. Intern. Med.* 68, 75-87

PARISH, W. E. (1974) Substances that attract eosinophils *in vitro* and *in vivo*, and that elicit blood eosinophilia. *Antibiot. Chemother.* 19, 233-270

PONZIO, N. M. & SPEIRS, R. S. (1974) Lymphoid cell dependence of eosinophil response to antigen. IV. Effects of *in vitro* X-irradiation on adoptive transfer of anamnestic cellular and humoral responses. *Proc. Soc. Exp. Biol. Med.* 145, 1178-1180

PRAKKEN, J. R. & WOERDEMAN, M. J. (1952) Mast cells in disease of the skin; their relation to tissue eosinophilia. *Dermatologica* 105, 116-124

ROBERTS, W. C., LIEGLER, D. G. & CARBONE, P. P. (1969) Endomyocardial disease and eosinophilia. A clinical and pathologic spectrum. *Am. J. Med. 46*, 28-42

RYTÖMAA, T. (1960) Organ distribution and histochemical properties of eosinophil granulocytes in rat. *Acta Pathol. Microbiol. Scand. 50*, Suppl. 140

SCHRIBER, R. A. & ZUCKER-FRANKLIN, D. (1975) Induction of blood eosinophilia by pulmonary embolization of antigen-coated particles: the relationship to cell-mediated immunity. *J. Immunol. 114*, 1348-1353

SEILER, G., WESTERMAN, R. A. & WILSON, J. A. (1969) The role of specific eosinophil granules in eosinophil-induced experimental encephalitis. *Neurology 19*, 478-488

SHINER, M., BALLARD, J. & SMITH, M. E. (1975) The small-intestinal mucosa in cow's milk allergy. *Lancet 1*, 136-140

SPRY, C. J. F. (1971) Mechanism of eosinophilia. V. Kinetics of normal and accelerated eosinopoiesis. *Cell Tissue Kinet. 4*, 351-364

VERCAUTEREN, R. & PEETERS, G. (1952) On the presence of an anti-histaminicum in isolated eosinophilic granulocytes. *Arch. Int. Pharmacodyn. 89*, 10-14

WALDMANN, T. A., WOCHNER, R. D., LASTER, L. & GORDON, R. S., JR (1967) Allergic gastroenteropathy. A cause of excessive gastrointestinal protein loss. *N. Engl. J. Med. 276*, 761-769

WALLS, R. S., BASTEN, A., LEUCHARS, E. & DAVIES, A. J. S. (1971) Mechanisms for eosinophilic and neutrophilic leucocytoses. *Br. Med. J. 3*, 157-159

WALLS, R. S. & BEESON, P. B. (1972a) Mechanism of eosinophilia. IX. Induction of eosinophilia in rats by certain forms of dextran. *Proc. Soc. Exp. Biol. Med. 140*, 689-693

WALLS, R. S. & BEESON, P. B. (1972b) Mechanism of eosinophilia. VIII. Importance of local cellular reactions in stimulating eosinophil production. *Clin. Exp. Immunol. 12*, 111-119

WASSERMAN, S. I., GOETZL, E. J. & AUSTEN, K. F. (1975) Inactivation of slow reacting substance of anaphylaxis by human eosinophil arylsulfatase. *J. Immunol. 114*, 645-649

WRIGHT, R. & TRUELOVE, S. C. (1966) Circulating and tissue eosinophils in ulcerative colitis. *Am. J. Dig. Dis. 11*, 831-846

ZUCKER-FRANKLIN, D. (1971) Eosinophilia of unknown etiology: a diagnostic dilemma. *Hosp. Practice 6*, 119-127

Discussion

Lachmann: You discussed evidence of mast cell factors being neutralized by eosinophil factors. Frank Austen has recently added a further factor by reporting that eosinophils contain phospholipase D, which would destroy the phospholipid platelet-activating factor (Kater *et al.* 1976). It is a novel report, since this enzyme is normally associated with cabbages and spinach rather than with mammalian tissue!

Perhaps you or Dr Ogilvie would comment on the work of Anthony Butterworth and his colleagues (1975) showing that the cell that kills the schistosomula of schistosomiasis in allergic reactions is in fact the eosinophil? If this is so, then even if the IgE antibodies and the mast cell are not directly involved in worm expulsion, perhaps they are acting indirectly by attracting eosinophils. Dr Beeson has said that their capacity to produce eosinophilia may be drawing an important effector cell to the site of infection.

Ogilvie: It is fair to mention that the first suggestion that schistosomules die as the result of eosinophil attack was published in histological studies of the fate of *Schistosoma japonicum* in the skin of monkeys made immune by several infections of irradiated cercariae (Hsü *et al.* 1974, 1975). Butterworth *et al.* (1975) in *in vitro* studies of immunity to *S. mansoni* in man found that peripheral leucocytes from people without helminth infections would kill *S. mansoni* schistosomules coated with IgG antibodies from infected individuals, and the functional cell appears to be the eosinophil. These studies are supported by the work of Mahmoud *et al.* (1975*a*) who showed that the immunity of mice to invading *S. mansoni* was obliterated by giving the mice anti-eosinophil antiserum at the time of a reinfection. This phenomenon may be important in many helminth infections. The original observation of eosinophil adherence to helminths coated with IgG antibodies was made by Higashi & Chowdhury (1970) in Bombay, working with human antiserum and the invading stage of the filarial nematode parasite *Wuchereria bancrofti*. Dr C. D. Mackenzie and I became interested in this recently, and we are working on a model using eosinophils and other inflammatory cells from normal rats. Dr Mackenzie has been able to show that there is attachment of rat eosinophils to the surface of various helminths; this attachment is mediated by specific antibody and does not seem to be dependent on complement. A sequence of changes in the morphology of the eosinophils parallels cell attachment and also various forms of damage to the parasites, particularly to *S. mansoni*. It seems from this work that there is selective antibody-mediated attachment of this particular cell type which is deleterious to the parasites. The class of antibody involved in this reaction is of course of much interest; however, so far the antibody has not been identified, but it is unlikely to be IgE (C. D. Mackenzie, unpublished results 1976).

Beeson: That is true *in vitro*, but not in tissue sections. We were never impressed that the eosinophil was in direct contact with the parasite, in sections.

Ogilvie: *T. spiralis* may not be a good parasite with which to observe this phenomenon *in vivo*. Recent studies with *S. japonicum* show large numbers of eosinophils around parasites invading the skin of immune monkeys (Hsü *et al.* 1974, 1975).

Lachmann: Do you think the eosinophil is what is dislodging *Nippostrongylus*?

Ogilvie: As far as the adult stages found in the lumen of the gut are concerned, I think expulsion is not by direct attack as can be shown *in vitro* but perhaps indirectly by, for example, the release of prostaglandins (Hubscher 1975). I believe it is possible that the tissue stages of helminths may be attacked directly by eosinophils/macrophages, etc.

Rosen: It needs emphasizing that in Butterworth's system immune serum must be present for the eosinophils to kill the schistosomula, which raises the question of the demonstration of the Fc receptor on the eosinophil: I believe such has been made?

Lachmann: Fc receptors on guinea pig eosinophils have been demonstrated in Robin Coombs' laboratory (Butterworth *et al.* 1976) and on human eosinophils by Tai & Spry (1976). They do indeed have very nice Fc receptors, but they are rather more particular than neutrophils about the species of Ig which they bind. Thus the guinea pig eosinophils do not react with rabbit IgG whereas they do with pig IgG. Normal human eosinophils behave similarly, whereas the immature eosinophils found in patients with eosinophilia have Fc receptors more similar to those of neutrophils and do react with rabbit IgG.

Rosen: Does the receptor have the same specificity that the human monocyte has for IgG1 and IgG3?

Lachmann: Tai & Spry (1976) have found that it does.

Rosen: The human monocyte Fc receptor also has considerable species specificity.

Pepys: Human eosinophils and basophils also have C3 receptors (Pepys & Butterworth 1974).

Ogilvie: One of the surprising things we have found is that not only do eosinophils (and macrophages and neutrophils) but also mast cells adhere very firmly to the surface of parasites (C. D. Mackenzie, unpublished 1976). Do you think, Dr Beeson, that eosinophils exist in what one might call an 'activated state', as macrophages do?

Beeson: There is growing evidence that even in the circulation, in hypereosinophilic states from any cause, eosinophils appear to have been activated, as judged by degranulation and vacuolization. Tai & Spry (1976) and others (Connell 1968; Saran 1973) have been finding in many different kinds of eosinophilia evidence that the cells in the circulation have been engaged in some activity.

Rosen: In the work John David did with Butterworth they were able to show that cytochalasin would stop the schistosomicidal activity of the eosinophil. Inhibitors of prostaglandin synthesis or of protein synthesis did not prevent this activity. Obviously, therefore, granule release is necessary for the eosinophil's K cell-like activity.

Lachmann: How similar is the schistosomula to *Nippostrongylus* in its structure?

Ogilvie: They are totally different. Whereas the surface of a nematode has an amorphous collagen-like structure, the surface of the schistosomula is an ordinary plasma membrane.

Booth: Another situation in which eosinophilia is found is fungal infection, particularly fungal endocarditis. I don't know how that fits in, in relation to the morphological differences between the infecting organisms.

Beeson: That is the exception. In terms of what are commonly thought to be the infections, fungal infections and even tuberculosis may sometimes be the cause of an eosinophilic response.

Our studies in animals and reports in the clinical literature suggest that a granulomatous type of response is one of the keys. The pathology associated with eosinophilia is a granuloma. It is an occasional response to fungal infection, just as it is an occasional response to cancer. Out of ten cases of coccidioidomycosis, only one will show marked eosinophilia, and the rest will show none.

Mayrhofer: It is possible to adsorb antigens onto particles such as bentonite, inject those and produce granulomata in the lungs, and I wondered whether this produced eosinophilia and whether it would be a good model for demonstrating specificity?

Beeson: Schriber & Zucker-Franklin (1975) have done exactly that with better-defined antigens than we were using. They used human gamma globulin on a latex particle large enough to be arrested in the lung and obtained an eosinophilic response, a secondary response to a second injection, and no secondary response to a different antigen.

Ogilvie: Mahmoud *et al.* (1975*b*) have shown in studies of the granulomata that occur in the lungs of animals given an intravenous injection of schistosome eggs that about half the cells are eosinophils. Both eosinophils and enormous numbers of mast cells or basophils are also found at the site of ectoparasite attachment on the skin. Allen (1973) and B. Bagnall (personal communication 1975) showed that guinea pigs infested with ticks have massive reactions consisting of eosinophils and basophils at the site of the bites, and the ticks seem to die of an overwhelming basophilic diarrhoea!

Beeson: Humans with scabies also show eosinophilia.

Evans: I did not agree with your inclusion of necrotizing vasculitis among the conditions which do *not* produce eosinophilia, Dr Beeson. It is not uncommon to see cases of Wegener's granulomatosis who have both necrotizing vasculitis and a severe degree of eosinophilia.

Beeson: If you look at all cases of necrotizing vasculitis, only those with pulmonary involvement develop eosinophilia. Patients with peripheral neuropathy and other manifestations are not likely to have an associated eosinophilia.

Lehner: Other granulomas, such as histocytosis X and eosinophilic granuloma, are very rich in eosinophils. We don't know the aetiology of histocytosis X at all. What part do these large numbers of eosinophils play?